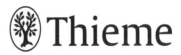

Handbook of Reconstructive Flaps

Matthew M. Hanasono, MD, FACS
Professor
Reconstructive Microsurgery Fellowship Program Director
Department of Plastic Surgery
The University of Texas MD Anderson Cancer Center
Houston, Texas

Charles E. Butler, MD, FACS
Chairman
Professor of Plastic Surgery
Department of Plastic Surgery
Charles B. Barker Endowed Chair in Surgery
The University of Texas MD Anderson Cancer Center
Houston, Texas

227 illustrations

Thieme
New York • Stuttgart • Delhi • Rio de Janeiro

Library of Congress Cataloging-in-Publication Data is available from the publisher

Names: Hanasono, Matthew M., editor. | Butler, C. E. (Charles E.), editor.
Title: Handbook of reconstructive flaps / [edited by]
   Matthew M. Hanasono, Charles E. Butler.
Description: New York : Thieme, 2020. | Includes bibliographical
   references and index.
Identifiers: LCCN 2019058772 (print) | LCCN 2019058773 (ebook) |
   ISBN 9781626235953 (hardback) | ISBN 9781626238602 (ebook)
Subjects: MESH: Surgical Flaps | Reconstructive Surgical
   Procedures--methods
Classification: LCC RD120.8 (print) | LCC RD120.8 (ebook) |
   NLM WO 610 | DDC 617.9/5--dc23
LC record available at https://lccn.loc.gov/2019058772
LC ebook record available at https://lccn.loc.gov/2019058773

Important note: Medicine is an ever-changing science undergoing continual development. Research and clinical experience are continually expanding our knowledge, in particular our knowledge of proper treatment and drug therapy. Insofar as this book mentions any dosage or application, readers may rest assured that the authors, editors, and publishers have made every effort to ensure that such references are in accordance with **the state of knowledge at the time of production of the book.**

Nevertheless, this does not involve, imply, or express any guarantee or responsibility on the part of the publishers in respect to any dosage instructions and forms of applications stated in the book. **Every user is requested to examine carefully** the manufacturers' leaflets accompanying each drug and to check, if necessary in consultation with a physician or specialist, whether the dosage schedules mentioned therein or the contraindications stated by the manufacturers differ from the statements made in the present book. Such examination is particularly important with drugs that are either rarely used or have been newly released on the market. Every dosage schedule or every form of application used is entirely at the user's own risk and responsibility. The authors and publishers request every user to report to the publishers any discrepancies or inaccuracies noticed. If errors in this work are found after publication, errata will be posted at www.thieme.com on the product description page

Some of the product names, patents, and registered designs referred to in this book are in fact registered trademarks or proprietary names even though specific reference to this fact is not always made in the text. Therefore, the appearance of a name without designation as proprietary is not to be construed as a representation by the publisher that it is in the public domain.

Thieme Publishers New York
333 Seventh Avenue, New York, NY 10001 USA
+1 800 782 3488, customerservice@thieme.com

Thieme Publishers Stuttgart
Rüdigerstrasse 14, 70469 Stuttgart, Germany
+49 [0]711 8931 421, customerservice@thieme.de

Thieme Publishers Delhi
A-12, Second Floor, Sector-2, Noida-201301
Uttar Pradesh, India
+91 120 45 566 00, customerservice@thieme.in

Thieme Publishers Rio de Janeiro, Thieme Publicações Ltda.
Edifício Rodolpho de Paoli, 25º andar
Av. Nilo Peçanha, 50 – Sala 2508,
Rio de Janeiro 20020-906 Brasil
+55 21 3172-2297 / +55 21 3172-1896
www.thiemerevinter.com.br

Cover design: Thieme Publishing Group
Typesetting by DiTech Process Solutions, India

Printed in USA by King Printing Company, Inc.   5 4 3 2 1

ISBN   978-1-62623-595-3

Also available as an e-book:
eISBN   978-1-62623-860-2

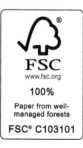

FSC
www.fsc.org
100%
Paper from well-managed forests
FSC® C103101

We dedicate this book to our mentors, families, and patients. To our mentors, our sincerest thanks for all that you have taught us. To our families, we thank you for your constant support and bringing meaning to the work that we do. To our patients, we are inspired by and stand in awe of your bravery and humanity. We have written this book for our students, residents, and fellows. We hope that the information contained herein will not only help you to learn, but also capture your imagination and that you will one day take reconstructive surgery far beyond anything we can imagine.

Matthew M. Hanasono, MD
Charles E. Butler, MD

Contents

Contents

Videos

Preface

We have both been honored to practice surgery at The University of Texas MD Anderson Cancer Center during our careers. MD Anderson Cancer Center is recognized as one of the top cancer treatment centers in the world. However, what we are especially proud of is our Reconstructive Microsurgery Fellowship Program. Both of us have served as program directors of this fellowship and Dr. Butler is now chair of the department. As such, we have had the privilege of overseeing the training of individuals who have gone on to become some of the world's top reconstructive surgeons. At the time of this writing, over 150 individuals have graduated from our program. An equally impressive, though not mutually exclusive group, are those who have belonged to our faculty at one time or another, many of whom have been promoted to leadership positions at some of our nation's top academic institutions. Teachers and former students have come together with great enthusiasm to produce the text you currently have in your hands.

The goal of this book is to provide a review of the key points involved in dissection of the most commonly utilized pedicled and free reconstructive flaps today. Additionally, we have included chapters on lymphovenous bypass and vascularized lymph node transfers from the groin and supraclavicular region because microsurgical treatment of lymphedema has become a significant part of many of our clinical practices in recent years. Rather than creating an encyclopedic text, of which there are already a number of excellent ones, we envisioned a portable handbook that can be studied right before dissecting a reconstructive flap that highlights all of the important components of the procedure. It is our hope that this text will find its way into the backpacks and briefcases of everyone who is in the process of learning reconstructive surgery. We also believe that this text will be a useful refresher for the seasoned veteran who are about to perform an unfamiliar or infrequently used flap.

The authors were tasked with highlighting pertinent anatomy, indications for usage, and preoperative considerations for each flap or procedure discussed, followed by a concise step-by-step description of the operative setup and the actual procedure itself, including donor site closure. The emphasis was to focus on the high impact points of the procedure and to include a combination of very clear diagrams and high-quality illustrative photos from actual surgeries. Along these lines, we have included a "Pearls and Pitfalls" section to each chapter outlining key concepts and critical nuances in surgical technique or patient management. We acknowledge that there is more than one "right" way to perform any given surgery, but hope that the reader will find the techniques we present, which have been refined by countless hours in the operating room, to be practical and reliable.

Matthew M. Hanasono, MD
Charles E. Butler, MD

Acknowledgments

We sincerely thank all of our contributors for their excellent work. We hope that this book conveys our collective passion for reconstructive surgery and restoring peoples' lives. Equally, we hope that it conveys the spirit of camaraderie and respect not only among those who have learned and taught at MD Anderson Cancer Center but all who belong to the brotherhood and sisterhood of reconstructive microsurgery. To our readers, we would appreciate your feedback on this textbook and look forward to incorporating your suggestions in future editions. Such is the dynamic nature of our field that we have little doubt that the next iteration of this book will contain many new techniques and modifications that have yet to be dreamed of as this volume goes to press and welcome the challenge of starting over again.

Contributors

David M. Adelman, MD, PhD
Associate Professor
Department of Plastic Surgery
The University of Texas MD Anderson Cancer Center
Houston, Texas

Andrew Michael Altman, MD
Clinical Assistant Professor
Division of Plastic Surgery
Department of Surgery
Baylor Scott & White Health
Texas A&M University Health Science Center College of Medicine
Temple, Texas

Blair M. Barton, MD
Resident
Otolaryngology – Head and Neck Surgery
Tulane University
New Orleans, Louisiana

Donald P. Baumann, MD, FACS
Professor
Department of Plastic Surgery
The University of Texas MD Anderson Cancer Center
Houston, Texas

Charles E. Butler, MD, FACS
Chairman
Professor of Plastic Surgery
Department of Plastic Surgery
Charles B. Barker Endowed Chair in Surgery
The University of Texas MD Anderson Cancer Center
Houston, Texas

David S. Cabiling, MD
Assistant Professor
Department of Plastic Surgery
The Ohio State University
Columbus, Ohio

Christopher A. Campbell, MD, FACS
Associate Professor
Department of Plastic Surgery
University of Virginia Health System
Charlottesville, Virginia

Martin J. Carney, MD
Resident Physician
Division of Plastic Surgery
Yale New Haven Hospital
New Haven, Connecticut

David W. Chang, MD, FACS
Professor
Section of Plastic and Reconstructive Surgery
Department of Surgery
The University of Chicago Medicine and Biological Sciences
Chicago, Illinois

Edward I. Chang, MD, FASC
Associate Professor
Department of Plastic Surgery
The University of Texas MD Anderson Cancer Center
Houston, Texas

Eric I-Yun Chang, MD, FACS
Associate Professor
Division of Plastic Surgery
Program Director, Reconstructive Microsurgery Fellowship
Surgical Oncology
Fox Chase Cancer Center
Philadelphia, Pennsylvania

Albert H. Chao, MD
Assistant Professor
Department of Plastic Surgery
The Ohio State University
Columbus, Ohio

Sydney Ch'ng, MBBS, PhD, FRACS
Associate Professor
Institute of Academic Surgery at Royal Prince Alfred Hospital
The University of Sydney
New South Wales, Australia

Mark W. Clemens, MD, FACS
Associate Professor
Department of Plastic Surgery
The University of Texas MD Anderson Cancer Center
Houston, Texas

Noopur Gangopadhyay, MD
Assistant Professor
Division of Plastic Surgery
Ann & Robert H. Lurie Children's Hospital of Chicago
Northwestern University Feinberg School of Medicine
Chicago, Illinois

Patrick B. Garvey, MD, FACS
Professor
Department of Plastic Surgery
The University of Texas MD Anderson Cancer Center
Houston, Texas

Deepak Gupta, MD
Assistant Professor
Division of Plastic Surgery
Department of Surgery
University of California San Diego
San Diego, California

Kevin Hagan, MD
Associate Professor, Plastic Surgery
Vanderbilt University Medical Center
Nashville, Tennessee

Matthew M. Hanasono, MD, FACS
Professor
Reconstructive Microsurgery Fellowship Program Director
Department of Plastic Surgery
The University of Texas MD Anderson Cancer Center
Houston, Texas

Summer E. Hanson, MD, PhD, FACS
Associate Professor
Director of Translational Research
Department of Plastic Surgery
The University of Texas MD Anderson Cancer Center
Houston, Texas

Christian P. Hasney, MD, FACS
Attending Physician
Otohrinolaryngology and Communication Sciences
Ochsner Health System
New Orleans, Louisiana

Aladdin H. Hassanein, MD, MMSc
Assistant Professor
Division of Plastic Surgery
Indiana University School of Medicine
Indianapolis, Indiana

Victor J. Hassid, MD, FACS
Associate Professor
Department of Plastic Surgery
The University of Texas MD Anderson Cancer Center
Houston, Texas

Suhail K. Kanchwala, MD
Associate Professor of Surgery
Division of Plastic Surgery
Hospital of the University of Pennsylvania
Philadelphia, Pennsylvania

Sahil K. Kapur, MD
Assistant Professor
Department of Plastic Surgery
The University of Texas MD Anderson Cancer Center
Houston, Texas

Ergun Kocak, MD
Plastic Surgeon
Midwest Breast and Aesthetic Surgery, Inc.
Gahanna, Ohio

Jeffrey H. Kozlow, MD, MS
Associate Professor (Clinical Track)
Section of Plastic Surgery
University of Michigan
Ann Arbor, Missouri

Howard N. Langstein, MD
Chief
Division of Plastic and Reconstructive Surgery
University of Rochester
Rochester, New York

Rene D. Largo, MD
Assistant Professor
Department of Plastic Surgery
The University of Texas MD Anderson Cancer Center
Houston, Texas

Gordon K. Lee, MD, FACS
Professor
Director of Microsurgery
Division of Plastic and Reconstructive Surgery
Stanford University School of Medicine
Stanford, California

Michelle Lee, MD
Plastic Surgeon
PERK Plastic Surgery
Beverly Hills, California

Samuel Lin, MD, MBA
Associate Professor
Program Director
BIDMC/Harvard Plastic Surgery Residency Program
Divisions of Plastic Surgery and Otolaryngology
Beth Israel Deaconess Medical Center
Harvard Medical School
Boston, Massachusetts

Alexander F. Mericli, MD
Assistant Professor
Department of Plastic Surgery
The University of Texas MD Anderson Cancer Center
Houston, Texas

Brian Moore, MD, FACS
Chair
Otohrinolaryngology and Communication Sciences
Ochsner Health System
New Orleans, Louisiana

Mauricio A. Moreno, MD
Associate Professor
Department of Otolaryngology, Head and Neck Surgery
University of Arkansas for Medical Sciences
Little Rock, Arizona

Amanda Murphy, MD
Resident
Department of Plastic Surgery
Dalhousie University
Halifax, Nova Scotia, Canada

Sara A. Neimanis, MD
Resident Physician
Division of Plastic and Reconstructive Surgery
University of Rochester
Rochester, New York

Anson Nguyen, MD
Plastic Surgeon
Scott & White Memorial Hospital
Temple, Texas

Laurence S. Paek, MD, CM, MSC, FRCSC
Assistant Professor
Plastic Surgery Service
Department of Surgery
Centre Hospitalier de l'Université de Montréal
Montreal, Quebec
Canada

Sameer A. Patel, MD, FACS
Associate Clinical Professor
Program Director
Temple University Hospital Plastic Surgery Residency
Division of Plastic and Reconstructive Surgery
Department of Surgical Oncology
Fox Chase Cancer Center
Philadelphia, Pennsylvania

Geoffrey L. Robb, MD, FACS
Professor of Plastic Surgery
Department of Plastic Surgery
The University of Texas MD Anderson Cancer Center
Houston, Texas

Justin M. Sacks, MD, MBA
Assistant Professor
Director, Oncological Reconstruction
Codirector, Microsurgery Fellowship
Department of Plastic and Reconstructive Surgery
Johns Hopkins School of Medicine
Baltimore, Maryland

Michel Saint-Cyr, MD
Director
Division of Plastic Surgery
Vice Chairman
Surgical Services
Wigley Professor in Plastic Surgery
Baylor Scott & White Medical Center
Temple, Texas

Mark Schaverien, MBChB, MD, MSc, Med, MRCS, PGCert(FLM), FRCS(Plast)
Assistant Professor of Plastic Surgery
Department of Plastic Surgery
The University of Texas MD Anderson Cancer Center
Houston, Texas

Jesse C. Selber, MD, MPH
Associate Professor
Department of Plastic Surgery
The University of Texas MD Anderson Cancer Center
Houston, Texas

Basel Sharaf, MD, DDS, FACS, FRCDC
Assistant Professor
Division of Plastic Surgery
Mayo Clinic
Rochester, Minnesota

Deana Shenaq, MD
Chief Resident
Department of Plastic and Reconstructive Surgery
The University of Chicago
Chicago, Illinois

Amanda K. Silva, MD
Microsurgery Fellow
Department of Plastic and Reconstructive Surgery
New York University
New York, New York

Geoffroy C. Sisk, MD
Assistant Professor
Department of Plastic and Reconstructive Surgery
The Ohio State University
Columbus, Ohio

Roman J. Skoracki, MD
Division Chief
Oncologic Plastic Surgery
The Ohio State University
Columbus, Ohio

Pankaj Tiwari, MD
Plastic Surgeon
Midwest Breast and Aesthetic Surgery, Inc.
Gahanna, Ohio

Jon Ver Halen, MD, FACS
Private Practice
Ver Halen Aesthetics and Plastic Surgery
Colleyville, Texas

Mark Villa, MD
Associate Professor
Department Plastic Surgery
The University of Texas MD Anderson Cancer Center
Houston, Texas

Jason G. Williams, MD, Med, FRCSC
Associate Professor
Department of Surgery
Dalhousie University
Halifax, Nova Scotia, Canada

Stacy Wong, MD
Plastic Surgeon
Department of Surgery
Division of Plastic Surgery
Baylor Scott & White Health
Temple, Texas

Liza C. Wu, MD, FACS
Associate Professor
Division of Plastic Surgery
University of Pennsylvania Health System
Philadelphia, Pennsylvania

Peirong Yu, MD, FACS
Professor
Department of Plastic Surgery
The University of Texas MD Anderson Cancer Center
Houston, Texas
Thomas Jefferson University Hospital
Philadelphia, Pennsylvania

Part 1

Head and Neck

1 Local Flaps of the Scalp

Victor J. Hassid

Abstract

This chapter examines the protocol used and the challenges involved in reconstructing the scalp by local flap surgery. Specific surgical concerns involved in the use of local flaps (e.g., the presence of hair, the convex shape of the skull) are discussed, including indications, anatomy, preoperative considerations, and a tested, viable technique that meets the reconstructive challenges in a way that results in the best possible outcome for the patient.

Keywords: scalp reconstruction, reconstructive ladder, local flaps, soft-tissue layers, vascular supply, innervation

1.1 Introduction

Scalp reconstruction techniques have advanced significantly throughout the years. Techniques have evolved from healing by secondary intention to complex microsurgical reconstruction, in order to resurface exposed calvarium. In the late 1600s, perforation of bare cranium was recommended as a means to promote development of granulation tissue and subsequent epithelialization. This method of scalp reconstruction, following the reconstructive ladder, subsequently advanced to skin grafting techniques, to local flaps, to use of tissue expansion, and to microsurgical reconstruction. Scalp reconstruction has always presented specific surgical challenges, secondary to its thick and inelastic nature, the presence of hair, its convex shape, and the fact that it is the only structure that provides native cranial coverage.

1.2 Typical Indications

- Cutaneous defects following oncological resection.
- Traumatic defects.
- Radiation necrosis of the calvarium.
- Unacceptable appearance of alopecia or scarring.

1.3 Anatomy

Scalp anatomy can be divided into three different elements: (1) soft-tissue layers, (2) vascular supply, and (3) innervation.[1,2] The layers include skin (3–8 mm thick), subcutaneous tissue (vessels, lymphatics, nerves), galea aponeurotica (continuous with the frontalis and occipitalis muscles and with the temporoparietal fascia, strength layer), loose areolar tissue (subgaleal fascia), and pericranium (dense adherence to calvarium) (▶ **Fig. 1.1**).

The vascularity of the scalp is based on arterial branches and vena comitantes of the internal and external carotid systems, which are divided into four distinct vascular territories. The anterior territory is supplied by the **supraorbital** (through supraorbital notch/groove) and **supratrochlear arteries** (more medial origin, approximately 2 cm lateral to midline), which are terminal branches of the internal carotid system. The lateral territory (largest territory) is supplied by terminal branches of the external carotid system, the **superficial temporal**

arteries, which bifurcates at the level of the superior helix, into frontal and parietal branches. The posterolateral territory (smallest territory) is supplied by the **posterior auricular arteries** (external carotid artery). The posterior territory is supplied by the **occipital arteries** (cephalad to nuchal line) and perforating branches of the trapezius and splenius capitis muscles (caudal to nuchal line) (▶ **Fig. 1.2**).

Sensory innervation is supplied by **three trigeminal nerve divisions, cervical spinal nerves, and branches from the cervical plexus**. The **supraorbital nerve** has a superficial and a deep branch. The superficial branch pierces the frontalis muscle and innervates the skin of the forehead and anterior hairline region.

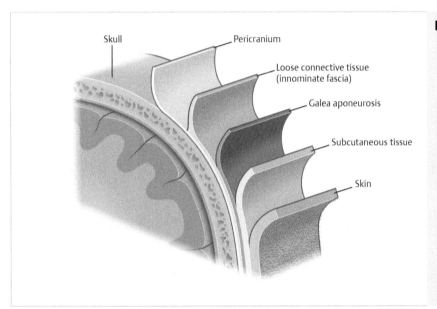

Fig. 1.1 Layers of the scalp.

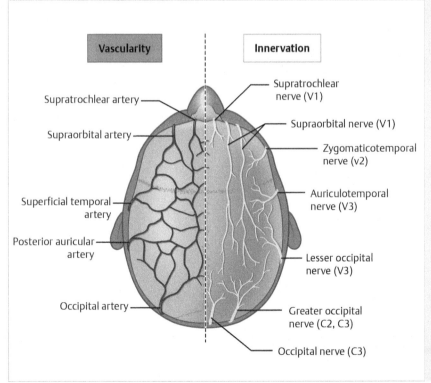

Fig. 1.2 Scalp vascularity and innervation.

The deep branch runs superficial to pericranium until the level of the coronal suture, at which point it pierces the aponeurotic layer, approximately 0.5 to 1.5 cm medial to the superior temporal line, to innervate the frontoparietal scalp. The **zygomaticotemporal nerve** (from maxillary division of trigeminal) innervates a small area lateral to the eyebrow, up to the superficial temporal crest. The **auriculotemporal nerve** (from mandibular division of trigeminal) supplies the lateral scalp. The **greater and lesser occipital nerves** (from the dorsal rami of cervical spinal nerves and the cervical plexus, respectively) innervate the occipital territory (▶Fig. 1.2).

Motor innervation is provided by the **frontal branch of the facial nerve** (courses superficial to superficial layer of deep temporal fascia) and the **posterior auricular branch of the facial nerve** (anterior and posterior auricular muscles, occipitalis muscle) (▶Fig. 1.2).

During dissection of local scalp flaps, great consideration should be made to preserve blood supply, based on vessel location, as well as normal hair bearing characteristics, since hair is the most visible feature of the scalp.

1.4 Variations

- Main variations of local scalp flaps include different designs, such as advancement and rotational flaps.[3]
- No variations exist in the flap components, which should include all scalp anatomic layers, except pericranium. Subgaleal dissection is performed.
- One to three separate scalp flaps can be raised, depending on the location, type, and size of the defect, as well as the vascular anatomy. For centrally located scalp defects, two rotation flaps can be designed to pivot from opposite or the same direction. A three-flap technique was described by Orticochea; another technique using three separate flaps is the "pinwheel" technique, which includes elevation of separate rotation flaps equally positioned adjacent to the defect and rotated in the same direction.
- Scalp flaps, including only skin and subcutaneous fat require sharp surgical dissection through a "nonanatomic" plane, are associated with more difficult hemostasis and higher risk for hair follicle injury. Therefore, they are generally not recommended.

1.5 Preoperative Considerations

It is of critical importance to consider etiology/location of scalp defect and exposed structures, available skin laxity, previous scalp incisions, and patient comorbidities when planning scalp reconstruction. Previous radiation to scalp can negatively impact the availability of any local reconstructive options, since it usually results in surrounding fibrotic scalp tissue. Previous scalp surgery and incision placement may have compromised the adjacent vascular territories, therefore limiting their use. Surrounding skin laxity and appropriate planning in regard to anticipated point of maximum tension, affect the orientation and design of local scalp flaps. Need for adjuvant therapies, such as radiotherapy, should be taken into consideration, in order to provide a reliable, long-lasting, early result and allow the patient to proceed with additional treatment.

Patient comorbidities, expectations, risks, and complications could affect the final reconstructive plan, in terms of extent and type of surgery planned. These should be discussed with the patient.

1.6 Positioning and Skin Markings

Supine, lateral, or prone positioning are the best positions for most applications. The use of Mayfield Swivel Horseshoe Headrest (Integra Lifesciences, Saint Priest, France) may be helpful in many cases, in order to allow better exposure. Furthermore, rotating the surgical bed away from anesthesia allows easy access to all areas of the scalp. The entire scalp should be draped into the surgical field, as well as other operative sites, such as the groin and/or thighs, which could serve as donor sites for skin grafting of the scalp donor site defect.

Previous scalp incisions and available surrounding skin laxity should be taken into consideration for appropriate flap design and skin markings. Rotational scalp flaps should be designed 4 to 6 times as long as the scalp defects. If appropriate, multiple rotation flaps can be designed based on surrounding skin laxity (e.g., "Yin–Yang" flaps), thus distributing wound closure tension over a larger scalp area (▶ Fig. 1.3).

Advancement flaps, although of limited use secondary to scalp inelasticity, can be designed to repair small (< 3 cm) defects in the lateral scalp, where the scalp tissue is relatively loose (▶ Fig. 1.4).

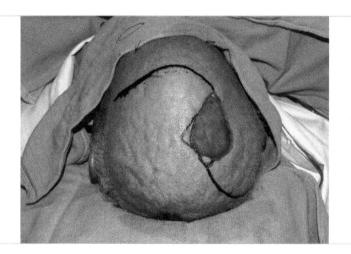

Fig. 1.3 Scalp-acquired soft-tissue defect, following wide local excision of cutaneous malignancy; "Yin–Yang" flaps designed.

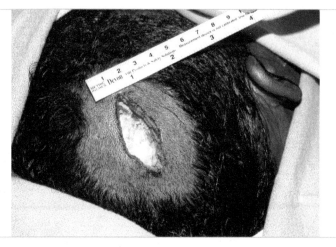

Fig. 1.4 Scalp-acquired soft-tissue defect amenable to reconstruction with advancement flaps.

1.7 Operative Technique

Following appropriate markings and Doppler identification of the course of scalp arteries—if needed—local anesthetic containing dilute epinephrine is injected along the proposed flap and the incision margin, in order to optimize hemostasis and facilitate subgaleal dissection through hydro-dissection. After waiting for appropriate amount of time for the hemostatic effect to take place, the open wound edges are debrided, if necessary, and an incision is made, based on preoperative markings. The designed scalp flaps are widely undermined along the avascular loose areolar tissue plane. Care should be taken in performing electrocautery onto the cut scalp edges, in order to prevent follicular damage and subsequent alopecia. The skin incision is beveled to parallel the direction of hair follicle growth.

To facilitate additional rotation and advancement, galeal scoring can be performed, being cautious of overlying vasculature, perpendicular to the direction of desired tissue gain. The galea can be incised at 1-cm intervals and the flap can be assessed following each score for tissue advancement (▶ **Fig. 1.5**). Consider scoring the galea sharply in order to avoid inadvertent thermal injury to the scalp arteries, which run superficially to the galea layer. A back-cut, extending from the base of the flap, can be performed to decrease tension on the closure; however, care should be taken not to compromise the flap's vascularity, secondary to decrease in flap width.

1.8 Donor Site Closure

Extensive undermining of the adjacent scalp tissue is usually necessary to decrease tension on the closure. Following placement of a small caliber Blake or Jackson–Pratt drain (if necessary), the flap is inset in layers. It is pivoted into the defect and the leading border is sutured in place, followed by the curvilinear part of the flap (▶ **Fig. 1.6a, b**). Approximation of the galea layer is important, since this is the strength layer of the scalp. If the scalp donor site defect cannot be primarily closed, it should be reconstructed with a full- or split-thickness skin graft, and appropriate bolster dressing should be used to cover it (▶ **Fig. 1.6c**).

Avoid excising the resulting standing cutaneous deformities, since majority of those usually resolve with time. Excising them at the time of reconstruction could affect the flap's vascularity. If necessary, those can be addressed at a later date.

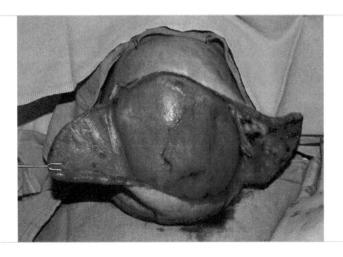

Fig. 1.5 "Yin–Yang" flaps widely undermined and galea scoring performed for additional tissue gain.

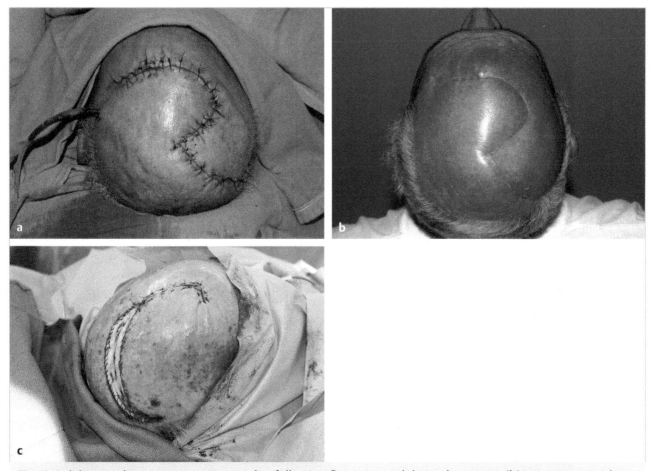

Fig. 1.6 **(a)** Immediate postoperative results, following flap inset and drain placement. **(b)** Long-term results. **(c)** Application of skin graft to cover donor site defect, in case of large scalp rotational advancement flap.

1.9 Pearls and Pitfalls

- The greatest amount of scalp mobility occurs in the parietal regions, where the temporoparietal overlies the temporalis fascia.
- Try to preserve the deep branch of the supraorbital nerve to avoid scalp numbness of the frontoparietal scalp.
- Take into consideration existing scalp incisions, potentially violating vascular territories.
- Design large rotational flaps, at least 4 to 6 times the width of the defect.
- Make a back-cut if necessary, if concerned about tension on the closure. Also, consider skin grafting scalp donor site defect.

References

[1] Leedy JE, Janis JE, Rohrich RJ. Reconstruction of acquired scalp defects: an algorithmic approach. Plast Reconstr Surg 2005;116(4):54e–72e
[2] Leedy JE. Scalp and calvarial reconstruction. In: Janis JE, ed. Essentials of Plastic Surgery. St. Louis, MO: Quality Medical Publishing; 2007
[3] Hoffmann JF. Reconstruction of the scalp. In: Baker SR, ed. Local Flaps in Facial Reconstruction. 2nd ed. Philadelphia, PA: Mosby; 2007

2 Paramedian Forehead Flap

Mark Villa

Abstract

The use of the paramedian forehead flap is the technique of choice for the reconstruction of nasal defects. This is because the forehead flap can provide a large volume of reliable, aesthetically pleasing skin for both external coverage and nasal lining when there is a partial or complete loss of the nose. Due to the nose's complex anatomy and functional importance (including airway patency and sense of smell), reconstructing it is a special challenge. This chapter describes the sequential steps necessary to perform this reconstruction in a way that results in optimum aesthetic and functional outcomes.

Keywords: paramedian forehead flap, oblique flap designs, anatomic landmarks, pedicle

2.1 Introduction

The paramedian forehead flap is commonly used for the reconstruction of nasal defects because of its excellent color and texture match as well as its proximity to the nose. First described in an Indian medical treatise called the Sushuruta Samita in the 6th century BC, the paramedian forehead flap is the result of a long process of anatomic investigation and surgical refinement of the technique by such pioneers as Lisfranc, Dieffenbach, Gillies, Converse, Millard, Burget, and Menick.[1] In particular, Menick and Burget both provide extensive, detailed descriptions of the approach to nasal reconstruction with the paramedian forehead flap.[2,3]

Whether the nasal defect under consideration consists of partial or complete loss of the nose, the forehead flap can provide a large volume of reliable, aesthetically pleasing skin for external coverage as well as nasal lining, if needed.

Nasal reconstruction is one of the most challenging tasks in facial reconstruction because of the nose's complex, subtle surface anatomy and contours, as well as its functional importance with regard to airway patency and the sense of smell. The use of the paramedian forehead flap must be undertaken with careful consideration of the defect to be reconstructed, how the operations will be staged, and what, exactly, will be done at each stage. Failure to consider the reconstruction appropriately can result in a poor aesthetic outcome or, worse, reconstructive failure that results in the patient's appearance being worse than it was before the surgery.

2.2 Typical Indications

The forehead flap can be used to resurface the entire nasal skin or just portions of it. Though the paramedian forehead flap is used most commonly for nasal reconstruction, it may be used for other soft-tissue deficits of the central face and eyelids.

2.3 Anatomy

The vasculature of the forehead includes the supraorbital, supratrochlear, infratrochlear, and dorsal nasal arteries, which are terminal branches of the ophthalmic artery that arises from the internal carotid artery. (Recall that the trochlea is the "pulley" attached to the nasal bone that redirects the tendon of the superior oblique muscle and, therefore, its vector, allowing it to perform its primary functions of depression and intorsion of the eyeball.) Additional branches of the facial artery, including the angular artery, contribute to the extensive plexus that forms anastomoses with both ipsilateral and contralateral vessels to supply the tissues of the forehead.

The **supratrochlear artery** (▶ Fig. 2.1) is the primary blood supply for the paramedian forehead flap. It branches off the **ophthalmic artery** and travels within the orbit, pierces the orbital septum, and comes around the orbital rim at the supratrochlear notch. The vessel then heads superiorly, accompanied by the supratrochlear nerve, to supply the forehead. As the vessel comes around the orbital rim, it enters a plane between the corrugator muscle deeply and the frontalis muscle superficially.[4] It is important to know the position of the artery superficial to both the periosteum and the corrugator muscle to allow for safe, consistent dissection of the supratrochlear artery below the level of the orbital rim.[5] Small veins run parallel to the course of the arteries.

As the supratrochlear artery travels superiorly, its course soon becomes more superficial as it traverses the frontalis muscle to run in a plane just deep to the dermis, where it remains as it makes its way to the level of the hairline and beyond.[4]

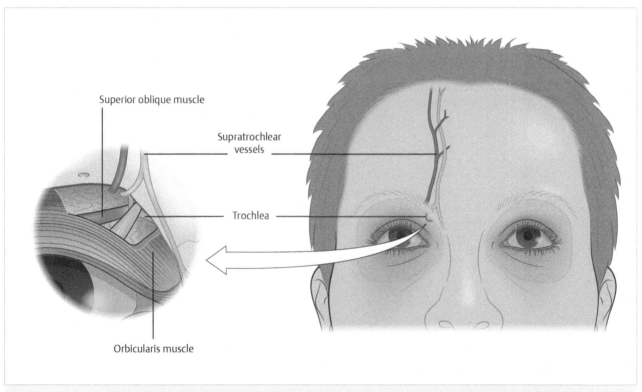

Superior oblique muscle

Supratrochlear vessels

Trochlea

Orbicularis muscle

Fig. 2.1 The supratrochlear vessels in relation to the trochlea at the upper, inner aspect of the orbit.

2.4 Variations

Avoid oblique flap designs as these can compromise the blood supply to the distal portions of the flap (▶ **Fig. 2.2b**).

2.5 Preoperative Planning

Planning is of paramount importance to the ultimate success of nasal reconstruction using the paramedian forehead flap. Any reconstruction of the nose must take into account the size, depth, location, and nature of the defect, including the type(s) of tissues absent. The defect must also be adequately prepared. This can include removing scar tissue and previous attempts at closure in a mature wound and taking into account swelling or local anesthetic injections

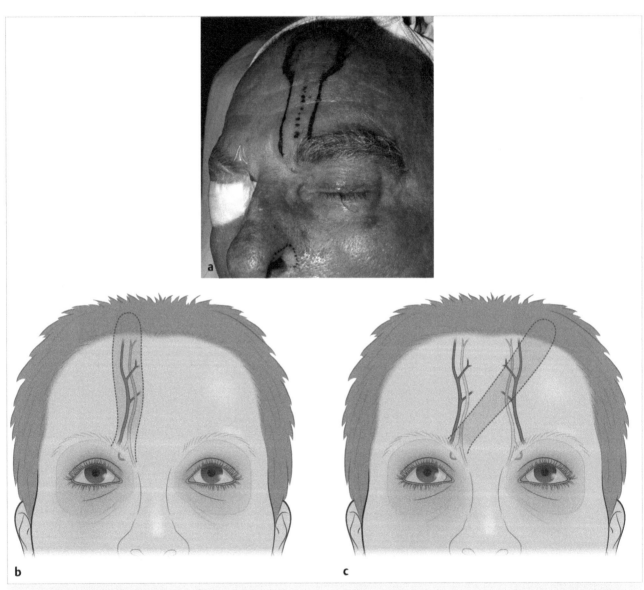

Fig. 2.2 (a) The flap design extending vertically from the orbit to the hairline, encompassing the supratrochlear vessels. The flap may extend beyond the hairline if extra length is needed. (b,c) Demonstrates an oblique flap design for added length showing how this fails to incorporate the supratrochlear vessel axially, converting the distal portion of the flap to a random pattern flap and potentially compromising its viability. ([a] is provided courtesy of Matthew M. Hanasono.)

in a fresh wound. Only when adequate preparation of the wound has occurred will the true extent of the defect be known.

2.6 Positioning and Skin Markings

Prior to making any incisions, the surgeon should mark various anatomic landmarks with ink. These include the course of the supratrochlear vessel (identified with a Doppler pencil), the hairline, the nasolabial folds, the facial midline, the subunits of the nose, and the upper lip.[2,3] The flap should be oriented with the template of the defect centered on the supratrochlear vessel once its course has been determined (▶ Fig. 2.2a). In general, the flap ipsilateral to the defect to be reconstructed is used.[6] To lengthen the flap, some have described designing the flap obliquely so that it travels at an angle across the forehead (▶ Fig. 2.2b). While this design may increase the length of the flap, it can compromise the blood supply to the distal aspect of the flap, as the axial vessel is no longer included in the distal portion. Instead, additional length may be safely obtained by extending the distal aspect of the flap into hair-bearing skin or more aggressively dissecting the base of the flap in the vicinity of the orbital rim.

A surgical sponge or an Esmarch bandage may be used to gauge the length of the pedicle and ensure that the flap reaches the defect under minimal tension. A template of the defect can be made at the time of the surgery. Unaffected subunits may be used for creation of the template, or the template may even be made preoperatively and sterilized if there is concern about the possible extent of resection.

Once the template has been created and marked on the forehead, 1% lidocaine with epinephrine may be injected into the forehead surrounding the flap to optimize hemostasis during flap dissection and donor site closure. Anesthetic with epinephrine *should not* be injected into the flap itself, as the blanching it causes will make it difficult to assess the vascularity of the flap. Anesthetic with epinephrine may also be injected around the defect but only after templates of the defect have been made because distortion of the tissues can occur.

2.7 Operative Technique

Once the periphery of the flap has been incised, dissection of the flap is undertaken from the distal to proximal end (▶ Fig. 2.3). The distal third of the flap should be raised in a subcutaneous plane, preserving the branches of the supratrochlear vessels located just deep to the dermis. If the distal aspect of the flap extends into hair-bearing skin, the bulbs of the hair follicles may be carefully trimmed with scissors at the time of flap dissection. Laser hair removal may be undertaken instead at a later date, but removal of hair follicles with a fine scissor under direct visualization may be more definitive.[3]

Dissection of the middle third of the flap is performed in the submuscular/subgaleal plane beneath the frontalis muscle, which protects the supratrochlear vessels that run superficial to the frontalis muscle at this level.

For the inferior third of the flap the plane of dissection changes to the subperiosteal plane. As noted before, the supratrochlear vessel travels between the corrugator and the frontalis after it comes around the orbital rim.[2] Staying in the subperiosteal plane at this level allows both the periosteum and the corrugator muscle to protect the vessel during this portion of the dissection.[4]

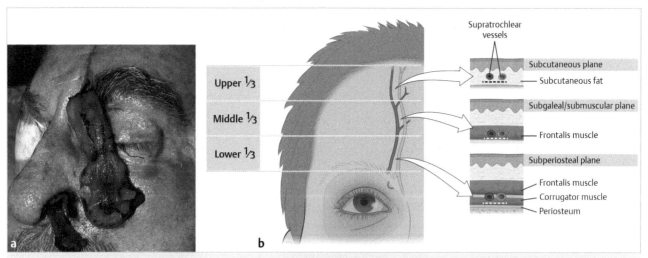

Fig. 2.3 **(a)** The flap after dissection and prior to inset. Muscle fibers are visible on the distal portion of the flap, as is a cartilage graft to be used for alar support. A nasal mucosal flap to be used for lining of the ala protrudes from the nare. **(b)** The left half shows the paramedian forehead flap divided into thirds, with the plane of dissection for each third. The right shows a cross section of the flap with the depth of the supratrochlear vessel shown for each third. ([a] is provided courtesy of Matthew M. Hanasono.)

The supratrochlear vessel travels out of the orbit, pierces the orbital septum, and comes around the orbital rim. It does not exit any bony foramen in the vicinity of the orbital rim, so there is no need to worry about transecting the vessel at this level as long as a careful subperiosteal dissection is performed.[5] This dissection may be carried down almost to the level of the medial canthus to provide additional length and a free point of rotation for the flap to reach the nose.

2.8 Donor Site Closure

Once the flap dissection is complete and the flap clearly reaches the defect under no tension, donor site closure can be undertaken (▶ **Fig. 2.4**). The forehead should be undermined in the subgaleal plane to the temporalis muscles bilaterally and extended superiorly under the hair-bearing skin to maximize the mobility of the skin available for donor site closure. Depending on the size of the flap and the laxity of the patient's forehead, primary closure of the entire donor site may be possible. For larger flaps, primary closure may be possible only for the inferior portion of the donor site. Portions that can't be closed primarily can be allowed to heal secondarily with dressing changes. This may take several weeks, and though it may look unpleasant while healing, the cosmesis of the donor site will ultimately be acceptable. It is incredibly important, however, to not allow the periosteum to dry out in those portions of the wound healing secondarily. Exposed calvarial bone will prolong wound healing and may necessitate further intervention to foster donor site healing.

Although the paramedian forehead flap may be used for single-stage reconstructions with the pedicle tunneled under the skin, it is more commonly used for two- and even three-stage reconstructions. Whether the reconstruction

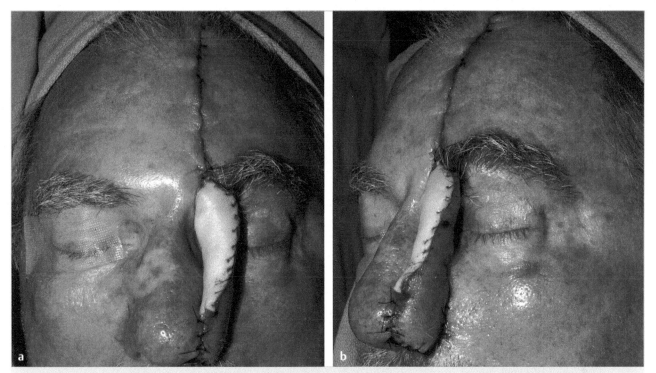

Fig. 2.4 The paramedian forehead flap after inset at the primary procedure. A full-thickness skin graft is present on the undersurface of the flap pedicle. (The image is provided courtesy of Matthew M. Hanasono.)

is two or three stages, the flap is generally allowed to heal for 3 to 4 weeks, in which time it will develop a blood supply from the recipient site. At this point, the pedicle should be temporarily occluded (with a cinched vessel loop, for example) to see how the distal portion of the flap responds. If the flap continues to look pink and healthy distally following pedicle occlusion, the pedicle can be safely divided. If the flap appears either pale or congested, one may consider delaying pedicle division to allow for further vascularization to occur.

Following division of the pedicle, the majority of the pedicle is excised and the base is carefully inset to restore and preserve the contour of the medial brow (▶**Fig. 2.5**).[3]

2.9 Pearls and Pitfalls

- Dissection of the upper third of the flap occurs in the subcutaneous plane, the middle third in the submuscular plane, and the inferior third in the subperiosteal plane.
- Oblique design of the flap can be less reliable secondary to not fully capturing the axial supratrochlear vessels
- *Do not* inject local anesthetic with epinephrine into the flap as it makes it more difficult to assess the flap.
- It is imperative that open areas on the forehead not be allowed to dry out as this can significantly prolong postoperative healing.

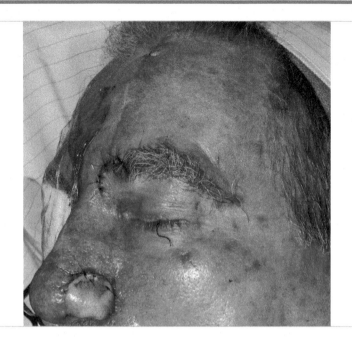

Fig. 2.5 The flap on the ala following division of the pedicle and final inset. (The image is provided courtesy of Matthew M. Hanasono.)

References

[1] Correa BJ, Weathers WM, Wolfswinkel EM, Thornton JF. The forehead flap: the gold standard of nasal soft tissue reconstruction. Semin Plast Surg 2013;27(2):96–103

[2] Menick FJ. Nasal Reconstruction: Art and Practice. Edinburgh: Saunders; 2008

[3] Burget GC, Menick FJ. Aesthetic Reconstruction of the Nose. St Louis, MO: Mosby-Year Book, Inc.; 1994

[4] Shumrick KA, Smith TL. The anatomic basis for the design of forehead flaps in nasal reconstruction. Arch Otolaryngol Head Neck Surg 1992;118(4):373–379

[5] Reece EM, Schaverien M, Rohrich RJ. The paramedian forehead flap: a dynamic anatomical vascular study verifying safety and clinical implications. Plast Reconstr Surg 2008;121(6):1956–1963

[6] Menick FJ. Aesthetic refinements in use of forehead for nasal reconstruction: the paramedian forehead flap. Clin Plast Surg 1990;17(4):607–622

3 Temporalis Muscle Flap

Summer E. Hanson

Abstract

The advancement of microsurgical techniques and free flap options have made free tissue transfer commonplace in reconstructive surgery. However, local tissue options in the head and neck often offer thin, pliable alternatives, wherein like is replaced with like, and donor site morbidity is minimal. The temporalis muscle flap is such an alternative for use in orbital reconstruction and facial reanimation. The number of defects and uses to which it can be put are examined in this chapter and proper techniques for its use are thoroughly discussed.

Keywords: temporalis muscle flap, intratemporal crest, deep temporal nerves, deep temporal artery, internal maxillary artery, temporal fat pad, eyelid sling

3.1 Introduction

The advancement of microsurgical technique and myriad free flap options available have made free tissue transfer commonplace in reconstructive surgery. However, local tissue options in the head and neck often offer thin, pliable alternatives to free tissue transfer, replacing like with like, and minimal donor site morbidity. The temporalis muscle flap is one such workhorse flap and is commonly used in orbital reconstruction and facial reanimation. It was first described in 1895 for temporomandibular joint ankylosis[1] and indications were quickly expanded to orbital and facial defects.[2] The temporalis muscle flap is useful for reconstructing defects of the periorbital region, maxilla, base of skull, palate, posterior oropharynx, and floor of mouth and tongue and includes immediate and delayed reconstruction.[3] Additionally, a split temporalis flap may be used as a sling for the lower eyelid and lip for facial paralysis. Dynamic movement is achievable through the third division of the trigeminal nerve (V3).

3.2 Typical Indications

- Periorbital defects/orbital exenteration.
- External cheek defects/facial resurfacing.
- Cranial base.
- Maxilla.
- Oral cavity.
  - Palate.
  - Floor of mouth.
  - Retromolar trigone.
  - Tonsilar fossa.
  - Pharyngeal defects.
- Facial reanimation.

3.3 Anatomy

The temporalis muscle is a flexible, fan-shaped Mathes and Nahai type III flap of moderate thickness (▶**Fig. 3.1**). It lies between the temporal fossa and the overlying **deep temporal fascia**. The layers of temporal fascia include

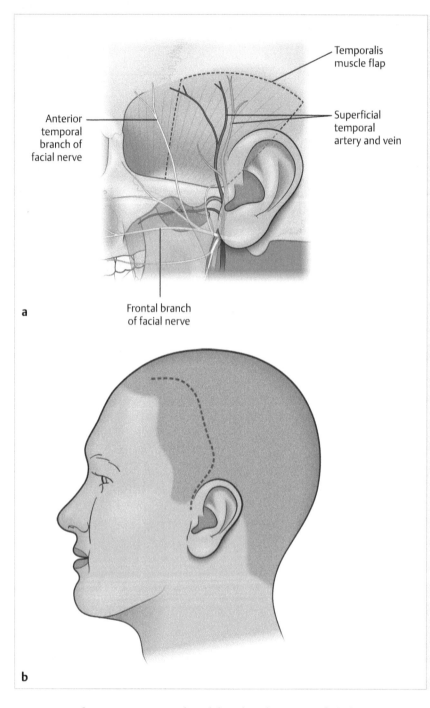

Anterior temporal branch of facial nerve

Temporalis muscle flap

Superficial temporal artery and vein

Frontal branch of facial nerve

a

b

Fig. 3.1 (a,b) Anatomy of the temporalis muscle.

the temporoparietal fascia, the superficial most layer, which is a continuation of the superficial aponeurotic system, and the deep temporal fascia, which invest the temporalis muscle and is further split into a superficial and deep layer. The temporalis originates at the infratemporal crest superiorly and inserts onto the coronoid process and anterior border of the mandibular ramus inferiorly. The muscle is 12 to 16 cm in length with a thickness of 0.5 to 1.0 cm.[4] It spans the lateral skull and passes beneath the zygomatic arch to elevate and retract the mandible. Additionally, the muscle provides contour of the upper lateral face.

The temporalis muscle is innervated by the **deep temporal nerves** from the mandibular branch of the trigeminal nerve. The blood supply to the temporalis muscle is two branches of the **deep temporal artery**, the anterior and posterior, arising from the pterygoid portion of the **internal maxillary artery**.[5] These enter the deep surface of the muscle medially just above its insertion. Accessory blood supply is from the middle temporal artery, originating from the superficial temporal artery within the temporoparietal fascia. This is usually sacrificed for muscle transfer. The robust blood supply of the scalp allows overlying skin and fascia to be included with the temporalis muscle; however, unlike a traditional myocutaneous flap, this composite represents a muscle flap and a separate fasciocutaneous flap.

3.4 Variations

- Muscle flap.
- Split muscle flap.
- Chimeric muscle flap with temporoparietal fascia flap.

3.5 Preoperative Considerations

The muscle flap is accessible through a hemicoronal incision, hidden in the hair bearing skin. The blood supply is reliable; however, the flap cannot be used if the ipsilateral internal maxillary or external carotid arteries have been sacrificed or compromised.

3.6 Positioning and Skin Markings

The temporalis muscle is palpated by forcibly clenching the jaw, with the insertion near the midpoint of the zygomatic arch. The superior margin is approximately halfway between the upper margin of the ear and the vertex. On the operating table, the head is positioned so that both sides of the head are easily accessed.

3.7 Operative Technique

A hemicoronal incision is made with a preauricular extension for exposure (▶ **Fig. 3.2a**). A rhytidectomy incision with superior extension may be used if a neck dissection is planned, as in ▶ **Fig. 3.2b**. Elevation of the scalp is carried out in a subaponeurotic plane, superior to inferior, directly on the deep temporal fascia until the superficial temporal fat pad is encountered. The dissection then transitions down to the deep layer of the deep temporal fascia, beneath the **temporal fat pad** to the level of the zygoma. At the zygomatic arch, a horizontal incision is made through the fat pad to the periosteum on the deep surface of the zygoma. The periosteum is incised and the scalp is further elevated from the preauricular region over the length of the zygoma to the orbital rim. This technique allows the temporal fat pad to remain with the scalp, protecting the temporal branch of the facial nerve and limiting hollowing when the muscle is transposed. To facilitate transposition to the orbit, a tunnel is created by drilling the lateral orbital wall (▶ **Fig. 3.2c**). Alternatively, to reach the oral cavity, a segment of the zygomatic arch is removed and a tunnel created bluntly between the temporal fossa, over the masseter and into the oral cavity. While the zygomatic arch may be replaced, the muscle fills the defect with little depression and the arch may cause unwanted compression of the flap. Split-thickness skin graft is usually used for coverage of the

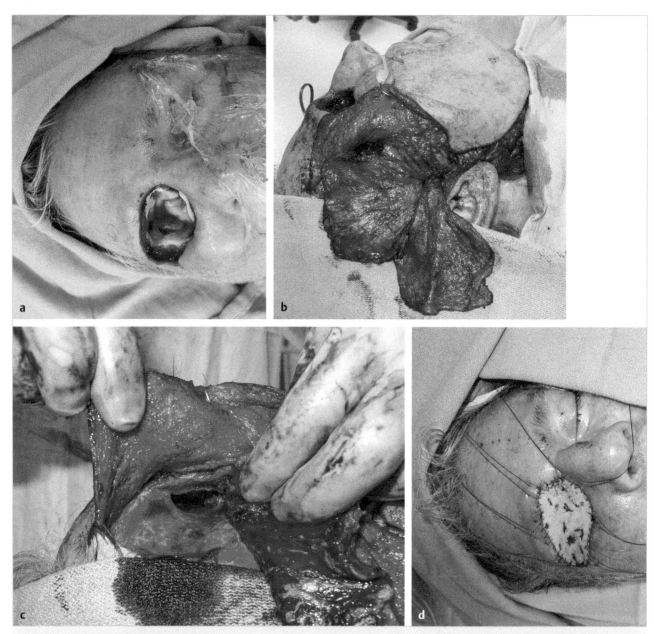

Fig. 3.2 (a) Defect following orbital exenteration for sebaceous cell carcinoma of the lacrimal gland. (b) Elevation of both temporalis muscle and temporoparietal fascia. (c) Tunnel to the lateral orbit to avoid pressure on the pedicle for transfer. (d) Inset of temporalis muscle flap with full-thickness skin graft.

muscle (▶**Fig. 3.2d**); however, the muscle surface reepithelializes well in the oral cavity. The longitudinal nature of the blood supply allows for splitting of the muscle into segments supplied by the anterior and posterior branches for dynamic reconstruction in facial paralysis.

3.8 Donor Site Care

Substantial elevation of the scalp is necessary for muscle flap dissection which may require small closed suction drains. The wound is closed in layers. Temporal hollowing is the most commonly cited aesthetic donor site complaint with the temporalis muscle flap. Preservation of the temporal fat pad or anterior third of muscle reduce hollowing in this region. Others have described minimizing the donor site deformity with pericranial flaps or alloplastic implant materials.

3.9 Pearls and Pitfalls

- The approach may be performed through a rhydidectomy incision with a temporal extension if parotidectomy or neck dissection is planned.
- Most defects require the full length of the muscle but not the full width. Sparing the anterior one-third minimizes significant hollowing of the temporal region.
- When the temporalis muscle is used to fill in orbital defects, a portion of the lateral orbital wall may be drilled to prevent compression of the pedicle.

References

[1] Lentz J. Resection du col du condyle avec interposition d'un lambeau temporal entre les surfaces de resction. Guerison Assoc Franc de Chirur (Paris) 1895;9:113–117

[2] Gilles HD. Plastic Surgery of the Face. London: Oxford University Press; 1920:54–55

[3] Hanasono MM, Utley DS, Goode RL. The temporalis muscle flap for reconstruction after head and neck oncologic surgery. Laryngoscope 2001;111(10):1719–1725

[4] Bradley P, Brockbank J. The temporalis muscle flap in oral reconstruction. A cadaveric, animal and clinical study. J Maxillofac Surg 1981;9(3):139–145

[5] Cheung LK. The vascular anatomy of the human temporalis muscle: implications for surgical splitting techniques. Int J Oral Maxillofac Surg 1996;25(6):414–421

4 Temporoparietal Fascia Flap

Basel Sharaf

Abstract

The Temporoparietal fascia flap (TPFF) is a valuable local flap in orbital, midface, ear, nasal, and oral reconstruction. The TPFF is one of the thinnest and most pliable vascularized flaps in the body. Other options in the microsurgeon's armamentarium when thin coverage is needed include the superficial circumflex iliac artery perforator flap (SCIP), serratus fascia/muscle flap, lateral arm fascia flap, and anteriolateral thigh fascia flap. This chapter discusses the indications, misconceptions, anatomy, preoperative considerations, and techniques involved in using the TPFF to achieve good outcomes.

Keywords: temporoparietal fascia flap, superficial temporal artery, superficial temporal vein, frontal branch of the facial nerve

4.1 Introduction

The temporoparietal fascia flap (TPFF) was described by Monks[1] and Brown[2] for eyelid and auricular reconstruction in 1898. The first free microvascular transfer of the TPFF was described by Smith for lower extremity coverage in 1980.[3] Since then, the flap has been used for several indications including head and neck and extremity reconstruction and remains the workhorse flap for microtia and ear reconstruction. The TPFF is a valuable local flap for periorbital, midface, ear, and oral reconstruction when thin and pliable vascularized tissue is required. Although other options of relatively thin vascularized tissue for extremity coverage have gained popularity over the past two decades, such as the superficial circumflex iliac artery perforator flap, serratus muscle/fascia flap, lateral arm flap, and anterior lateral thigh flap, the TPFF remains a useful flap in the reconstructive surgeon's armamentarium.

4.2 Typical Indications

The TPFF can be utilized in a pedicled fashion for coverage of lateral forehead, temporal, skull base and dura, orbital, cheek, maxillary, and palatal reconstruction. It remains the flap of choice for ear reconstruction and coverage of ear cartilage after trauma or in microtia reconstruction. A composite TPFF–osseous flap using a split outer calvarial bone has been described for craniofacial reconstruction. In this scenario, a generous cuff of fascia and pericranium is harvested beyond the dimension of the split calvarial bone graft and the graft is fixed to the overlying pericranium and TPFF with sutures to avoid shearing during manipulation. The TPFF has been favored in dorsal hand and foot coverage for its ability to allow thin vascular tissue coverage and tendon gliding. TPF–cutaneous (hair-bearing) flaps have been utilized for brow restoration and upper lip reconstruction (mustache in men). Careful design of the hair-bearing flap over the vascular pedicle and taking into consideration hair follicle orientation after flap rotation into the defect is paramount to allow hair growth in proper direction. However, advanced hair transplantation techniques have largely substituted this indication.

4.3 Anatomy

The TPFF nomenclature has been described inconsistently throughout the literature. This has created confusion in its anatomic descriptions. The TPF is located under the temporoparietal scalp and extends superiorly and posteriorly to the temporal fusion line (the origin of the temporalis muscle), anteriorly to the lateral orbital rim, and inferiorly to the zygomatic arch and supramastoid crest (▶Fig. 4.1). The TPF is a 2- to 3-mm thick, translucent and highly vascular distinct layer underneath the subcutaneous fat layer. In the temporal fossa, nine anatomic layers exist including from superficial to deep: the skin; the subcutaneous tissue; the temporoparietal fascia (TPF) (or superficial temporal fascia); the loose areolar layer (or innominate fascia); the superficial layer of the deep temporal fascia; the superficial temporal fat pad; the deep layer of the deep temporal fascia; the deep temporal fat pad; and the temporalis muscle.

The **superficial temporal artery** (STA) and **vein** (STV) run on or within the TPF and provide the vascular pedicle to the TPFF. The STA, one of the terminal branches of the external carotid artery, passes through the parotid gland posterior to the mandibular ramus prior to taking a more superficial course and piercing the TPF at the level of the tragus where it can be palpated. Handheld Doppler examination delineates its course. The STA bifurcates into an anterior (frontal) and posterior (parietal) branches 1 to 3 cm above the zygomatic arch. The artery is found anterior to the tragus within 0.5 to 1.5 cm distance and approximately 1 cm deep to the preauricular skin. The STA is tortuous

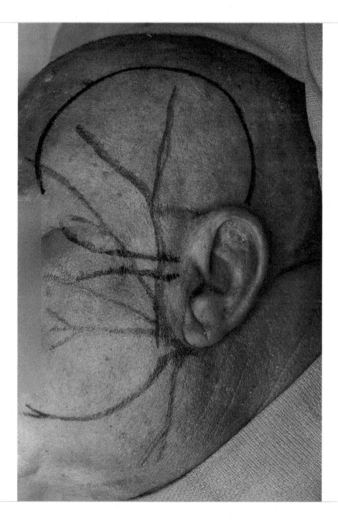

Fig. 4.1 The outline of the temporal fossa, zygomatic arch, approximate course of the superficial temporal vessels, and facial nerve branches are marked. The TPF becomes confluent with the galea aponeurotica at the superior temporal line. The STA bifurcates 2 to 3 cm above the zygomatic arch.

and release of this tortuosity may add an extra 1 to 2 cm of length to the pedicle. The mean diameter of the STA at the zygomatic arch is 1 to 2 mm. The STA lies anterior to the STV. The STA may be hypoplastic or have an anomalous course in patients with certain craniofacial anomlaies such as hemifacial microsomia, Treacher-Collins syndrome or Romberg's hemifacial atrophy. The **frontal branch of the facial nerve** crosses over the zygomatic arch within the loose areolar layer (innominate fascia) where it remains for a distance of 1.5 to 3.0 cm above the superior border of the arch (▶ **Fig. 4.1**). The auriculotemporal nerve travels posterior to the STA in the preauricular crease and can be preserved or included in flap dissection if sensory innervation to the flap is needed. During TPF flap elevation, attention should be paid to the frontal branches of the facial nerve, which course obliquely across the zygomatic arch along a line connecting the tragus to the lateral brow. Up to three frontal nerve branches at the level of zygomatic arch may be present, with the most posterior branch reported at 24 mm from the tragus and the most anterior branch within 42 mm from the tragus.[4] Dissection should be limited to within a 2.4 cm distance from the tragus to prevent injury to the frontal nerve branches.

The temporalis muscle fascia (also known as the deep temporal fascia) splits above the zygomatic arch into two leaflets: the superficial layer of the deep temporal fascia, which is adherent to the lateral zygomatic arch periosteum, and the deep layer of the deep temporal fascia, which runs medial (deeper) to the zygomatic arch. The temporal fat pad is located between the superficial and deep layers of the deep temporal fascia. The middle temporal artery arises from the STA at the level of the zygomatic arch where it can be seen on the temporalis muscle fascia. Proximal dissection of the STA to include the middle temporal artery allows for elevation of bilayered fascial flap containing the TPFF and the deep temporal fascia. This provides two vascularized surfaces to assist in greater area of wound coverage or in tendon gliding (▶ **Fig. 4.3g,h**).

4.4 Variations

- Fascial flap (is most common).
- Fasciocutaneous flap for hair-bearing tissue reconstruction (brow, mustache).
- Bilayered TPFF–deep temporal fascia flap for tendon/extremity coverage.
- Composite TPFF–osseous flap.
- Prelaminated TPFF–cartilage flap for tracheal reconstruction.
- Prelaminated TPFF–skin graft for oral/nasal lining.
- Prelaminated TPFF–fat graft for facial contour correction.

4.5 Preoperative Considerations

Doppler examination of the STA is important to determine the reliability of this flap. Prior ligation or embolization of the external carotid artery, prior coronal scalp incisions in the STA territory, ablative neck surgery sacrificing the external carotid artery or STA, and radiation to the STA area are contraindications to using this flap. Furthermore, anomalous course or hypoplasia of the STA have been reported in certain congenital craniofacial syndromes. Additional imaging (Duplex Ultrasound or CTA) maybe required in such cases.

The vascularity of the TPFF based on the STA extends to the midline of the cranium. Flap dimensions of up to 12 × 14 cm can be elevated. Careful assessment of flap reach to the intended area of reconstruction using a template is recommended. Temporary removal of the zygomatic arch may improve flap reach for maxillary, posterior nasal, or oral reconstruction by an extra 1 to 2 cm. Furthermore, proximal dissection of the vascular pedicle below the tragus can also improve flap reach; however, this places the facial nerve at risk of injury. Identification of the facial nerve branches within the parotid gland may be necessary in this scenario. The TPF can be advanced into skull base defects and dural reconstruction for cerebrospinal fluid leaks by advancing it from the temporal to the infratemporal fossa through a transpterygoid tunnel.[5]

4.6 Positioning and Skin Markings

The hair can be trimmed over the incisions. Alternatively, the entire scalp hair can be trimmed. The course of the STA is marked on the scalp after a hand-held Doppler examination. The patient is positioned in a supine manner and a horseshoe surgical headrest allows turning the head easily during flap elevation. Several incisions have been described to access the TPFF. A lazy S, zig-zag, Y, or T incision can be utilized. Scar alopecia at the T and Y incision junction has been reported in up to 8% of patients. The author's preference is to use a lazy S or zig-zag incision over the center of the TPF (▶ Fig. 4.2).

4.7 Operative Technique

The flap is elevated under general anesthesia. Local infiltration with dilute epinephrine solution (1:400,000) at the scalp incision facilitates hemostasis

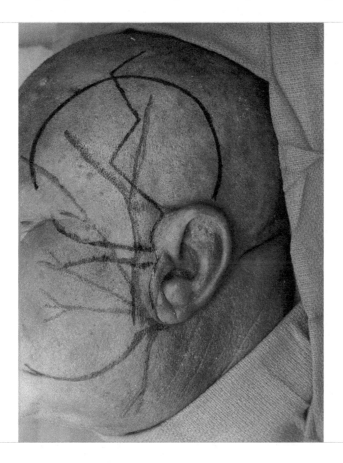

Fig. 4.2 A preauricular incision is extended superiorly in a zig-zag fashion over the center of the TPF.

during flap elevation, although not essential. When scalp infiltration is done, it is important to do so over the distal flap area, avoiding injection near the main vascular pedicle. If free flap transfer is planned, use of papaverine prior to flap division will help reverse residual vasoconstrictor effect. Bipolar cautery is helpful during flap elevation. Flap elevation is started distally under loupe magnification. The scalp flaps are retracted anteriorly and posteriorly to facilitate TPFF flap elevation. The TPFF is found just underneath the scalp hair follicles. Small perforating branches to the scalp are cauterized with bipolar cautery (▶ **Fig. 4.3a**). Leaving the subcutaneous fat on the scalp flaps helps minimize injury to the hair follicles. Flap dissection past the temporal fusion line is more difficult as fibrous connections to the scalp exist in this area. After the scalp flaps have been elevated anteriorly and posteriorly, the TPFF flap dimensions are marked using a template. It is recommended to raise a larger flap than required as some minor primary contraction of the TPF occurs after

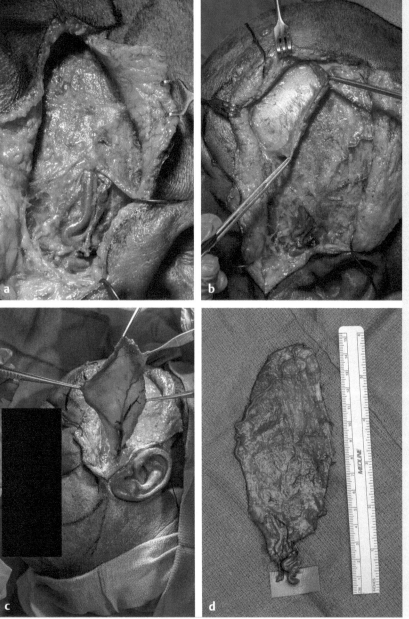

Fig. 4.3 **(a)** The STA and STV are identified in the pretragal area and the TPF is shown just underneath the scalp hair follicles. Small perforating branches to the scalp are shown and cauterized with bipolar cautery. **(b)** The TPFF is raised off the deep temporal fascia (temporalis muscle fascia). The loose areolar plane (arrow) is shown and makes for easy plane of dissection. **(c)** The TPFF is elevated and transilluminated. Note the translucent quality of the TPF and the branching pattern of the vascular pedicle showing the frontal and parietal branches of the STA. **(d)** A 14 × 7 cm TPFF is raised and the vascular pedicle is divided for free tissue transfer. The pedicle is approximately 3- to 4-cm long.

(*Continued*)

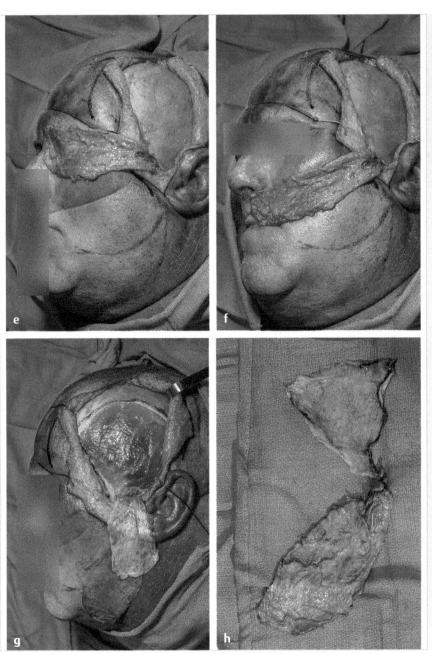

Fig. 4.3 (*Continued*) **(e)** The arc of rotation of the TPFF is demonstrated for orbital reconstruction, **(f)** cheek, midface, or oral reconstruction. **(g)** A bilayered TPFF–deep temporal fascia flap can be elevated. **(h)** This allows for greater surface area coverage if needed, or a bilayered coverage for tendon gliding in extremity reconstruction.

flap division. Staying 2 to 3 cm posterior to the anticipated course of the frontal branch of the facial nerve is important. The pedicle is then dissected more proximally after extending the scalp incision into the preauricular crease. If free TPF flap transfer is indicated, the pedicle is best dissected under the microscope. Small branches off the STA and STV can then be easily visualized and ligated using small hemoclips to aid in maintaining a bloodless field. If further pedicle length or caliber is needed, dissection can be extended more proximally below the tragus paying great attention to facial nerve branches in this area as the STA may lie within the parotid gland. Then the TPF is incised along its intended flap design and elevated off the loose areolar plane, where the deeper temporalis muscle fascia is visualized (►**Fig. 4.3b**). Flap elevation in this plane is quick and bloodless. The anterior branch of the STA is ligated at the anterior edge of the TPFF if needed. Likewise, the STA may need to be ligated superiorly at the superior extent of the TPF flap (►**Fig. 4.3c–h**).

4.8 Donor Site Closure

After meticulous hemostasis, the donor site incision is closed in two layers using monofilament for the deeper layer and running resorbable monofilament or staples for the skin. Closure is done over a suction or penrose drain. The drain should be positioned away from the vascular pedicle when the the TPFF is used as a pedicled flap. When hair-bearing scalp is not included, primary closure is performed easily. If hair-bearing scalp is included with the flap, attention to flap width is important to avoid undue tension during closure and alopecia at the incision.

4.9 Pearls and Pitfalls

- The most common complication after elevation of TPFF is alopecia. Meticulous dissection of the TPFF off the scalp's subcutaneous fat and preservation of hair follicles by judicious use of bipolar cautery is necessary to avoid this complication. Avoidance of unipolar cautery is recommended during flap elevation.
- Meticulous hemostasis during flap elevation is the key in avoiding blood-tinged operative field. Careful bipolar cautery use is recommended to avoid injury to the vascular pedicle which runs within or on the surface of the TPF.
- Prior radiation to the temporal scalp area may predispose it for ischemic injury after TPFF elevation and is a relative contraindication to using this flap.
- Anterior dissection of the TPFF should be limited to within 2.5 cm anterior to the tragus at the level of the zygomatic arch to prevent injury to the frontal branch of the facial nerve.

References

[1] Monks GH. The restoration of a lower lid by a new method. N Engl J Med 1898;139:385
[2] Brown WJ. Extraordinary case of horse bite: the external ear completely bitten off and successfully replaced. Lancet 1898;1:1533
[3] Smith RA. The free fascial scalp flap. Plast Reconstr Surg 1980;66(2):204–209
[4] Tayfur V, Edizer M, Magden O. Anatomic bases of superficial temporal artery and temporal branch of facial nerve. J Craniofac Surg 2010;21(6):1945–1947
[5] Fortes FS, Carrau RL, Snyderman CH, et al. Transpterygoid transposition of a temporoparietal fascia flap: a new method for skull base reconstruction after endoscopic expanded endonasal approaches. Laryngoscope 2007;117(6):970–976

5 Facial Artery Musculomucosal Flap

Matthew M. Hanasono

Abstract

The facial artery musculomucosal flap is a soft-tissue flap used for the reconstruction of modest-sized defects of the lips, oral cavity, oropharynx, and nasal cavity. The flap is strictly used as a pedicled flap, based on the facial artery and submucosal venous plexus. It may be inferiorly based or superiorly based, relying on retrograde flow through the facial artery. Indications for its use, anatomy, perioperative considerations, and the surgical techniques involved are clearly laid out in this chapter.

Keywords: facial artery, submucosal venous plexus, facial vein anteriorly, pterygold plexus, internal maxillary vein posteriorly, buccinator muscle, retromolar trigone

5.1 Introduction

The facial artery musculomucosal (FAMM) flap was first described by Pribaz et al in 1992.[1] This soft-tissue flap is used for reconstruction of modest sized defects of the lips, oral cavity, oropharynx, and nasal cavity.[2,3,4] The flap is strictly used as a pedicled flap, based on the facial artery and submucosal venous plexus. It may be inferiorly based or superiorly based, relying on retrograde flow through the facial artery.

5.2 Typical Indications

- Wet and vermillion lip reconstruction.
- Intraoral reconstruction of gingival, floor of mouth, and palatal defects.
- Nasal lining defects.

5.3 Anatomy

The **facial artery** is a branch of the external carotid artery. It ascends deep to the submandibular gland, and then passes superficially over the mandible at the antegonial notch. It follows an ascending and tortuous course toward the medial angle of the eye, at which point it is termed the angular artery. It forms anastomoses with the dorsal nasal branch of the ophthalmic artery and the infraorbital artery, a terminal branch of the maxillary artery, which allows the superiorly based FAMM flap to be based on retrograde flow.

A **submucosal venous plexus** connects to both the **facial vein anteriorly** and the **pterygoid plexus** and **internal maxillary vein posteriorly**, which serves as the venous drainage for the FAMM flap. Inclusion of the facial vein is not necessary.

The facial artery is lateral to the buccinator, levator anguli oris, and the lateral edge of the deep lamina of the orbicularis oris muscles and medial to the risorius, zygomaticus major, and superficial lamina of the orbicularis oris muscles. The FAMM flap, therefore, needs to include the mucosa, submucosa, part of the **buccinator muscle**, and the facial artery, was well as the submucosal venous plexus, to be viable (▶ **Fig. 5.1**).

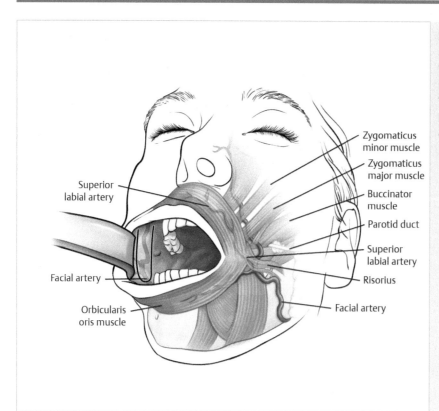

Fig. 5.1 Anatomy of the facial artery musculomucosal flap. The flap includes the buccal mucosa and buccinator muscle along with the facial artery. Several facial mimetic muscles are superficial to the facial artery.

Labels in figure: Zygomaticus minor muscle; Zygomaticus major muscle; Buccinator muscle; Parotid duct; Superior labial artery; Risorius; Facial artery; Superior labial artery; Facial artery; Orbicularis oris muscle

5.4 Perioperative Considerations

Ligation of the facial artery during neck dissection is a contraindication to inferiorly based FAMM flap use. Prior incisions in the buccal mucosa and soft tissues may also make the flap unreliable. The author has successfully used this flap in the setting of prior oral cavity irradiation.

5.5 Position and Markings

This flap is entirely intraoral. The course of the facial artery, from the **retromolar trigone** area to the ipsilateral **labial sulcus**, is traced with a hand-held Doppler ultrasound probe. The flap width is limited to a maximum of 2.5 to 3 cm (more commonly, 1–2 cm) to allow primary closure of the donor site. Care is taken to stay anterior to the parotid duct (also known as **Stensen's duct**), whose orifice is located across from the second maxillary molar. The anterior border of the flap should be kept at least 1 cm posterior to the oral commissure. The mouth is kept open during retraction with a retractor.

5.6 Operative Technique

For an inferiorly based flap, the dissection starts anterosuperiorly (▶ **Fig. 5.2**). The mucosa, submucosa, and buccinator muscles are incised to expose the facial artery, which resides within a layer of fatty tissue. The distal (superior) facial artery is identified then ligated and divided. The rest of the flap is then incised and dissection continues from superior to inferior. Alternately, an anterior incision 1 cm posterior to the oral commissure can be made and the **superior labial** artery can be traced posteriorly until it joins the facial artery. The **superior**

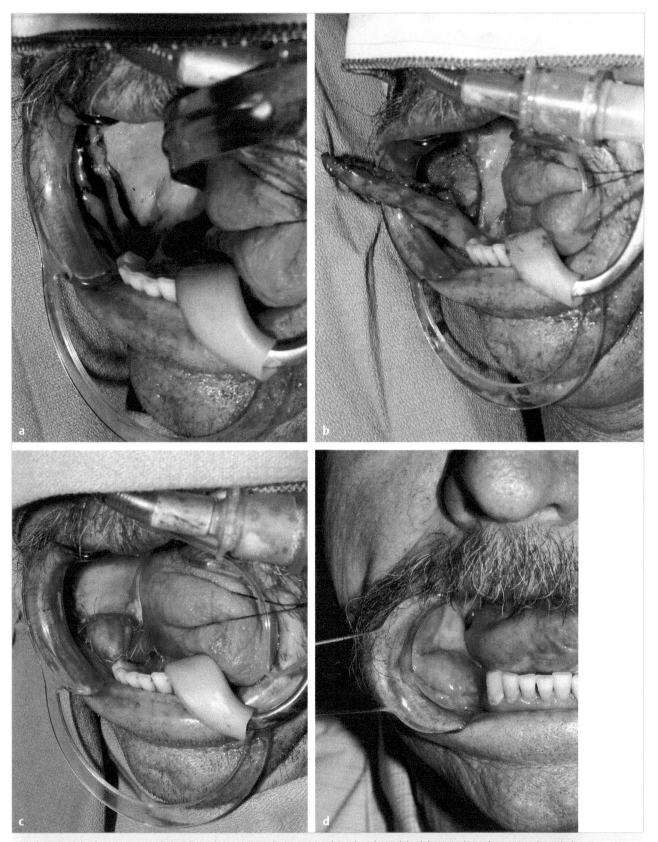

Fig. 5.2 **(a)** The course of the facial artery is determined with a hand-held Doppler ultrasound and the musculomucosal flap is centered over it. **(b)** An inferiorly based FAMM flap is elevated, including the mucosa and submucosa, the buccinator muscle, and the facial artery with a cuff of fibrofatty tissue. **(c)** The flap is inset into a gingival defect where the mandible was exposed. **(d)** Postoperative appearance after healing.

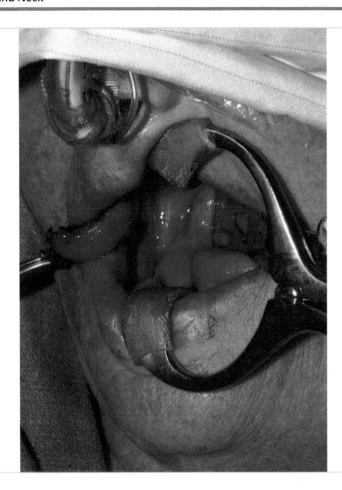

Fig. 5.3 A superiorly based FAMM flap based on retrograde blood flow via collateral circulation.

labial artery is then divided as it joins the facial artery and the facial artery is then followed superiorly until it is divided at the gingivolabial sulcus.

Care is taken to include a strip of the buccinator muscle and, more importantly, the facial artery. Frequent use of a Doppler ultrasound can be helpful in making sure the facial artery remains attached to the flap. Side branches of the artery and veins will need to be carefully ligated and divided. A long axial flap measuring 7 to 8 cm can be raised safely. The average flap thickness is about 1 cm.

If there is intervening intact mucosa between the proximal flap and the recipient defect, it may either be split and the entire flap laid into the enlarged defect, or a two-stage procedure may be performed with delayed pedicle base division of the FAMM flap performed about 2 to 3 weeks after initial flap elevation and inset.[3]

For a superiorly based flap, the dissection commences anteroinferiorly. Dissection proceeds from inferior to superior (▶ **Fig. 5.3**).

5.7 Donor Site Closure

A two-layered closure of the donor defect is performed with absorbable suture, approximating the buccinators muscle and mucosa. Care is taken to avoid interfering with the opening of the parotid duct. Drains are typically not needed.

5.8 Pearls and Pitfalls

- A Doppler ultrasound is very helpful in planning the flap and to make sure intraoperatively that the facial artery is included within the fatty soft tissues of the deepest layer of the flap.
- Because the artery lies deep to the buccinator muscle, a thin strip is included with the flap, causing the flap to be about 1-cm thick.
- Care needs to be taken to avoid interrupting the parotid duct during design and harvest of this flap.

References

[1] Pribaz J, Stephens W, Crespo L, Gifford G. A new intraoral flap: facial artery musculomucosal (FAMM) flap. Plast Reconstr Surg 1992;90(3):421–429

[2] Pribaz JJ, Meara JG, Wright S, Smith JD, Stephens W, Breuing KH. Lip and vermilion reconstruction with the facial artery musculomucosal flap. Plast Reconstr Surg 2000; 105(3):864–872

[3] Duranceau M, Ayad T. The facial artery musculomucosal flap: modification of the harvesting technique for a single-stage procedure. Laryngoscope 2011;121(12):2586–2589

[4] Ayad T, Xie L. Facial artery musculomucosal flap in head and neck reconstruction: A systematic review. Head Neck 2015;37(9):1375–1386

6 Lip Reconstruction with Abbe and Estlander Flaps

Mauricio A. Moreno

Abstract

The goals of lip reconstruction are functional and aesthetic. From the functional perspective, maintaining oral competence and preventing microstomia are probably the most critical to achieve. From the esthetic standpoint, it's important to maintain the integrity of the skin–vermillion junction, the height of the lip, and the symmetry in terms of length between the upper and lower lips. This chapter discusses the critical considerations involved in this delicate surgery, beginning with indications for the procedure, to anatomy, to the Abbe and Estlander flap options, to a step-by-step review of the operative technique that will give the best opportunity for achieving the desired outcome for the patient.

Keywords: Abbe flap, Estlander flap, superior labial artery, inferior labial artery, facial artery, facial nerve

6.1 Introduction

The goals of lip reconstruction are functional and esthetic. From the functional perspective, maintaining oral competence and preventing microstomia are probably the most critical to achieve. From the esthetic standpoint, it is important to maintain the integrity of the skin–vermillion junction, the height of the lip, and the symmetry in terms of length between the upper and lower lips. Given the anatomical characteristics of the lip, the principle or replacing "like with like" plays a major role in reconstruction, as no other tissue allows for a functional restoration of all three layers of the lip other than the lip itself. As such, primary advancement techniques (discussed in another chapter) represent the preferred method for reconstruction for defects smaller than 30% of the lip, without involvement of the oral commissure. While technically possible, attempting a primary advancement technique in defects larger than 30% will result in significant lip size asymmetry ("short lip" defect), which carries profound functional and cosmetic implications. In these scenarios, the Abbe and Estlander flaps— commonly referred as "lip switch" procedures—can achieve the same goal of full-thickness lip reconstruction though a vascularized transposition flap from the opposite lip.

6.2 Typical Indications

Indications for this reconstruction are full-thickness lip defects encompassing between one- and two-thirds of the lip, and that spare the oral commissure. Since this is a staged procedure, the patient's ability to cooperate and participate in his or her care must be considered for patient selection. In most cases, a V-shaped defect is preferable as it allows for partial primary closure, and for an easier inset of the flap. This morphology can be planned at the time of the resection, or achieved as a preliminary stage of the reconstruction.

6.3 Anatomy

The lip is a three-layered structure: skin, orbicularis oris muscle, and mucosa, with the vermillion covering its free edge. The **superior labial artery** provides the blood supply for the upper lip, and has terminal branches reaching the nasal septum and alae, while the **inferior labial artery** provides the blood supply for the lower lip. Both vessels originate from the ipsilateral **facial artery**, but anastomose in the midline to create a vascular continuum around the oral stoma (▶ **Fig. 6.1a**). The labial arteries are immediately posterior to the fibers of the orbicularis muscle in a horizontal plane located deep to the epithelium of the vermillion (▶ **Fig. 6.1b**). The superficial location and consistent anatomy of the labial vessels allow transposition of large segments of lip with minimal risk in terms of vascular insufficiency. The motor input to the orbicularis and all muscles of the lower third of the face is through the three lower branches of the **facial nerve**. In general, lip elevators are innervated by zygomatic and buccal branches, while depressors are innervated by the marginal mandibular branch. All lip switch flaps undergo temporary motor denervation that lasts for 6 to 18 months, but almost invariably recovers completely.[1] Sensory innervation of the upper lip is through the **infraorbital nerve** (a branch of V2), while the **mental nerve** (branch of V3) provides sensory innervation to the lower lip.

6.3.1 Abbe Flap

The concept of "lip switch" reconstruction has been sporadically reported in the medical literature since the 18th century,[2] but the technique was popularized by Abbe in 1899, who initially reported it for reconstruction of bilateral cleft lip defects.[3] Even though numerous variations to the technique have been described, conceptually, the procedure has remained unchanged for more than a century. Advantages of this approach include the symmetric distribution of tissue loss between both lips, and its ability to maintain the continuity and orientation of the orbicularis fibers, thus preserving its function as a sphincter. Being a staged procedure probably constitutes the main disadvantage of the technique.

6.4 Variations

- A bilateral cross lip procedure can be used for large, central defect of the lower lip. This approach is usually combined with crescentic advancement of the cheeks for closure of the donor sites.
- Another variation of the cross-lip approach is for reconstruction of entire aesthetic subunits, which has the advantage of improving the cosmetic outcome placing the incisions along the natural lines of the lower face (▶ **Fig. 6.2**).

6.5 Preoperative Considerations

Nasotracheal intubation—ideally on the opposite side—is highly recommended as it minimizes lip traction and avoids distortion of the vermillion morphology. Every patient should also be consented for adjunct procedures that may facilitate the closure of the defect.

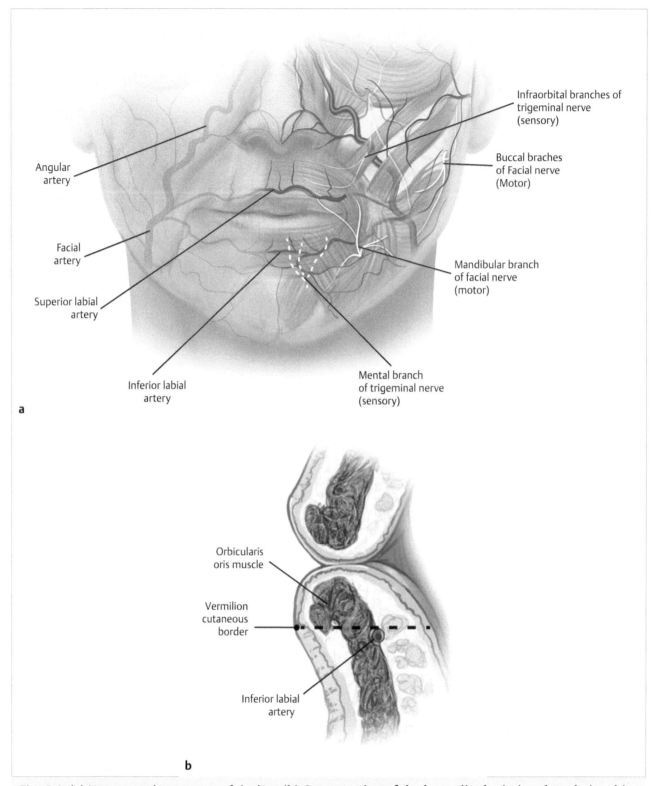

Angular artery

Facial artery

Superior labial artery

Inferior labial artery

Infraorbital branches of trigeminal nerve (sensory)

Buccal braches of Facial nerve (Motor)

Mandibular branch of facial nerve (motor)

Mental branch of trigeminal nerve (sensory)

a

Orbicularis oris muscle

Vermilion cutaneous border

Inferior labial artery

b

Fig. 6.1 **(a)** Neurovascular anatomy of the lips. **(b)** Cross-section of the lower lip depicting the relationship between the inferior labial artery and the orbicularis oris muscle.

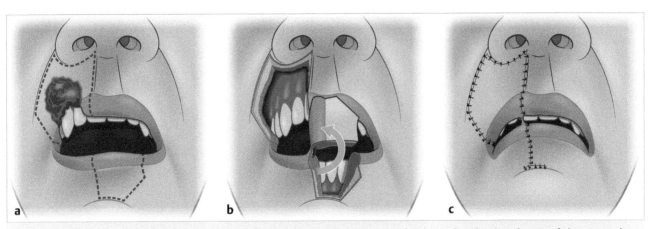

Fig. 6.2 (a-c) Variation of the cross-lip flap for reconstruction of the entire lateral esthetic subunit of the upper lip.

6.6 Positioning and Skin Markings

The patient is placed in supine position with the head elevated at 20 to 30 degrees. If a shoulder roll was placed for the ablative portion of the procedure, it is recommended to remove it prior to the reconstruction in order to avoid neck hyperextension and caudal lip retraction. A neutral position of the neck facilitates flap inset and donor site closure.

Careful marking of the skin is critical prior to performing any type of lip switch procedure. In the case of Abbe flaps, the vertical height and width of the defect are meticulously measured. The flap is designed in the opposite lip, with a width of half of the primary defect and placing its pivot point close to the medial aspect of the defect (▶ **Fig. 6.3**). This relationship is critical to evenly distribute tissue loss between both lips and prevent excessive tension at the pedicle.

For Estlander flaps, a triangular wedge of tissue is marked in the opposite lip and cheek, with approximately half of the defect width but maintaining the vertical height. The medial aspect of the flap, which contains the vascular pedicle, will serve as the pivot point and ultimately become the neocommissure.

6.7 Operative Technique

6.7.1 Abbe Flap

Once the skin margins are completed, a full-thickness lip flap is elevated starting on the lateral aspect (or the side opposite to the pivot point), taking special care to avoiding beveling of the incision. Electrocautery can be safely used for most of the procedure, except when dissecting close to the pedicle in the medial aspect of the flap. Overzealous dissection or thinning of the pedicle should be avoided, and is recommended to leave a thin cuff of muscle protecting the labial vessels. Prior to the translocation of the flap, meticulous hemostasis is achieved with bipolar electrocautery (▶ **Fig. 6.4**).

The flap is then rotated 180 degrees toward the defect, and the inset proceeds. All three layers are closed separately, with interrupted absorbable sutures for the muscular and mucosal planes, and nonabsorbable material for the skin. The first step is reapproximating the orbicularis muscle along the vermillion–cutaneous border on the medial aspect of the defect. This closure line is not routinely revised in the second stage, so meticulous alignment of these

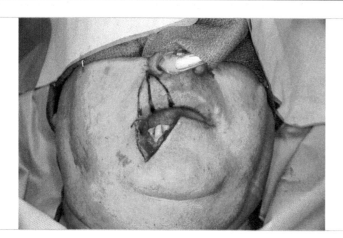

Fig. 6.3 Abbe technique used for reconstruction of an oncologic defect of the lower lip. The flap is designed in the upper lip with approximately half of the width of the primary defect.

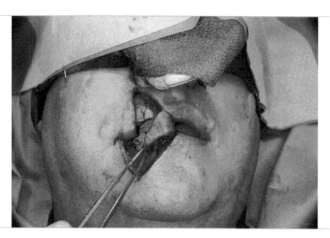

Fig. 6.4 The flap has been elevated and remains attached by the pedicle containing the labial artery; a cuff of orbicularis muscle protects the vessel.

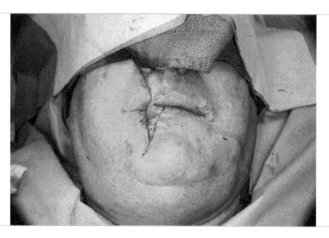

Fig. 6.5 Completed inset of deep muscular and mucosal layers. Note that defect was partially closed to perfectly match the height of the flap. The donor site has been partially reapproximated.

structures is paramount at this point. Subsequently, the rest of the flap is inset around its perimeter, leaving the lateral vermillion partially open to accommodate for the pedicle (▶ Fig. 6.5). Finally, the donor site is as described later, and the patient is discharged on soft mechanical diet and educated to avoid maneuvers that could pose a challenge to the tissue.

The second stage of the reconstruction is performed 2 to 3 weeks later (▶ Fig. 6.6a). The pedicle is transected and the redundant tissue is discarded. The open edges of the upper and lower lip are refreshed prior to completing a meticulous closure of the vermillion with thin, absorbable suture (▶ Fig. 6.6b).

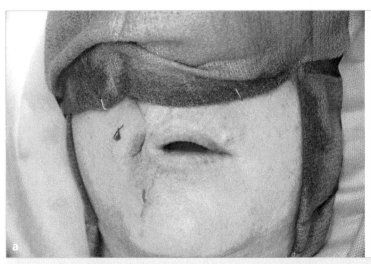
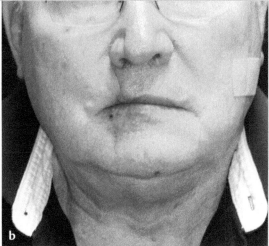

Fig. 6.6 **(a)** Appearance 3 weeks after the initial surgery. The flap is well healed and neovascularization has been achieved. At this point, the pedicle is transected and both lips are closed primarily. **(b)** Reconstruction appearance at 1 month postoperatively.

6.7.2 Estlander Flap

Estlander described this variation of the lip switch technique in 1872.[4] It involves rotating a triangular section of the labial tissue around a defect located in the commissure for a single-stage reconstruction. This creates a neocommissure that while functional, consistently has a blunting deformity, so a second-stage commissuroplasty may be required to improve cosmesis and function.

This flap is indicated for full-thickness defects of the lateral lip that are less than one-third of the total length and involve the oral commissure. This flap can be used to reconstruct defects of the upper or lower lip, but is more commonly used for the latter. In this setting, the superior incision can be continued along the nasolabial fold to facilitate the cheek advancement necessary for the donor site closure.

The surface markings are performed as described earlier (▶ **Fig. 6.7a**). The flap is elevated around its entire perimeter leaving the pedicle attachment intact, and with a cuff of muscle for protection. Once the tissue has been elevated, it is rotated medially into the defect and inset in three layers with absorbable suture for the mucosa and muscular layers, and nylon for the skin (▶ **Fig. 6.7b**). The folded pedicle becomes the neocommissure, which at this point is characteristically thick and blunt, but a good percentage of patients can achieve oral competence and appropriate lip function in this setting (▶ **Fig. 6.7c**). The second stage is performed not sooner than 2 to 3 weeks after the initial surgery. In contrast to the Abbe flap, the second stage is not mandatory, and is performed as needed to improve function or cosmesis.

6.8 Donor Site Closure

For Abbe flaps, closure of the donor site is only completed after at the second stage. In the first stage, the white lip is closed in three layers, using absorbable suture for the mucosal and muscular layers, and nylon for the skin. Part of the vermillion must be left unclosed to accommodate for the vascular pedicle. Over the following weeks, the pedicle will invariably become redundant, while the open wound in the lip will tend to heal by second intention. To account for these

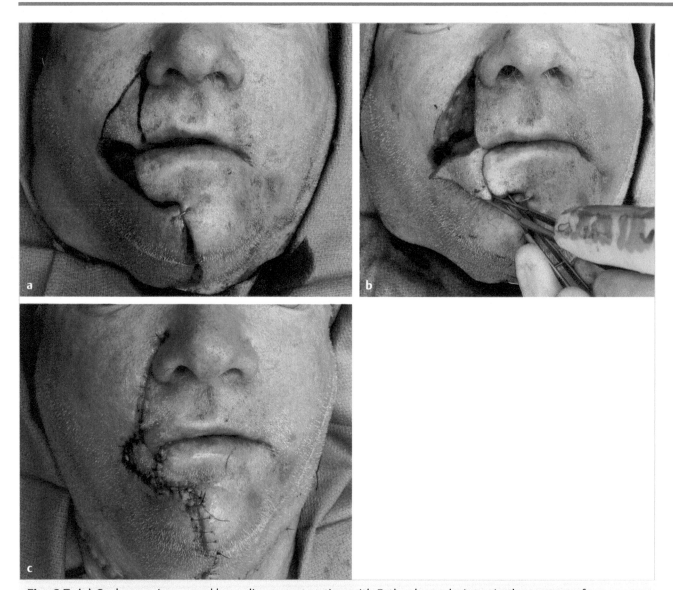

Fig. 6.7 **(a)** Oral commissure and lower lip reconstruction with Estlander technique, in the context of synchronic mandibular reconstruction. The flap is designed in the upper lip with the same vertical height as the defect, and the incision can be extended along the nasolabial fold to facilitate advancement and closure. **(b)** The flap has been elevated and is subsequently rotated medially to cover the lower lip defect. The vascular pedicle serves as a pivot point and will become the neocommissure. The flap is inset in three layers and the donor site is closed primarily by a check advancement. **(c)** Immediate postoperative appearance. This patient achieved good oral competence and overall function after the first stage, so the second stage was not performed.

changes, in the second stage of the reconstruction, the granulation tissue must be debrided and the redundant vermillion carefully excised. These steps are important to attain a cosmetically appealing result, as proceeding with a direct closure can lead to an unsightly protuberance in the free edge of the donor lip. Once perfect restoration of the vermillion–cutaneous junction has been achieved, the vermillion defect is usually closed in a single layer with fine absorbable suture.

Closure of an Estlander flap donor site is obtained by performing a medial check advancement and a three-layered closure, as previously described. This can be easily accomplished in patients with appropriate facial laxity. If primary advancement is inadequate—or if there is excessive tension at the suture line—additional cheek mobilization can be obtained by extending the incision along the nasolabial fold and removing Burrow's triangles.

6.9 Pearls and Pitfalls

- Patient selection is critically important; these techniques should not be considered for defects less than two-thirds of the lip.
- The width of the flap should always be half of the defect to minimize tension and maintain lip symmetry.
- Is important to design the flap in a plane perpendicular to the axis of the lateral lip and not to the horizontal plane, as this will result in an asymmetric donor site defect that is difficult to correct.
- When performing the second-stage closure of an Abbe flap donor site, debride the granulation tissue and excise the redundant pedicle. This maintains the aesthetic line of the lip and avoids an unsightly protuberance in the vermillion.

References

[1] Burget GC, Menick FJ. Aesthetic restoration of one-half the upper lip. Plast Reconstr Surg 1986;78(5):583–593

[2] Al-Benna S, Steinstraesser L, Steinau HU. The cross-lip flap from 1756 to 1898. Reply to "The Sabattini–Abbé flap: a historical note". Plast Reconstr Surg 2009;124(2):666–667, author reply 667–668

[3] Abbe R. A new plastic operation for the relief of deformity due to double harelip. Plast Reconstr Surg 1968;42(5):481–483

[4] Estlander JA. Eine mMethode aus der einen Lippe Substanzverluste der Anderen zu Erstetzen. Arch Klin Chir 1872;14:622

7 Karapandzic Flap

Sara A. Neimanis and Howard N. Langstein

Abstract

The Karapandzic flap is a method of reconstruction for acquired lip defects. It uses circumoral full-thickness rotation-advancement flaps in which the neurovascular supply to the orbicularis oris muscle is maintained. Due to its ability to provide a functional repair by preserving the neurovascular supply and restoring continuity of the perioral musculature, it remains an integral part of the lip reconstruction algorithm, employing one of the most important tenets of plastic surgery by replacing lost tissue with similar tissue. Every step involved in Karapandzic flap reconstruction is examined, from indications for surgery, to anatomy, to preoperative considerations, to the techniques necessary to achieve the desired outcome.

Keywords: Karapandzic flap, superior labial arteries, inferior labial arteries, facial nerve, infraorbital branch of the trigeminal nerve, mental branch of the trigeminal nerve

7.1 Introduction

The Karapandzic flap was first described as a method of reconstruction of acquired lip defects by Karapandzic in 1974.[1] It uses circumoral full-thickness rotation-advancement flaps in which the neurovascular supply to the orbicularis oris muscle is maintained. Due to its ability to provide a functional repair by preserving the neurovascular supply and restoring continuity of the perioral musculature, it remains an integral part of the lip reconstruction algorithm. It calls upon one of the most important tenets of plastic surgery by replacing lost tissue with similar tissue.

7.2 Typical Indications

- Full-thickness defects.
- Half to two-thirds defects of the upper lip.
- Defects up to three-fourths of the lower lip.
- Central or lateral defects.
- Defects involving commissure.

7.3 Anatomy

7.3.1 Musculature

A number of perioral and muscles of facial expression are involved in movement of the upper and lower lips (▶ **Fig. 7.1**). Oral sphincter function is accomplished by the orbicularis oris muscle. It consists of two parts: pars marginalis and pars peripheralis. The pars marginalis is mainly deep to the vermilion. The pars peripheralis originates deep to the pars marginalis and can be found beneath the cutaneous upper and lower lips.

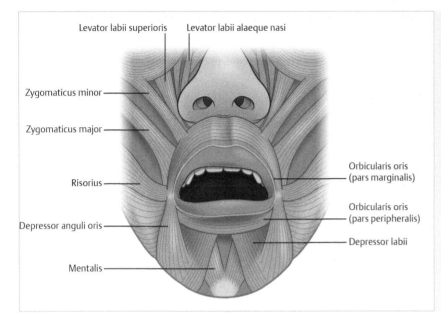

Fig. 7.1 Perioral musculature, including the orbicularis oris, which is raised in a Karapandzic flap.

The upper lip is elevated by the zygomaticus major and minor, the levator labii superioris, the levator labii superioris alaeque nasi, and the levator anguli oris. Lower lip depressors include the depressor anguli oris, depressor labii, and platysma. The mentalis contributes to lower lip movement by pushing it against the mandible, causing it to elevate.

The buccinator, along with the pharyngeal constrictors, control the lips by pushing them against the maxillary and mandibular teeth and gingiva. This is important in manipulating food within the oral cavity to allow for effective and safe eating.

The perioral muscles interdigitate to form the modiolus at the corners of the mouth.[2]

7.3.2 Blood Supply

The lips are supplied by the external carotid system. The facial artery branches from the external carotid. Approximately 1.5 cm lateral to the oral commissures it branches into the **superior and inferior labial arteries**, which supply the lips and the Karandanzic flap. The superior labial artery is found within 1 cm of the upper lip vermilion border. The inferior labial artery is usually found 4 to 13 mm from the lower lip vermilion border.

7.3.3 Innervation

Motor innervation to the perioral musculature is provided by the **facial nerve (CN VII)**. Sensory innervation is provided by the **infraorbital (V2)** and **mental (V3)** branches of the trigeminal nerve (CN V). All of the muscles are innervated on their deep surfaces except for the mentalis, buccinators, and levator labii superioris.

7.4 Preoperative Considerations

It is important to complete a thorough history and physical examination, documenting sensation, and motor function of the various CN V and VII distributions preoperatively. Total upper and lower lip "stock" should be assessed as well as tissue laxity which increase with advanced age. Prior lip resections should be investigated in detail. If the patient has had prior injuries or insult compromising these nerves, one should not expect a functional repair.

It is also important to consider whether or not the defect will be created at the time of reconstruction, as in a skin cancer resection with frozen sections, or if the patient will present with the defect, as in trauma or referral from a Mohs dermatologist.

7.5 Positioning and Skin Markings

The patient should be positioned supine. This operation can be performed using local or regional anesthetic or under general anesthesia. If general anesthesia is employed, nasal intubation should be chosen to prevent interference of the endotracheal tube in the operative site.

Markings should begin by squaring off the defect such that a right angle is created at the lip margin and continues to the base of the flap. The flap border should then be marked perpendicular to the initial marks and parallel to the lip margin.[3] This marking should be made at least 1 cm superior to the upper lip or 1.3 cm inferior to the lower lip to be sure the labial artery is captured. In lower lip defects one should attempt to place this incision in the mental crease. The marking should extend around the oral commissure and into the melolabial crease, maintaining equal distance from the lip margin throughout (▶Fig. 7.2a,b). Minor deviations in thickness when placing incisions in the melolabial crease are tolerated. In upper lip defects the incision is marked at the alar facial groove rather than the mental crease. One should anticipate a dog ear and can mark this on the on the outer circle, though it may require adjustments as the flap is inset (▶Fig. 7.3c).

7.6 Operative Technique

The incisions are carried out through skin and soft tissue, but are not made full-thickness as to preserve the neurovascular supply to the tissue and muscle. The muscle is then progressively incised until the neurovascular structures are identified and preserved. Incisions are carried through or at the periphery of the orbicularis oris, as this muscle must be released to allow for advancement into the defect. The other perioral muscles of facial expression may be divided from the orbicularis oris. Separate partial-thickness incisions are made through the mucosa on the deep surface to allow for its advancement. Unilateral or bilateral flaps may be used, though bilateral flaps allow for reconstruction of larger defects and provide better symmetry. Once the flaps are approximated with one another, or a unilateral flap approximates the existing lip tissue, with minimal tension, they are sutured into place. This is accomplished by using techniques of primary lip repair with careful approximation of the vermilion border and multilayered closure.[4]

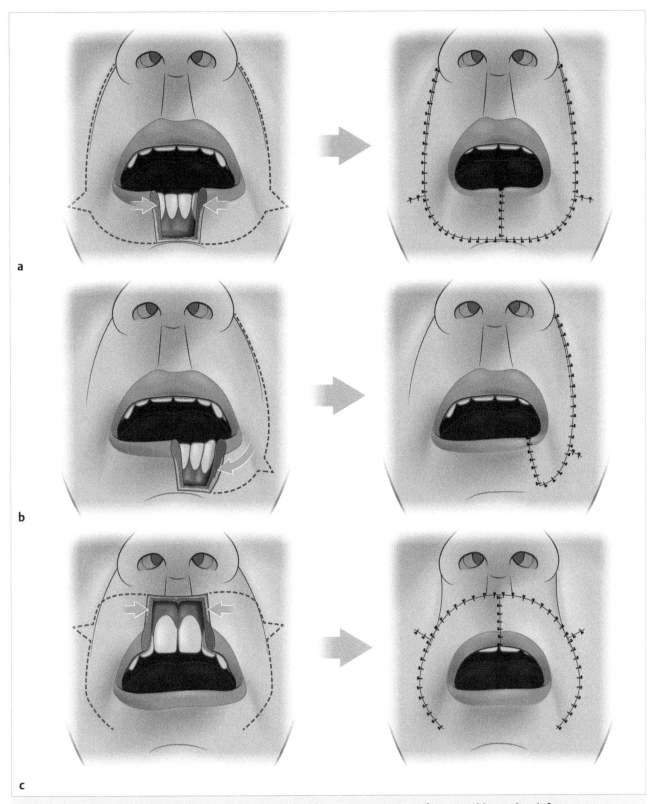

Fig. 7.2 **(a)** Markings for a bilateral Karapandzic flap for reconstruction of a central lower lip defect.
(b) Markings for unilateral Karapandzic flaps for reconstruction of a lateral lower lip defect. **(c)** Markings for bilateral Karapandzic flaps for reconstruction of a central upper lip defect. Note the Burow's triangles excised to eliminate dog ears.

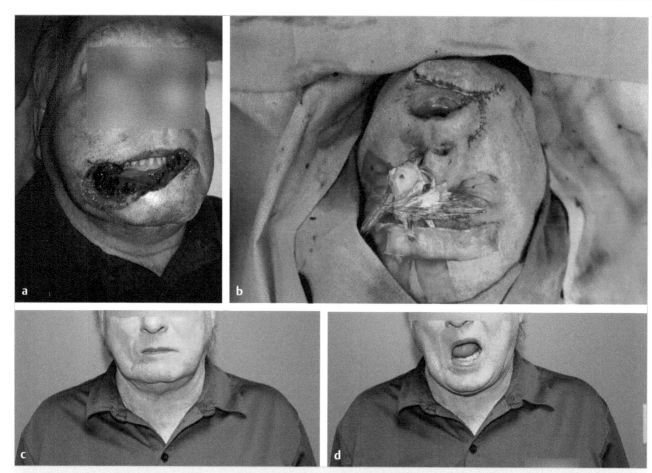

Fig. 7.3 **(a)** Large lower lip defect involving the right commissure after excision of squamous cell carcinoma. **(b)** Right Karapandzic flap inset at completion of case. **(c)** Patient several months postoperative with acceptable cosmetic and functional results. **(d)** Demonstrating widening of the adequate oral aperture over time.

7.7 Donor Site Closure

Attempt should be made to reattach the muscles of facial expression that have been divided with the orbicularis oris in the appropriate anatomic positions. The donor site should be closed in layers, approximating mucosa, muscles, and skin. Burow's triangles may need to be excised to treat dog ears.

7.8 Pearls and Pitfalls

- Consider the risk of microstomia prior to proceeding. The lips will stretch with time so some degree of microstomia may be acceptable. A secondary Abbe flap can also restore lip balance.
- Defects often appear larger than they are when orbicularis oris is divided and the tissue splays open. Most of these even very large defects can be reconstructed with Karapandzic flaps.
- Anticipate dog ears and additional Burow's triangle excisions.

References

[1] Karapandzic M. Reconstruction of lip defects by local arterial flaps. Br J Plast Surg 1974;27(1):93–97

[2] Thorne CH, ed. Grabb and Smith's Plastic Surgery. 7th ed. Philadelphia, PA: Lippincott Williams & Wilkins; 2014

[3] Ethunandan M, Macpherson DW, Santhanam V. Karapandzic flap for reconstruction of lip defects. J Oral Maxillofac Surg 2007;65(12):2512–2517

[4] Baker S. Local Flaps in Facial Reconstruction. 3rd ed. Philadelphia, PA: Saunders; 2014

8 Submental Island Flap

Blair M. Barton, Brian Moore, and Christian P. Hasney

Abstract

Reconstruction of postablative defects of the head and neck is complex and challenging. Free tissue transfer, in many cases, is the current standard for reconstruction for postablative and other orofacial defects, such as resection of low-grade cutaneous malignancies. This chapter discusses the surgical option involving the submental island flap. Indications for its propriety are listed, as well as anatomy, variations to the basic technique are covered, postoperative considerations are reviewed, and detailed instructions on the actual procedure are given. Specific attention is paid to the possibility that flaps may contain malignant submental nodes.

Keywords: submental island flap, submental artery, anterior belly of the digastric muscle, submental vein

8.1 Introduction to Submental Island Flap

Reconstruction of postablative defects of the head and neck is a complex, challenging, yet rewarding endeavor. It is the reconstructive surgeons' aim to restore both form and function to the greatest extent possible. Free tissue transfer, in many cases, is the current standard for reconstruction of postablative defects of the head and neck. Naturally, if a simpler reconstructive technique allows the restoration of form and function, that technique should be employed. One such option is the pedicled submental island flap (SIF). The SIF was initially described in 1993 by Martin[1] as a reliable alternative to more commonly employed techniques for reconstruction of postablative head and neck defects. Martin[1] demonstrated that the SIF was an excellent option for orofacial defects following resection of low-grade cutaneous malignancies.

8.2 Typical Indications

- Patients who refuse free tissue transfer.
- Patients with severe comorbidities.
- Patients with limited physiologic reserve.
- Patients with microvascular comorbidities that may result in free tissue transfer failure.

8.3 Anatomy

The SIF is based off the **submental artery**, which is a reliable branch of the **facial artery**. The submental artery arises deep to the submandibular gland and is roughly 1.0 to 1.5 mm in diameter.[2] It courses forward behind the body of the mandible and superficially across the mylohyoid muscle. At this point, the artery either continues superficial (30%) or deep (70%) to the **anterior belly of the digastric muscle**, terminating at the mandibular symphysis. The submental artery gives off several cutaneous perforators that pierce the platysma, forming a subdermal plexus that anastomoses to the contralateral submental artery approximately 90% of the time.[3] Venous drainage of the SIF is via the **submental vein** that drains into the **facial vein** (▶ Fig. 8.1).

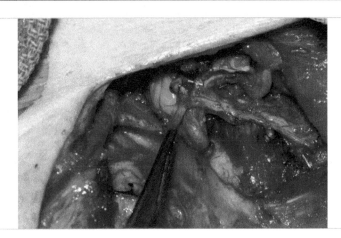

Fig. 8.1 The submental vessels branching off the facial artery, diving deep to the anterior belly of the digastric muscle and superficial to the mylohyoid.

8.4 Variations

The pedicle of the SIF is generally of adequate length to allow reconstruction of a variety of defects. However, if the flap is needed for reconstruction of defects superior to the lower two-thirds of the face, a number of adjunctive techniques may be utilized to achieve additional pedicle length:

- Division of the distal facial vessels: division of the facial vessels distal to the origin of the submental artery can provide up to 1 to 2 cm of additional length. The limitation of the pedicle length is then the submental vein. The submental or common facial vein can be divided and anastomosed to a suitable vein in close proximity to the recipient site if additional length is required for reconstruction.[4]
- Y–V procedure: there is often a communicating branch between the external jugular and the facial vein that tethers the pedicle. This anatomic configuration forms a Y pattern. The surgeon can ligate the trunk of the facial vein proximal to this communicating vessel. In so doing, the Y-shaped configuration is converted to a V shape. This maneuver may provide up to an additional 5 cm of length of the pedicle.[5]
- Reverse flow: by ligating the facial artery proximal to the origin of the submental artery the submental flap can be by retrograde arterial flow by the distal facial artery. It is worth noting that reverse flow through the venous system is prohibited by the presence of the valves allowing only for unidirectional flow. Should additional vein length be required, the vein should be transected and a microvascular anastomosis performed to a recipient vein proximate to the recipient site.
- Free flap: one of the major limitations of the submental pedicle flap is the limited arc of rotation of the pedicle, only reliably used in the reconstruction of the lower two-thirds of the face. The submental flap has been used for microvascular reconstruction due to its favorable pedicle diameter and length. The free submental flap has been utilized for reconstruction of lateral defects of the nose, treatment of lower extremity lymphedema, and forehead reconstruction.

8.5 Preoperative Considerations

While there are no absolute contraindications to performing a submental flap, there are some considerations that may preclude its use. Bulky lymphadenopathy in level I is a relative contraindication, even with meticulous dissection of the lymphatic tissue from the flap. The first priority of the head and neck surgical oncologist is to ensure that no residual malignant cells are introduced into the recipient site. Ligation or compromise of the facial vein on the ipsilateral side as the pedicle would prevent adequate venous drainage of the flap. Thus, in patients with a history of a prior neck dissection, one must consider that the facial vein has been ligated and may result in venous drainage issues resulting in flap compromise and postoperative wound complications.

8.6 Positioning and Skin Markings

A number of different methods of harvesting the submental flap have been previously described. Here, we describe the technique employed at our institution.

The patient is placed in the supine position with his or her neck in a neutral position or slightly extended. The upper limit of the flap is planned at the inferior border of the mandibular arch to avoid a visible scar and to prevent lip eversion. The length (medial–lateral dimension) of the flap is limited by the size of the defect needed to be reconstructed and, if needed, can be extended from one mandibular angle to the other (▶ Fig. 8.2a). The width (anterior–posterior dimension) is again limited by the size of the defect, and is maximally determined by the "pinch test," which assesses the feasibility of closing the incision primarily (▶ Fig. 8.2b). If a concomitant neck dissection is to be performed, an incision is planned extending from the proximal aspect of the skin paddle to a site just below the mastoid tip on the side that the neck dissection is to be performed. This incision is planned to lie within a natural skin crease when possible.

8.7 Operative Technique

The proximal aspect of the skin paddle and the neck incision is carried out with a number 15 blade. Sharp dissection then proceeds through the platysma muscle. A superiorly based subplatysmal flap is then elevated over the body of the mandible. If necessary, an inferiorly based subplatysmal flap is elevated to allow for exposure as dictated by the extent of the planned neck dissection. The submandibular gland is then removed in the standard fashion (▶ Fig. 8.3). The submental vessels are typically identified as they traverse the superior aspect of the submandibular gland. Several branches of the submental artery and submental vein supply the submandibular gland and must be ligated and divided. Once the submandibular gland resection is complete, the marginal mandibular nerve is identified and the level Ib lymph nodes are extirpated. These nodes typically lie inferior to the nerve and superior to the submental vessels. Great care is exercised to avoid injury to either the marginal mandibular nerve or submental vessels.

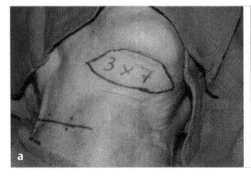 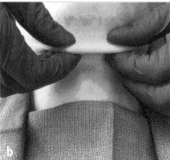

Fig. 8.2 (a) Typical markings for elevation of the submental flap. Incision can be extended laterally if a neck dissection planned, or a separate neck incision can be used. (b) The "pinch test" to determine maximum width and feasibility of primary closure.

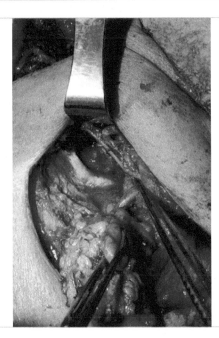

Fig. 8.3 Excision of the submandibular gland to reveal the submental vessel.

Following level Ib lymphadenectomy, the remainder of the skin paddle is incised. Sharp dissection proceeds through the platysma muscle. The remainder of flap harvest is then carried out from the distal skin paddle toward the proximal skin paddle and submental vascular pedicle. With the platysma divided, the flap is elevated in the subplatysmal plane. The contralateral anterior belly of the digastric and mylohyoid muscle is identified. The mylohyoid is then bluntly dissected away from the underlying geniohyoid and divided with electrocautery in the midline. Once the transverse fibers of the mylohyoid are divided, the vertically oriented fibers of the geniohyoid are identified in the depths of the field. Next, the attachments of the anterior belly of the digastric and mylohyoid to the hyoid bone are bluntly dissected away from the hyoid and divided with electrocautery. Blunt dissection with a Kitner dissector is then carried out over the surface of the geniohyoid separating the attachments to the mylohyoid up to the level of the mandible. The superior attachments of the platysma, anterior belly of the digastric and mylohyoid to the mandible are then divided with electrocautery. Care is taken to err toward the mandible in order to avoid inadvertent injury to the delicate cutaneous perforators that may be traversing the anterior belly of the digastric or mylohyoid. Finally, the remainder of the vascular pedicle is dissected and any additional branches of the pedicle are ligated until the skin paddle is able to reach the recipient site in a tension-free manner (▶ **Fig. 8.4**).

8.8 Donor Site Closure

The donor site can, in most cases, be closed primarily. If additional undermining is required, it should be performed on the cervical side of the incision, in order to prevent lower lip eversion. The cervical skin can be sutured to the hyoid bone to ensure the cervicomental angle is maintained.

8.9 Pearls and Pitfalls

- Early identification of the submental vessels and the marginal mandibular nerve is the key for successful flap elevation.

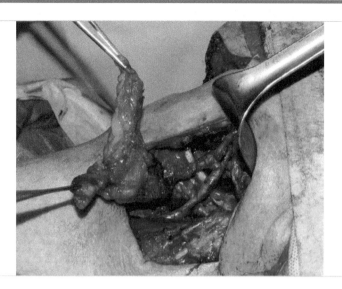

Fig. 8.4 Freed submental flap with intact pedicle. Adequate dissection of the pedicle is necessary to ensure tension-free closure.

- If a concomitant neck dissection is planned, the submental incision can be extended laterally and allow for the submental flap to be used as an interpolated flap.
- Meticulous dissection of the pedicle is necessary to achieve a safe oncologic resection and allow for a tension-free closure.
- Review of the preoperative computed tomography is essential to determine if the facial vein drains into the internal jugular vein or the external jugular vein.

8.10 Oncologic Safety

One of the primary concerns raised in the use of the SIF is the incorporation of potentially malignant submental nodes into the substance of the flap. Tumors of the anterior oral cavity may spread through the lymphatic channels to the nodes overlying the anterior belly of the digastric and mylohyoid and, as such, the SIF has the potential to transpose microscopic disease from the in situ location of the submental nodes to the recipient site.

Howard and colleagues reported their 10-year experience in using the submental flap for reconstruction of oral cavity cancer defects with respect to the oncologic safety of the technique. They reported on 50 patients undergoing resection of oral cavity malignancies with SIF reconstruction. All 50 patients were clinically and radiographically N0 in levels Ia and 1b preoperatively. Occult metastases were identified in level I in five patients. They reported no local recurrence rates associated with the submental flap.[6]

With the technique described earlier, it is feasible to resect the entirety of level Ia. Aggressive extirpation of this nodal basin will, at least theoretically, place the cutaneous perforators at a greater risk of injury than would incorporation of these nodes into the flap. With this consideration in mind, it has become our practice to forego the use of the submental flap in those with anterior oral cavity cancers requiring bilateral neck dissection. In these patients, comprehensive removal of the level I nodes is of critical oncologic importance. Again, unless a perforator dissection is performed, aggressive dissection of levels Ia and Ib carries a significant likelihood of injury to the cutaneous perforators to the submental skin paddle. It is our belief that, in these cases, free tissue transfer is the most sensible choice from both an oncologic and reconstructive standpoint.

References

[1] Martin D, Pascal JF, Baudet J, et al. The submental island flap: a new donor site. Anatomy and clinical applications as a free or pedicled flap. Plast Reconstr Surg 1993;92(5):867–873

[2] Faltaous AA, Yetman RJ. The submental artery flap: an anatomic study. Plast Reconstr Surg 1996;97(1):56–60, discussion 61–62

[3] Abouchadi A, Capon-Degardin N, Patenôtre P, Martinot-Duquennoy V, Pellerin P. The submental flap in facial reconstruction: advantages and limitations. J Oral Maxillofac Surg 2007;65(5):863–869

[4] Sterne GD, Januszkiewicz JS, Hall PN, Bardsley AF. The submental island flap. Br J Plast Surg 1996;49(2):85–89

[5] Multinu A, Ferrari S, Bianchi B, et al. The submental island flap in head and neck reconstruction. Int J Oral Maxillofac Surg 2007;36(8):716–720

[6] Howard BE, Nagel TH, Donald CB, Hinni ML, Hayden RE. Oncologic safety of the submental flap for reconstruction in oral cavity malignancies. Otolaryngol Head Neck Surg 2014;150(4):558–562

9 Supraclavicular Cutaneous Pedicled Flap

Eric I-Yun Chang

Abstract

The supraclavicular cutaneous pedicled flap has become popular for use in the reconstruction of complex head and neck defects. It was first used as an island flap, but with the advent of microvascular free tissue transfer, a multitude of additional flap options have emerged. Additionally, this pedicled flap can be utilized not only for salvage after a failed free flap but also as the primary option for head and neck reconstruction. In this chapter, the entire spectrum of surgical considerations for supraclavicular cutaneous pedicle flap surgery is covered, from indications, to anatomy, to preoperative considerations, to operative techniques. A variation involving the extended fasciocutaneous flap is also included.

Keywords: supraclavicular artery, supraclavicular nerve, transverse cervical artery, middle third of the clavicle, acromioclavicular joint, third and fourth cervical nerves

9.1 Introduction

The supraclavicular cutaneous pedicled (SCP) flap has been recently popularized for reconstruction of complex head and neck defects. The flap was first described by Mutter in 1842 and clinically used by Kazanjian and Converse in 1949.[1] Further anatomical studies were performed by Mathes and Vasconez in 1979 and later refined by Lambery and Cormack in 1983.[2] The SCP flap was reintroduced as an island flap in 1997 by Pallula.[3] With the advent of microvascular free tissue transfer, a multitude of additional flap options emerged. However, the SCP flap can be utilized not only for salvage after a failed free flap but also as the primary option for head and neck reconstruction.

9.2 Typical Indications

- Intraoral and glossectomy defects.
- Pharyngeal defects.
- Skull base defects involving the temporal bone and mastoid region.
- Cutaneous defects of the lower face and neck.
- Sternal wounds.

9.3 Anatomy

The SCP flap is an axial fasciocutaneous flap based on the **supraclavicular artery**. The supraclavicular artery is a branch of the **transverse cervical artery**, which lies in the posterior triangle of the neck bordered by the sternocleidomastoid muscle, clavicle, and trapezius muscle. The transverse cervical vessels originate from the thyrocervical trunk, which is a branch of the subclavian artery and can consistently be identified along the **middle third of clavicle**. The transverse cervical vessels give rise to the supraclavicular vessels, which are typically located 2 cm posterior to the posterior border of the clavicle. The main pedicle runs perpendicular to the transverse cervical vessels toward the **acromioclavicular joint** and proceeds over the deltoid muscle, traversing the line connecting the olecranon and the acromion tip.[1,4]

The **supraclavicular nerve** from the **third and fourth cervical nerves** allow the SCP flap to be a sensate flap. The main nerve branch originates from the posterior aspect of the sternocleidomastoid muscle along the midpoint of the muscle belly. These nerves emerge from the deep fascia from a location separate from the main vascular pedicle. As the nerves travel along the length of the flap, a major anterior nerve branch can often be identified running toward the clavicle approximately 1 to 2 cm posterior to the supraclavicular vessels. Smaller nerve branches (range: 2–5) can often be identified, which may be seen along the more posterior and distal aspects of the flap.[2]

9.4 Variations

Extended fasciocutaneous flap with supercharge to posterior circumflex humeral vessels.[4]

9.5 Preoperative Considerations

Preoperative imaging and radiographic studies are typically not necessary for flap elevation. The main supraclavicular pedicle is identified with a Doppler probe and the flap is centered along the course of the vascular pedicle. The SCP flap generally may be harvested up to 5 cm beyond the most distal point where a Doppler signal can be identified, if additional flap length is necessary.[5]

9.6 Positioning and Skin Markings

The patient is placed supine on the operating table with the ipsilateral arm abducted. The posterior border of the clavicle and sternal notch are marked in order to identify the origin of the transverse cervical vessels. The course of the supraclavicular artery is identified with a Doppler probe and marked. The dimensions of the defect are marked and transposed onto the shoulder centered along the course of the main vascular pedicle (▶ Fig. 9.1).

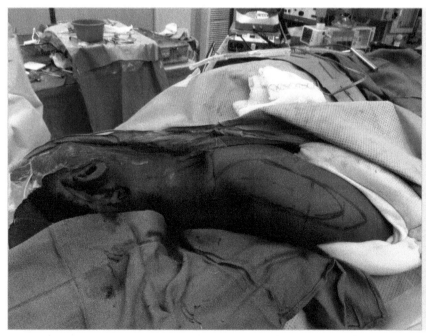

Fig. 9.1 Preoperative markings of the SCP flap with the course of the supraclavicular artery identified with the Doppler probe and the skin paddle centered over the vessel.

9.7 Operative Technique

The course of the supraclavicular artery is identified with the Doppler probe and the size of the flap is marked centered over the previously marked pedicle. The skin incisions are made and dissection proceeds through the subcutaneous tissues. The fascia is incised and flap elevation proceeds below the level of the fascia and above the musculature in a distal to proximal direction. The vascular supply to the distal aspect of the SCP flap is superficial, which facilitates elevation in the subfascial plane. The deltoid muscle is easily dissected from the undersurface of the flap. As the dissection proceeds proximally toward the clavicle, the supraclavicular artery should be identified and preserved. The muscle fibers of the trapezius are more adherent than those of the deltoid and may require additional blunt dissection (▶ Fig. 9.2).

After flap elevation nears the main vascular pedicle, a distinct layer of white fascia is encountered. The fascia surrounds the supraclavicular artery and transverse cervical artery and is carefully divided in order to achieve additional flap length (▶ Fig. 9.3). The pedicle is dissected from the undersurface of the platysma muscle. The Doppler probe can be useful in helping to identify the course of the pedicle, which does not need to be completely visualized. The soft tissues surrounding the supraclavicular artery may be preserved to protect the vascular pedicle from injury. The nerve branches can be identified beneath the platysma muscle along with the supraclavicular artery. There nerves may be preserved in order to maintain sensation to the SCP flap.

Once the flap has been completely elevated, a wide tunnel is created between the defect within the head and neck region and the shoulder, if necessary. In most cases, a portion of the skin paddle is preserved to allow flap insetting, while the remainder of the flap is deepithelialized and buried beneath the skin bridge (▶ Fig. 9.4).

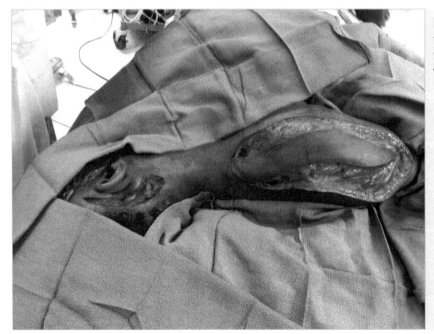

Fig. 9.2 The SCP flap is elevated off the trapezius and deltoid muscles in the subfascial plane to protect the vascular pedicle.

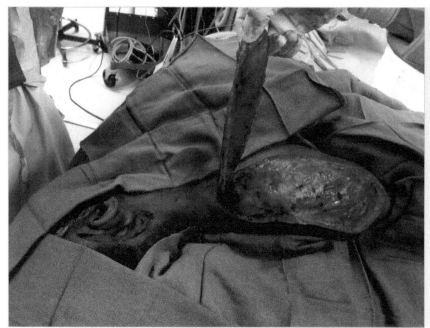

Fig. 9.3 The layer of white investing fascia surrounding the supraclavicular vessels has been divided in order to increase the length of the flap.

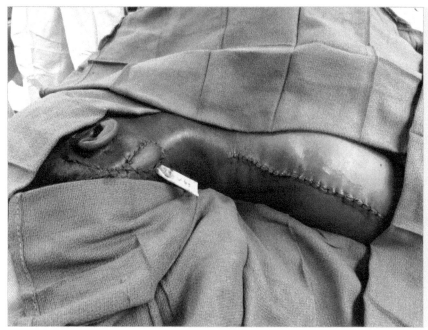

Fig. 9.4 The proximal portion of the flap is deepithelialized and tunneled beneath the skin bridge for reconstruction of the defect.

9.8 Donor Site Closure

The donor site along the shoulder and proximal arm can often be closed primarily after wide undermining of the surrounding soft tissues. If primary closure is not possible, which typically occurs along the shoulder region for flaps greater than 5 cm in width, skin grafting will be required.

9.9 Pearls and Pitfalls

- The course of the pedicle should be identified with the Doppler and marked, so that the flap is centered along the markings.
- The thin layer of white investing fascia around the pedicle should be carefully divided in order to obtain greater length of the flap.

References

[1] Chiu ES, Liu PH, Friedlander PL. Supraclavicular artery island flap for head and neck oncologic reconstruction: indications, complications, and outcomes. Plast Reconstr Surg 2009;124(1):115–123

[2] Sands TT, Martin JB, Simms E, Henderson MM, Friedlander PL, Chiu ES. Supraclavicular artery island flap innervation: anatomical studies and clinical implications. J Plast Reconstr Aesthet Surg 2012;65(1):68–71

[3] Pallua N, Machens HG, Rennekampff O, Becker M, Berger A. The fasciocutaneous supraclavicular artery island flap for releasing postburn mentosternal contractures. Plast Reconstr Surg 1997;99(7):1878–1884, discussion 1885–1886

[4] Vinh VQ, Van Anh T, Ogawa R, Hyakusoku H. Anatomical and clinical studies of the supraclavicular flap: analysis of 103 flaps used to reconstruct neck scar contractures. Plast Reconstr Surg 2009;123(5):1471–1480

[5] Di Benedetto G, Aquinati A, Pierangeli M, Scalise A, Bertani A. From the "charretera" to the supraclavicular fascial island flap: revisitation and further evolution of a controversial flap. Plast Reconstr Surg 2005;115(1):70–76

Part 2

Chest

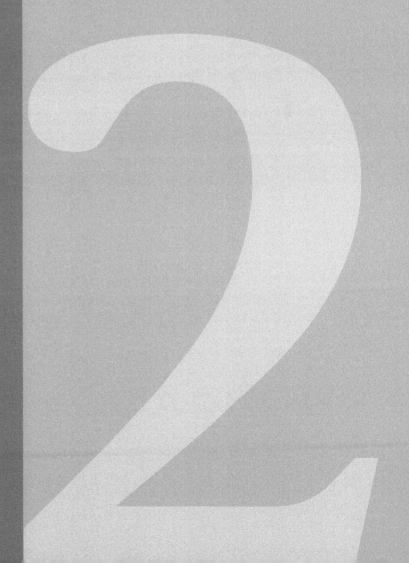

10 Internal Mammary Artery Perforator Flap

Peirong Yu

Abstract

The pectoralis major muscle (myocutaneous flap) remains a popular flap for head and neck reconstruction, especially when muscle is needed. The internal mammary artery perforator flap is less well known, but it is a valuable option when used as a pedicled flap. For head and neck reconstruction, the internal mammary artery perforator flap may provide superior color match compared to other donor sites, is easy to dissect, and flap elevation can usually be completed within thirty minutes. It is particularly useful in high-risk patients who may not tolerate a free flap reconstruction. As a free flap, it can be used for facial resurfacing, but is limited by a short pedicle and small size if primary closure of the donor site is planned. In this chapter, the steps involved in using the internal mammary artery perforator flap are clearly delineated, beginning with typical indications, anatomy, preoperative considerations, and operative technique. A variation in which this flap is useful as a modest-sized flap is also included.

Keywords: internal mammary artery perforator flap, internal mammary artery, subclavian artery, superior epigastric artery

10.1 Introduction

Local and regional flaps from the upper chest are traditionally limited to the deltopectoral flap and the pectoralis major flap. The former has been largely abandoned due to its significant donor site morbidity and the need for surgical delay in most cases. The pectoralis major muscle or myocutaneous flap remains a popular flap for head and neck reconstruction, especially when muscle is needed. The internal mammary artery perforator (IMAP) flap is less well known. This flap was first described in the literature in 2006 for tracheostoma reconstruction by Yu et al.[1] Neligan et al conducted injection studies and reported their clinical use of this flap in 2007.[2] More recently, Saint–Cyr's group reported the three-dimensional (3D) perforator anatomy using injections and 3D computed tomography (CT) scan of cadaveric specimens.[3] More anatomic and clinical cases have since been reported.[4,5,6] The IMAP flap is a valuable option when used as a pedicled flap. For head and neck reconstruction, the IMAP flap may provide superior color match compared to other donor sites, especially flaps from the thigh. This flap is very easy to dissect and the flap elevation can usually be completed within 30 minutes. Therefore, it is particularly useful in high-risk patients who may not tolerate a free flap reconstruction. As a free flap, the IMAP flap can be used for facial resurfacing, which provides excellent color match, but is limited by a short pedicle and small size if primary closure of the donor site is planned.

10.2 Typical Indications

The best indication for the IMAP flap is a cutaneous defect in the lower neck and upper chest, making it an excellent choice for tracheostoma reconstruction.

10.3 Anatomy

The **internal mammary** artery originates from the **subclavian artery** and travels along the sternal border on each side of the sternum. The average distance between the artery and the sternal border is approximately 1.5 cm.[7] It continues to descend as the **superior epigastric artery** in the upper abdomen and nourishes the upper part of the rectus abdominis muscle. In its path along the sternal border, the internal mammary artery sends out several perforators through the intercostal space to the chest skin (►**Fig. 10.1**). The more proximal perforators are usually larger than distal perforators as with other perforators in the body. The dominant IMAP is usually the one located in the second intercostal space.[3,4,5,6] Cadaveric studies found that the mean perforator diameter was 1.50 mm (range: 1.0–2.2 mm) in the first intercostal space, 1.83 mm (range: 1.3–2.4 mm) in the second intercostal space, and 1.47 mm (range: 1.3–1.7 mm) in third intercostal space.[3] Similar findings were reported in clinical series.[8,9] The author's own clinical experience shows that the IMAP arteries at the second intercostal space range from 1 to 1.5 mm and the perforator veins, 1.5 to 2 mm in diameter.

Based on the injection study, IMAPs in the first intercostal space perfuse to the level of the clavicle and lateral mammary fold in all cases and inferiorly to the level of the xiphisternum one-third of the time.[3] IMAPs in the second intercostal space had a territory reaching the clavicle and xiphisternum in four of six cases and the lateral mammary fold in all cases. IMAPs in the third intercostal space reached the clavicle in only 40%, the xiphisternum in 60%, and the lateral mammary fold in 80% of the cases. When the superior IMAPs (first and second interspaces) were injected, the perfusion territory was more horizontally oriented whereas it took an inferolateral orientation when the inferior IMAPs (third to seventh interspaces) were injected. This is useful information for flap

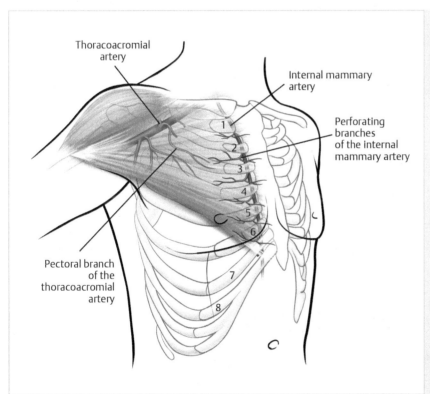

Fig. 10.1 The internal mammary artery and vein travel along the sternal border and send out perforators through each intercostal space to the skin.

design. In clinical practice, however, the second intercostal IMAP is most useful since it is dominant, reaches the neck more easily, and a horizontal design results in an inconspicuous donor site scar.

10.4 Variations

- IMAP free flap: useful as a modest sized flap with good color match to the facial skin.

10.5 Preoperative Considerations

A history of coronary artery bypass surgery with the left internal mammary artery precludes the use of this flap. Preoperative imaging studies are not indicated except in patients with a history of major anterior chest wall surgeries and/or radiotherapy. A CT angiogram may be obtained in these patients to evaluate the patency of the internal mammary artery and its perforators.

10.6 Positioning and Skin Markings

Harvest is performed in the supine position. The second and third ribs at the sternal border are identified. The IMAPs at the second and third intercostal spaces lateral to the sternal border are evaluated with a hand-held Doppler device. The IMAP in the second intercostal space is usually the largest and also closer to the head and neck. If the Doppler signal in the second intercostal space is significantly weaker than that at the third intercostal space, the latter should be considered. An elliptical flap is outlined with the central axis of the flap in a horizontal orientation, parallel to the ribs. Depending on the skin laxity, the flap width can be 5 to 8 cm to allow primary closure of the donor site. The medial limit of the flap is the anterior midline and the lateral limit is the midaxillary line. The superior border of the flap is just above the second rib, which is then curved to the axilla (▶ Fig. 10.2). No part of the flap should extend beyond

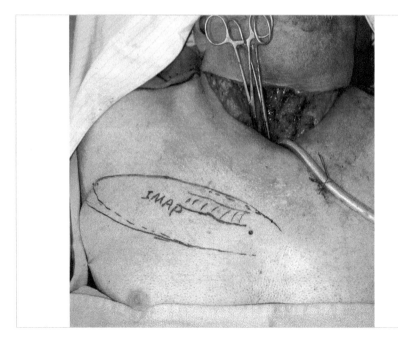

Fig. 10.2 The IMAP flap is usually based on the perforator at the second intercostal space. The flap is designed in a horizontal orientation parallel to the ribs. The distal end of the flap can extend 2 to 3 cm beyond the anterior axillary line.

the deltopectoral groove. The inferior incision is usually just below the third rib, depending on the flap width.

Clinically, the width of the flap is usually limited to 6 to 8 cm for primary closure of the donor site and maximal length is needed for the arc of rotation. The author's personal experience suggests that a single IMAP from the second intercostal space is able to carry a narrow (6 cm) and long (20 cm from the perforator) flap that extends 2 to 3 cm beyond the anterior axillary fold into the axilla.

10.7 Operative Techniques

The medial half of the superior incision is made first down to the fascia; subfascial dissection proceeds inferiorly with a pair of tenotomy scissors until the internal mammary perforator vessels are identified (▶ Fig. 10.3a). The perforator vessels do not need to be skeletonized unless it is used as a free flap. Once

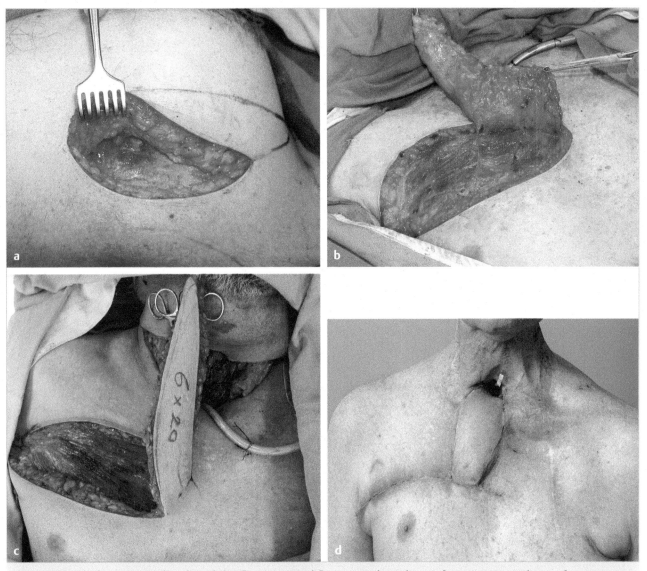

Fig. 10.3 **(a)** The superior border of the flap is incised first to explore the perforators. Once the perforators are identified, the rest of the flap is incised. **(b)** Small intercostal perforators may be encountered laterally. These vessels can be safely divided. **(c)** Once the flap is islanded, it is rotated up to reach the neck defect. **(d)** Donor site can usually be closed primarily.

the perforators are located, the rest of the flap is incised. Perforators either from the lateral thoracic artery or intercostal artery may be encountered in the lateral aspect of the flap. These perforators can be safely divided without compromising the flap perfusion (▶Fig. 10.3b). If needed, the pectoralis major muscle attachments cephalad to the perforators are divided to increase the length of the vascular pedicle. The flap is then rotated to reconstruct the neck defect, either through a subcutaneous tunnel or by dividing the narrow skin bridge between the donor site and the neck defect (▶Fig. 10.3c,d). The viability of the very distal end of the flap is confirmed by active bleeding from the skin edge. The donor site is then closed primarily.

When used as a free flap, the internal mammary artery and vein may need to be included to obtain more pedicle length and larger diameter vascular pedicle (▶Fig. 10.4a). The rib cartilage above the perforator is removed to facilitate the dissection of the internal mammary vessels. If a large flap is needed and the donor site cannot be closed primarily, a thoracodorsal artery perforator flap or skin graft can be used to close the chest donor site (▶Fig. 10.4b–e). For circumferential tracheal reconstruction, bilateral IMAP flaps may be needed to form a tube (▶Fig. 10.4f–h).

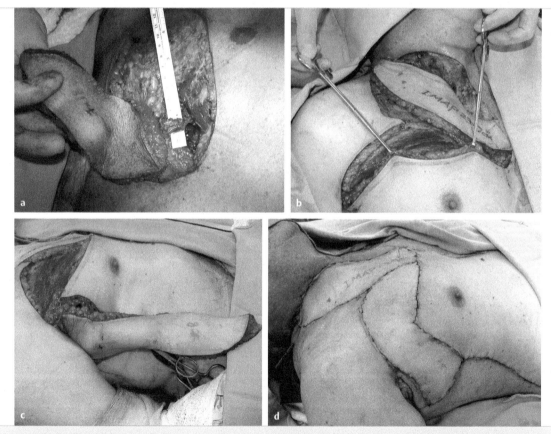

Fig. 10.4 (a) When the IMAP is used as a free flap, the main internal mammary vessels are dissected out proximally to obtain a longer and larger sized pedicle. **(b)** When a large IMAP flap is needed and the donor site cannot be closed primarily, **(c)** a thoracodorsal artery perforator flap **(d)** can be used as a pedicled island flap to cover the IMAP donor site.

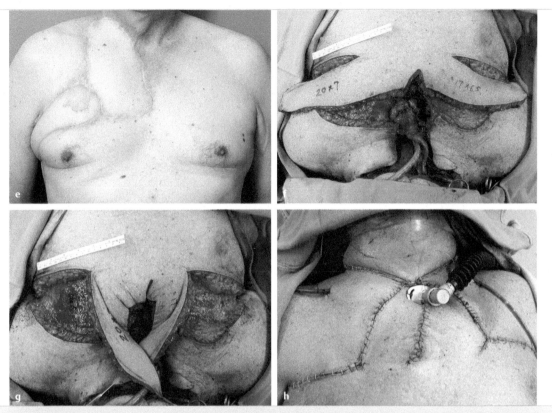

Fig. 10.4 (*Continued*) (**e**) with minimal donor site morbidity (**f**) for circumferential tracheal reconstruction. Bilateral IMAP flaps may be needed to form a tube bilateral IMAP flaps are dissected out. (**g**) Both IMAP flaps are rotated up to reach the neck. (**h**) The two IMAP flaps are sewn together to form a tube for circumferential tracheal reconstruction.

10.8 Donor Site Closure

The donor site can usually be closed primarily. If necessary, a thoracodorsal artery perforator flap (▶ **Fig. 10.4b**) or lateral split latissimus myocutaneous flap can be used to close the donor site.

10.9 Pearls and Pitfalls

- The perforators in the second intercostal space are usually largest.
- When based on the second intercostal space, the flap design should be horizontal and the tip of the flap may extend just beyond the anterior axillary fold.
- The flap should not extend above the clavicle or over the deltoid region.
- When used as a free flap, the internal mammary vessels should be included to obtain a larger and longer pedicle.

References

[1] Yu P, Roblin P, Chevray P. Internal mammary artery perforator (IMAP) flap for tracheostoma reconstruction. Head Neck 2006;28(8):723–729

[2] Neligan PC, Gullane PJ, Vesely M, Murray D. The internal mammary artery perforator flap: new variation on an old theme. Plast Reconstr Surg 2007;119(3):891–893

[3] Wong C, Saint-Cyr M, Rasko Y, et al. Three- and four-dimensional arterial and venous perforasomes of the internal mammary artery perforator flap. Plast Reconstr Surg 2009;124(6):1759–1769

[4] Schmidt M, Aszmann OC, Beck H, Frey M. The anatomic basis of the internal mammary artery perforator flap: a cadaver study. J Plast Reconstr Aesthet Surg 2010;63(2):191–196

[5] Schellekens PP, Paes EC, Hage JJ, van der Wal MB, Bleys RL, Kon M. Anatomy of the vascular pedicle of the internal mammary artery perforator (IMAP) flap as applied for head and neck reconstruction. J Plast Reconstr Aesthet Surg 2011;64(1):53–57

[6] Schellekens PP, Hage JJ, Paes EC, Kon M. Clinical application and outcome of the internal mammary artery perforator (IMAP) free flap for soft tissue reconstructions of the upper head and neck region in three patients. Microsurgery 2010;30(8):627–631

[7] Ninković MM, Schwabegger AH, Anderl H. Internal mammary vessels as a recipient site. Clin Plast Surg 1998;25(2):213–221

[8] Munhoz AM, Ishida LH, Montag E, et al. Perforator flap breast reconstruction using internal mammary perforator branches as a recipient site: an anatomical and clinical analysis. Plast Reconstr Surg 2004;114(1):62–68

[9] Hamdi M, Blondeel P, Van Landuyt K, Monstrey S. Algorithm in choosing recipient vessels for perforator free flap in breast reconstruction: the role of the internal mammary perforators. Br J Plast Surg 2004;57(3):258–265

11 Pectoralis Major Muscle/Myocutaneous Pedicled Flap

Matthew M. Hanasono

Abstract

Because of its versatility and reliability, the pectoralis major myocutaneous pedicled flap served as the workhorse flap for the majority of head and neck oncologic defects, until microvascular free flaps became commonplace. The pectoralis major muscle and myocutaneous pedicled flaps are still favored for many thoracic defects, as well as a backup in head and neck reconstruction in the event of a free flap loss, wound dehiscence, or fistula, and in combination with a free flap for reconstruction of extensive defects. This chapter takes the surgeon through every phase of the operative procedure, beginning with indications for use, anatomy, preoperative considerations, and surgical techniques. A section on variations lists deviations from the standard flap procedure.

Keywords: thoracoacromial artery, lateral thoracic artery, internal mammary artery, anterior intercostal artery, lateral pectoral nerve, medial pectoral nerve

11.1 Introduction

The pectoralis major myocutaneous (PMMC) pedicled flap was first described for head and neck reconstruction by Ariyan in 1979.[1] Because of its versatility and reliability, this flap served as the workhorse flap for the majority of head and neck oncologic defects encountered until microvascular free flaps became commonplace. The pectoralis major muscle and myocutaneous pedicled flaps are still favored for many thoracic defects as well as a backup in head and neck reconstruction in the event of a free lap loss, wound dehiscence, or fistula and in combination with a free flap for reconstruction of extensive defects.

11.2 Typical Indications

- Cutaneous defects of the neck and lower face.
- Hypopharyngeal defects, either as a muscle flap reinforcement of a primary pharyngeal closure or a myocutaneous patch for a partial pharyngeal defect.
- Oral and oropharyngeal defects.
- Sternal wounds, either by detaching the humeral insertions and advancing the pectoralis major muscles medially, or, sometimes, by dividing the thoracoacromial pedicle, using the internal mammary perforators as a blood supply, and turning one or both muscle flaps over (these techniques are not discussed further here).[2]
- Axillary and shoulder defects.

11.3 Anatomy

The pectoralis major muscle is a fan-shaped muscle that abducts and internally rotates the humerus. It originates on the anterior surface of the medial half of the clavicle, the anterior surface of the lateral half of the sternum, costal cartilages from the second to the sixth rib, and the aponeuorosis of the external oblique muscle. The pectoralis major converges laterally toward a tendon that inserts into the crest of the **greater tubercle of the humerus**.

The dominant blood supply of the pectoralis major muscle is the **thoracoacromial artery** and secondary blood supply includes the **lateral thoracic artery** and branches of the **internal mammary artery** as well as perforating branches of the **anterior intercostal arteries** (▶ Fig. 11.1). The thoracoacromial artery divides into **pectoral, clavicular, acromial, and deltoid** branches inferior to the middle third of the clavicle. The pectoral branch is the dominant blood supply to the muscle.

The lateral thoracic artery follows the lateral border of the pectoralis minor muscle and supplies the lateral part of the pectoralis major muscle. The venous drainage is via paired venae comitantes that accompany the arteries. The main blood supply to most of the skin overlying the pectoralis major muscle comes from the perforating branches of the internal mammary artery in the second through sixth intercostal spaces, medially, and the perforating branches of the third through sixth anterior intercostal arteries, laterally. These perforators are connected to the thoracoacromial artery pedicle via anastomotic "choke" vessels. The pectoral branch of the thoracoacromial artery also supplies small perforating branches to the skin overlying its course, although the artery dissipates at about the level of the fourth rib.

The **lateral and medial pectoral nerves** are the motor nerve supply to the pectoralis major muscle. They are named for their origin from the brachial plexus rather than the anatomic location of the portion of the muscle they supply. Thus the lateral pectoral nerve enters the pectoralis major muscle on its deep surface about 3 cm medial to the medial pectoral nerve. The nerves are

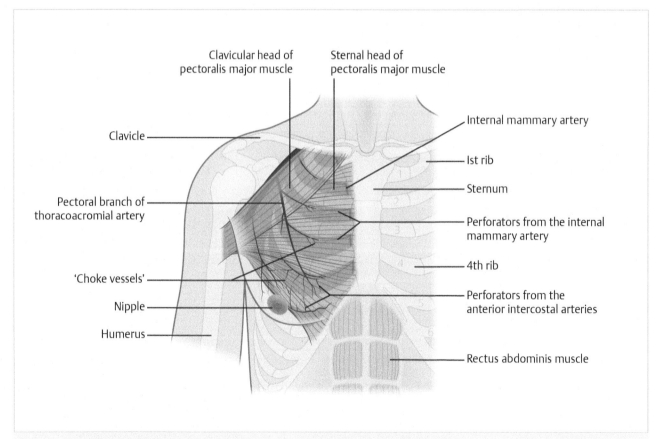

Fig. 11.1 Vascular anatomy of the pectoralis major muscle and overlying skin.

usually divided during flap harvest to prevent unwanted contraction and maximize arc of rotation. This flap is usually not harvested as a sensate flap.

11.4 Variations

- Myo-osseous or an osteomyocutaneous flap by including the fifth rib.
- Myo-osseous or osteomyocutaneous flap by including the lateral sternal bone via thoracoacromial connections with the internal mammary artery perforators.[3]
- Myo-osseous flap by including clavicular head via the clavicular branch of the thoracoacromial artery.
- Two separate muscle flaps, one based on the pectoral branch of the thoracoacromial artery and one based on the lateral thoracic artery.

11.5 Preoperative Considerations

In obese patients and in women due to the presence of the breast, a skin paddle may be excessively bulky and harvesting of a PMMC flap may also significantly distort the breast shape. In such cases, consideration should be given to performing a pectoralis major muscle flap and covering it with a split- or full-thickness skin graft. An alternative would be to center the skin paddle superomedially over the internal mammary perforators in the third intercostal space, where there is usually less soft-tissue bulk.[4]

However, designing the skin paddle in a more proximal location shortens the reach of the flap. While a reliable skin paddle could also be designed directly over the thoracoacromial artery, such a flap would have even less reach.

11.6 Positioning and Skin Markings

Supine positioning is best for most applications. The course of the thoracoacromial artery can be estimated by drawing a line from the acromion to the xiphoid process. If a pectoralis muscle flap is being elevated, an incision within the inframammary fold in women, or along the inferior border of the pectoralis major muscle in men, is planned. If a PMMC flap is being elevated, surgical dissection of the muscle is performed through the skin paddle incision.

In addition to the access afforded by an inframammary incision (in the pectoralis muscle flap) or the skin paddle incision (in the PMMC flap), it is often helpful to make a counter incision, just below and parallel to the clavicle when the flap is used in head and neck reconstruction for surgical exposure. While a vertical or oblique incision could be made over the pectoralis muscle, the recommended transverse incisions are preferable since they preserve the skin over the second and third intercostal spaces, which could be used for a deltopectoral or internal mammary artery perforator flap.

In order to design a myocutaneous flap with maximal reach of the skin paddle from the origin of the thoracoacromial artery, the skin paddle is usually centered over the inferior portion of the pectoralis major muscle, outside the vascular territory of the musculocutaneous perforating branches of the thoracoacromial artery. The skin paddle is, therefore, usually supplied by the musculocutaneous perforating branches of the anterior intercostal blood vessels of the fourth, fifth, and sixth costal interspaces, which communicate with the thoracoacromial artery via choke vessels that dilate in response to interruption of the primary blood supply (▶ Fig. 11.2a). Centering the skin paddle over the fourth intercostal space where the largest perforators typically occur results in

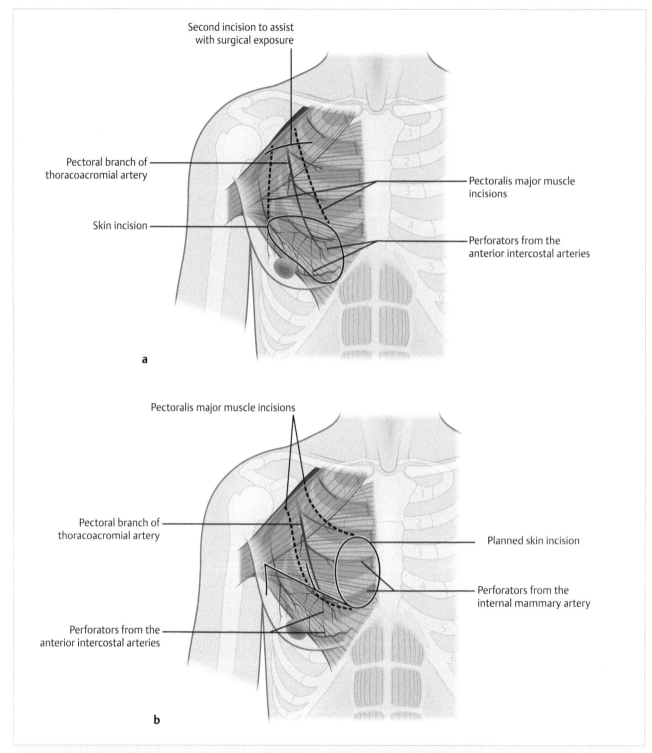

Fig. 11.2 **(a)** Skin markings for a PMMC pedicled flap with a distal skin paddle centered over intercostal artery perforators arising from the fourth intercostal space. The planned muscular incisions are indicated by the broken lines. **(b)** Skin markings for a PMMC pedicled flap with a superomedial skin paddle centered over the internal mammary artery perforator arising from the third intercostal space. This skin paddle design may be useful in patients with larger breasts or substantial subcutaneous fat. Note that the incisions depicted feature a Z-plasty closure that reduces distortion of the breast.

a high degree of reliability and should not extend more than a few centimeters beyond the borders of the muscle. As mentioned earlier, in obese patients and in women with moderate to large breasts, skin paddle may also be placed over the medial portion of the pectoralis major muscle, which is primarily supplied by perforating branches of the internal mammary artery, also connected to the thoracoacromial artery via choke vessels (▶Fig. 11.2b).[5]

11.7 Operative Technique

After the incision around the skin island (if any) is made, the rest of the chest skin is elevated from the underlying muscle. The muscle is then detached and raised from the chest wall. The pectoralis major is easily dissected from the pectoralis minor muscle in an avascular plane. Care is taken to ligate rather than cauterize musculocutaneous perforating blood vessels arising from the intercostal spaces, since these communicate directly with the skin paddle after they course through the thickness of the muscle (▶Fig. 11.3). The thoracoacromial pedicle should be identified early, on the undersurface of the muscle, and protected from injury.

The proximal muscle is divided with electrocautery above the skin island (if any) and the muscle portion of the flap is "narrowed" overlying the pedicle (▶Fig. 11.4). This detaches the flap from both the humerus laterally and the sternum medially. Proximally, minimal muscle needs to be left over the pedicle, and, in fact, the pedicle can be completely dissected from the muscle with appropriately delicate technique to minimize bulk. The lateral thoracic

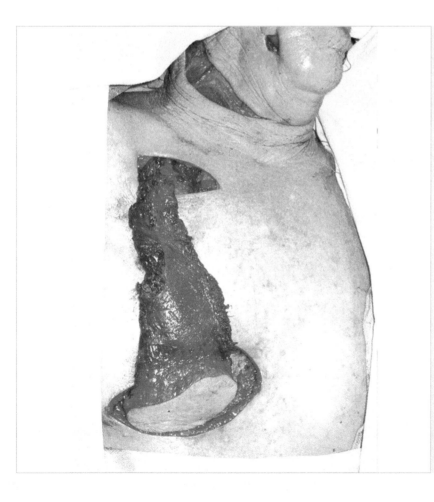

Fig. 11.3 Elevated PMMC pedicled flap. Note that the very little proximal muscle is included in the flap to minimize a proximal bulge in the neck.

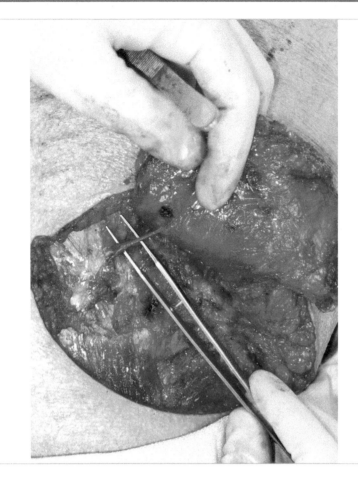

Fig. 11.4 Elevation of the PMMC pedicled flap showing the intercostal perforating blood vessels, arising from the interspace between the fourth and fifth ribs, adjacent to the nipple. These vessels should be ligated rather than cauterized to avoid injury to the blood supply to the skin paddle.

blood vessels lie lateral to the thoracoacromial vessels and do not need to be included with the flap if the maximum arc of rotation is required to reach the defect. The medial and lateral pectoral nerves are also divided.

The skin bridge between the donor site incisions and the defect is elevated, creating a wide tunnel for the pedicle. Muscle-only flaps and myocutaneous flaps where the skin paddle is used to reconstruct an intraoral or intraluminal pharyngeal defect can be transposed into the defect such that the deep surface of the muscle comes to lie superficially (▶ **Fig. 11.5a**). Myocutaneous flaps are usually rotated up to 180 degrees if the skin paddle is needed for an external defect of the chest wall or head and neck (▶ **Fig. 11.5b,c**).

11.8 Donor Site Closure

Substantial undermining is often necessary when a wide skin paddle (> 5 cm) is included with the flap. If the donor site wound cannot be closed primarily, skin grafting of the donor site may be necessary. Skin grafts over the costal cartilages and ribs may take poorly and healing may be prolonged.

11.9 Pearls and Pitfalls

- For the longest arc of rotation, the skin paddle of the PMMC pedicled flap should be centered over the fourth intercostal space.

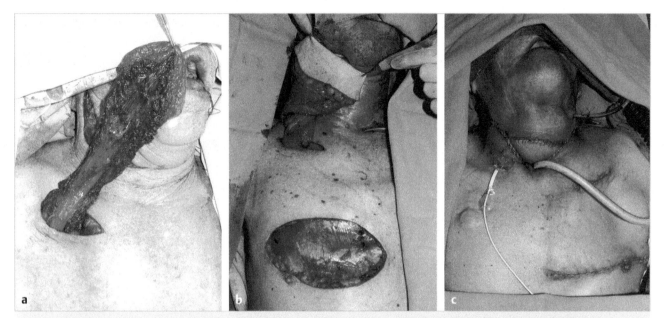

Fig. 11.5 **(a)** Turnover of right PMMC pedicled flap for an oral reconstruction so that the skin paddle faces intraorally. **(b)** Counter-clockwise rotation of a right PMMC pedicled flap for a cutaneous neck reconstruction. **(c)** Postoperative appearance of a different patient following left PMMC pedicled flap reconstruction after laryngopharyngectomy. Bulkiness in the proximal neck is minimized by including only a modest amount of muscle around the proximal pedicle. Note that a deltopectoral or internal mammary artery perforator flap is still possible.

- In obese patients and in women, a skin paddle centered medially over the third intercostal perforating branch of the internal mammary artery may allow the harvest of thinner skin paddles. Otherwise, consider performing a pectoralis muscle flap covered with a skin graft instead.
- Only a small cuff of proximal muscle around the vascular pedicle should be included in the flap design to minimize an unsightly bulge as well as contracture that can limit movement.

References

[1] Ariyan S. The pectoralis major myocutaneous flap. A versatile flap for reconstruction in the head and neck. Plast Reconstr Surg 1979;63(1):73–81

[2] Ascherman JA, Patel SM, Malhotra SM, Smith CR. Management of sternal wounds with bilateral pectoralis major myocutaneous advancement flaps in 114 consecutively treated patients: refinements in technique and outcomes analysis. Plast Reconstr Surg 2004;114(3):676–683

[3] Green MF, Gibson JR, Bryson JR, Thomson E. A one-stage correction of mandibular defects using a split sternum pectoralis major osteo-musculocutaneous transfer. Br J Plast Surg 1981;34(1):11–16

[4] Rikimaru H, Kiyokawa K, Inoue Y, Tai Y. Three-dimensional anatomical vascular distribution in the pectoralis major myocutaneous flap. Plast Reconstr Surg 2005;115(5):1342–1352, discussion 1353–1354

[5] Rikimaru H, Kiyokawa K, Watanabe K, Koga N, Nishi Y, Sakamoto A. New method of preparing a pectoralis major myocutaneous flap with a skin paddle that includes the third intercostal perforating branch of the internal thoracic artery. Plast Reconstr Surg 2009;123(4):1220–1228

12 Trapezius Muscle/Myocutaneous Flap

Deepak Gupta and Matthew M. Hanasono

Abstract

The trapezius flap has been used to reconstruct the soft tissue of the neck and protect the carotid arteries from blowout. Myocutaneous versions can be based either on the inferior muscle fibers and descending blood supply posteriorly or on the superior fibers on the ascending blood supply (cervicohumeral). It has also less commonly been harvested with the scapular spine as an osteomyocutaneous flap. With the improvements in microsurgical free tissue transfer, the trapezius flap has largely fallen out of favor, but it remains an option for reconstruction of the trunk, head, neck, face, and less commonly, the oral cavity, when microsurgical reconstruction is not available. It is typically used as a pedicled flap for locoregional reconstruction but has also been used as a free flap. This chapter offers valuable guidance to any surgeon who chooses this option for his or her patient, beginning with typical indications, to anatomy, to the preoperative considerations, to the operative techniques. Variations to the procedure are also listed and illustrated.

Keywords: levator scapulae muscle, rhomboid major muscle, rhomboid minor muscle, latissimus dorsi muscle, spinal accessory nerve, transverse cervical artery, thyrocervical trunk, occipital artery, dorsal scapular artery

12.1 Introduction

The trapezius flap was first described in a single-center case series published in 1971 and was used to reconstruct the soft tissue of the neck and protect the carotid arteries from blowout.[1] Myocutaneous versions can be based either on the inferior muscle fibers and descending blood supply posteriorly[2,3] or superior fibers on the ascending blood supply (cervicohumeral).[4,5] It has also less commonly been harvested with the scapular spine as an osteomyocutaneous flap.[6] With the improvements in microsurgical free tissue transfer, the trapezius flap has largely fallen out of favor, but remains an option for reconstruction of the trunk, head, neck, face, and less commonly, oral cavity, when microsurgical reconstruction is not available. It is typically used as a pedicled flap for locoregional reconstruction, but has also been used as a free flap.[7]

12.2 Typical Indications

- Coverage of skull: the arc of rotation allows for occipital skull coverage. Further dissection of the pedicle can extend its reach to the temporal skull.
- Head and neck reconstruction: after parotidectomy or for coverage of carotid and jugular vessels. Less commonly, may also be used for mandibular reconstruction or reconstruction of the oral cavity including floor of mouth or buccal lining.
- Coverage of spinal hardware: the flap can be used to cover both the cervical and thoracic vertebral columns and/or hardware, either as a muscle flap or a myocutaneous flap.
- Coverage of shoulder, sternum, or axilla wounds.

12.3 Anatomy

The trapezius muscle is a flat, fan-shaped muscle of the posterior trunk. It is located in the upper back and neck and is the most superficial muscle at its location. The **levator scapulae muscle** lies deep to the superior portion. In its midportion and inferiorly, the **rhomboid major and minor muscles**, and the **latissimus dorsi muscle** lie deep to the trapezius.

The trapezius has three functional regions: the **superior region** (descending part), which supports the weight of the arm; **the middle region** (transverse part), which retracts the scapulae; and the **inferior region** (ascending part), which medially rotates and depresses the scapulae (▶ **Fig. 12.1**). The superior fibers of the trapezius have origins at the external occipital protuberance and medial third of the superior nuchal line of the occipital bone of the skull. From here, they continue to originate inferiorly along the ligamentum nuchae and spinous process of C7. The superior fibers insert on the posterior aspect of the lateral third of the clavicle. The middle fibers originate from the spinous processes of C7 to T4 and insert on the spine of scapula and acromion. The inferior fibers originate from the spinous processes of T4 to T12 and insert on the spine of the scapula. If the scapula is fixed, the superior fibers will laterally flex the neck (unilateral muscle action) or extend the neck (bilateral muscle action).

The trapezius muscle is innervated by the **spinal accessory nerve (cranial nerve XI)**. A shoulder droop deformity results from muscle denervation. Preservation of the superior fibers during flap harvest will maintain shoulder stability and prevent drooping.

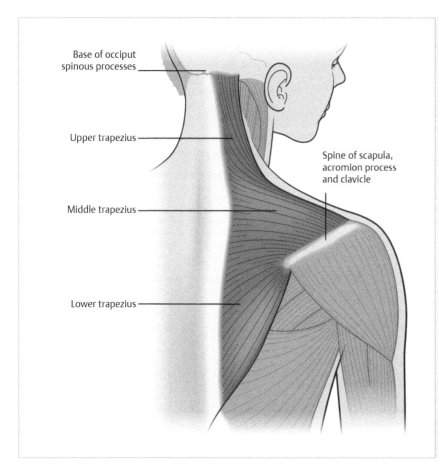

Fig. 12.1 The trapezius is a flat, fan-shaped muscle of the upper back. It has origins at the occipital skull, C7, T1 to T12 and inserts at the clavicle, acromion, and scapular spine. The trapezius can be thought of as having superior, middle, and inferior thirds. In general, most flaps will employ the middle and inferior thirds. The superior fibers should be preserved for shoulder and scapular stability.

Base of occiput spinous processes

Upper trapezius

Spine of scapula, acromion process and clavicle

Middle trapezius

Lower trapezius

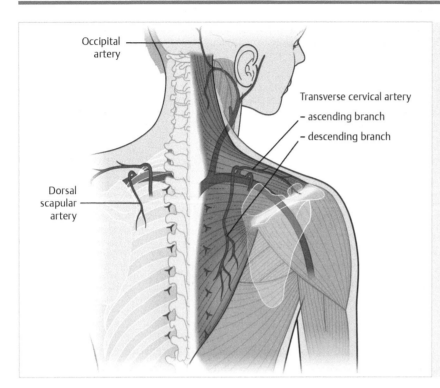

Occipital artery

Transverse cervical artery
– ascending branch
– descending branch

Dorsal scapular artery

Fig. 12.2 The trapezius has one dominant pedicle and several minor pedicles. The transverse cervical artery originates from the thyrocervical trunk.

The dominant vascular pedicle to the trapezius muscle is the **transverse cervical artery**. It originates in the anterior inferior neck usually from the **thyrocervical trunk** and has both ascending and descending branches. The trapezius also receives minor contributions from branches of the **occipital artery**, which originates from the external carotid artery, and dorsal scapular artery, which usually originates from the subclavian artery or, occasionally, shares an origin with the transverse cervical artery. The **dorsal scapular artery** (also known as the deep branch of the transverse cervical artery) runs under the rhomboid muscles and sends a branch to the trapezius between the rhomboid major and minor muscles. This vessel is lateral and basically runs parallel to the descending branch of the transverse cervical artery and can be used to support the trapezius muscle or myocutaneous flap alone or along with the descending branch of the transverse cervical artery. There are also minor contributions from posterior intercostal arteries, which originate from the descending aorta (▶ **Fig. 12.2**).

12.4 Variations

- Standard flap: used in the majority of cases and is typically muscle only or myocutaneous and is based on the descending branch of the transverse cervical artery with or without the dorsal scapular artery. The flap is vertical in design (▶ **Fig. 12.3**).
- Turnover flap: the transverse cervical artery may be divided so the muscle can be turned over for spinal coverage. This flap is based on the posterior branches of the intercostal vessels.
- Osteomyocutaneous: the superior fibers have vascularized connections to the lateral/superior spine of the scapula. The middle and inferior fibers have vascularized connections to the medial/inferior spine of the scapula. A 10 × 2 cm segment of scapular spine can be harvested with the flap for use in mandibular reconstruction.

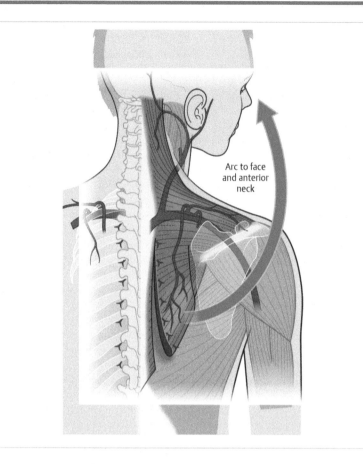

Fig. 12.3 The trapezius myocutaneous flap is designed either on the descending or ascending branch of the transverse cervical artery.

Arc to face and anterior neck

12.5 Preoperative Considerations

If extensive neck dissection has been performed, attention should be paid to the patency of the transverse cervical vessels. This should be confirmed before undertaking the harvest of the flap.

Shoulder droop due to spinal accessory (cranial nerve XI) nerve injury or actual loss of the superior portion of the trapezius muscle is a painful and debilitating complication of trapezius harvest. The superior fibers of the trapezius should be spared from dissection as they will maintain shoulder stability and scapular position. If the spinal accessory nerve will be sacrificed (e.g., for cancer), it should be grafted to restore function.

The trapezius flap has greatest reach as a vertical design based on the descending branch of the transverse cervical artery. If the trapezius is needed to reach a far distance, careful attention should be given to the design of the flap. Any skin paddle that is used should be limited to a maximum of 15 cm below the tip of the scapula, as skin below this may not possess adequate perfusion.

12.6 Positioning and Skin Markings

The standard vertically oriented flap is discussed further here. A skin island up to 20 × 8 cm can be supported on the middle and inferior fibers of the trapezius muscle flap. This skin island can be located and marked between the posterior trunk midline (located by palpation of the spinous processes between C7 and T12) and the medial, vertical, border of the scapula (▶ **Fig. 12.4**). The top of the skin island should be marked at the midpoint of the height of the scapula.

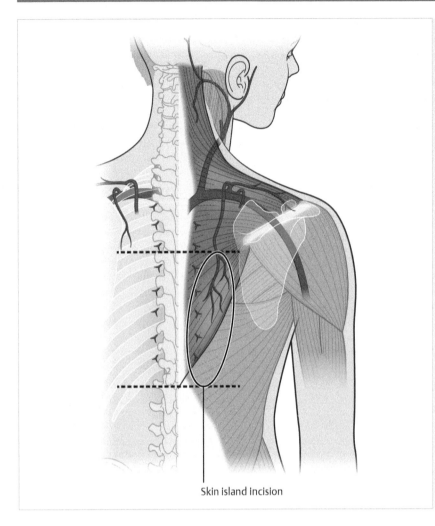

Fig. 12.4 The most common design of the trapezius flap is the vertical skin island myocutaneous flap. It is marked between the midline of the back and the medial border of the scapula. The top of the skin island should be marked at the midpoint of the height of the scapula. The bottom of the skin island should be marked either at the inferior tip of the trapezius (T12), below the tip of the trapezius (may depend on the dorsal scapular artery), or at a point located halfway between the tip of the scapula and the posterior superior iliac crest.

Skin island incision

The bottom of the skin island should be marked either at the inferior tip of the trapezius (T12), 10 cm (ideally) to 15 cm (maximum) below the tip of the scapula, or at a point located halfway between the tip of the scapula and the posterior superior iliac crest, depending on the design and the need. It is best to mark surface landmarks in standing or sitting position, as once the patient is prone or lateral, the scapula will rotate and distort the muscle territory. If a myocutaneous flap is being elevated, the remainder of the muscle dissection can be performed through the skin island incision (▶Fig. 12.4).

If a muscle-only flap is to be designed, it can be accessed through any number of incisions including median, paramedian, oblique, transverse, or others, again depending on the design or the area to be reached.

12.7 Operative Technique

In most cases, the trapezius flap will be used for immediate reconstruction of the head and neck region. As such, it is advantageous to prep and drape both surgical fields together to avoid a position change. The patient is placed in either the lateral decubitus or prone position for elevation of the vertical trapezius

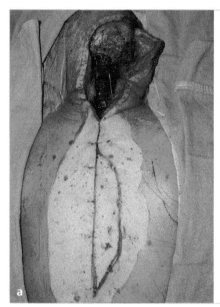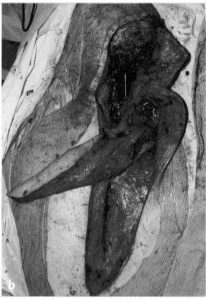

Fig. 12.5 This patient underwent vertical myocutaneous trapezius flap, based on the descending branch of the transverse cervical artery, for coverage of occiput, skull base, and cervical spine. **(a)** The inferior tip of the flap is 10 cm below the scapular tip. **(b)** After elevating the flap, detaching its medial and lateral attachments, and dividing the muscle over the proximal pedicle, it was rotated medially to reach the recipient site.

flap. Assuming a myocutaneous flap is needed, the procedure begins with incision of the skin island. Dissection continues until the muscle fascia is reached. The fascia is incised.

In preparation for transposition of the flap, one must determine whether the flap will be passed through a tunnel between the recipient and donor sites, or if an additional incision is required to connect the two. If a tunnel is chosen, it must be created subcutaneously above the trapezius muscle and should be wide enough not to compress the transposed flap. Any undue compression can lead to venous congestion and partial or complete flap failure. If the donor and recipient sites are to be connected by an incision, this can be either closed primarily after transposition of the flap or closed with inset of the flap into the incision and/or possible skin graft.

We prefer to start distally (inferiorly) and continue the muscle dissection superiorly in the submuscular plane, which is mostly avascular (▶Fig. 12.5). The medial origins are detached from the spinous processes. Laterally, the muscle fibers of the inferior and middle thirds are divided.

The plane proceeds over the rhomboideus major (inferior) and rhomboideus minor (superior) muscles. Between these muscles is the most frequent location to encounter the emergence of the dorsal scapular artery. Note that the flap can be based on either the descending branch of the transverse cervical artery or the dorsal scapular artery or both. If the dorsal scapula artery blood supply is to be included with the flap, then the distal artery that runs beneath the rhomboid major muscle needs to be ligated and the rhomboid minor muscle needs to be divided for maximal reach (▶Fig. 12.6). Dividing the dorsal scapular artery can reduce the blood supply to the flap, but increases its arc of rotation and reach.

Some muscle can typically be divided around the pedicle, thereby reducing its bulk and facilitating this point of rotation. A small amount of muscle is usually left in place to reduce tension on the pedicle, but, if needed, the pedicle can be meticulously dissected and all the muscle divided, resulting in a true island flap.

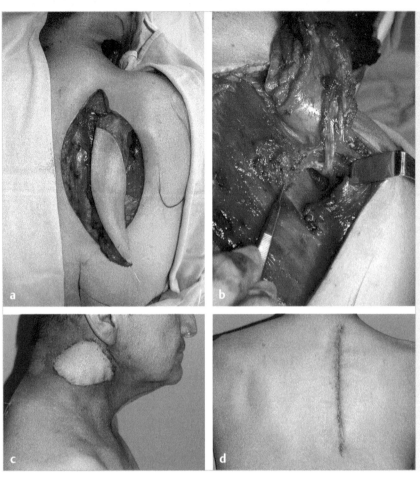

Fig. 12.6 This patient underwent vertical myocutaneous trapezius flap for closure of a lateral neck defect. **(a)** The inferior tip of the flap is about 10 cm below the scapular tip. **(b)** The upper rhomboid minor was divided to free the dorsal scapular artery, which served as the primary blood supply for this flap. **(c)** The flap was passed through a wide subcutaneous tunnel to the recipient site. **(d)** The donor site was closed primarily.

12.8 Donor Site Closure

The donor site can usually be closed primarily over a closed suction drain. The subcutaneous plane can be undermined laterally to allow advancement of the skin to the midline. Caution should be exercised in undermining across the midline as this may eliminate the possibility of a contralateral trapezius myocutaneous flap skin island in the future, should the need arise. A skin graft may also be used for closure of the donor site if the skin paddle width is more than about 5 to 6 cm. Skin grafts, however, may have a higher rate of partial or complete failure in this area because of their location on the posterior trunk and significant shear in this area from shoulder movement.

12.9 Pearls and Pitfalls

- A vertically designed trapezius myocutaneous flap is most common. Particular attention should be paid to the location of the inferior tip of the skin island and its perfusion.
- The trapezius myocutaneous flap can usually be passed through a tunnel to the recipient site in the head and neck region. Ensure the tunnel is wide enough such that the pedicle (muscle) is not compressed. The point of rotation should also be checked for kinking of the pedicle.
- For the longest arc of rotation, the dorsal scapular pedicle should be divided. This may be associated with reduced perfusion of the distal tip of the skin island of the vertical myocutaneous flap.

References

[1] Jaques DA, Hovey LM, Chambers RG. Carotid artery protection by means of a trapezius muscle flap. Am J Surg 1971;122(6):744–747

[2] Mathes SJ, Nahai F. Muscle flap transposition with function preservation: technical and clinical considerations. Plast Reconstr Surg 1980;66(2):242–249

[3] Baek SM, Biller HF, Krespi YP, Lawson W. The lower trapezius island myocutaneous flap. Ann Plast Surg 1980;5(2):108–114

[4] Demergasso F, Piazza MV. Trapezius myocutaneous flap in reconstructive surgery for head and neck cancer: an original technique. Am J Surg 1979;138(4):533–536

[5] McCraw JB, Magee WP Jr, Kalwaic H. Uses of the trapezius and sternomastoid myocutaneous flaps in head and neck reconstruction. Plast Reconstr Surg 1979;63(1):49–57

[6] Dufresne C, Cutting C, Valauri F, Klein M, Colen S, McCarthy JG. Reconstruction of mandibular and floor of mouth defects using the trapezius osteomyocutaneous flap. Plast Reconstr Surg 1987;79(5):687–696

[7] Mardini S, Chen HC, Salgado CJ, Chen KT, Tsai FC, Feng GM. Extended trapezius myocutaneous free flap for the reconstruction of a foot defect lacking adjacent recipient vessels. J Reconstr Microsurg 2004;20(8):599–603

13 Paraspinous Muscle Pedicled Flap

Andrew Michael Altman

Abstract

The paraspinous muscle complex can be utilized as a flap and advanced medially to provide robust vascularized muscle coverage of the spine at the midline in cases of difficult wounds and prophylactically in cases of spinal surgery at high risk for healing problems. Paraspinous muscle flaps can be used at all levels of the spine. The morbidity of this flap is low, the learning curve is gentle, and its efficacy in treating challenging spine surgery problems is great. Accordingly, this is a technique that is a welcome tool available to the reconstructive surgeon. This chapter delves into the crucial surgical concerns in the use of the paraspinous muscle pedicled flap, ranging from typical indications, to anatomy, to preoperative considerations, to surgical techniques. Three variations for this option are also listed.

Keywords: spinalis muscle, longissimus muscle, iliocostalis muscle, dorsal branch of the intercostal vessel

13.1 Introduction

The paraspinous muscle complex can be mobilized and advanced medially to provide robust vascularized muscle coverage of the spine at the midline in cases of difficult wounds and prophylactically in cases of spinal surgery at high risk for healing problems.[1,2,3,4,5] Paraspinous muscle flaps can be used at all levels of the spine. The morbidity of this flap is low, the learning curve is gentle, and the efficacy in treating challenging spine surgery problems is great. Accordingly, this is a technique that is a welcome tool in the array at the disposal of the reconstructive surgeon.

13.2 Typical Indications

- Coverage of spinal wounds that have failed to heal or have exposed hardware.
- Prophylactic coverage of the spine immediately following spinal surgery in patients with risk factors for wound healing complications.

13.3 Anatomy

The paraspinous muscle complex is made up of the **spinalis muscle, the longissimus muscle, and the iliocostalis muscle** moving progressively more lateral. This complex runs parallel to the spine on each side. Their function is to stabilize the spine. The space occupied by this complex is from the spinous processes medial to the lateral level where the ribs begin to change their angle to an anterior-sloping inclination.

From superficial to deep as one approaches the spine are the skin, subcutaneous tissue, and superficial fascia. Trapezius muscle fibers are then encountered relatively superficially in the cervical and upper thoracic levels. Additionally, the rhomboids (minor and major) are encountered from rostral to caudal respectively in the cervical region. Confluent with the level of the trapezius, at the thoracolumbar levels, is the thoracolumbar fascia, which invests the insertions of the latissiumus dorsi muscle onto the spine. Deep to the latissiumus dorsi muscle is the serratus posterior inferior muscle caudally and the serratus posterior superior muscle cephalad. The paired serratus posterior superior muscles are situated just deep to the rhomboid muscles in the cervical range and extend more cephalad on their trajectory to the spinous processes at the midline. Deep to the trapezius muscle in the cervical region is the splenius capitis muscle cephalad and then the extension referred to as the splenius cervicis muscle more cadual. The trapezius, serratus posterior superior and inferior, rhomboids (minor and major), and latissiumus dorsi muscles, as described earlier, constitute the relatively more superficial muscle envelope of the back at the midline and paramedian zone. Deep to these muscles are the paraspinous muscles. These muscles fuse into continuity and constitute the erector spinae complex at the lumbosacral region. The deep muscles of the back are collectively termed the transversospinalis muscles; they are the paired semispinalis muscles, multifidus muscles, and rotatores muscles, from superficial to deep, respectively. These are of less clinical significance in the present context because they are generally not in a position to be mobilized for spinal coverage.

The paraspinous muscles are skeletal muscles having origins and insertions as follows: the spinalis muscles originate at the spinous processes of the lower vertebral levels and insert at the spinous processes of the superior vertebral levels and the skull base; the longissiumus muscles originate at the transverse processes of the caudal vertebral levels and insert at the transverse processes at the superior vertebral levels and the mastoid process; the iliocostalis muscles originate at the sacrum and the iliac crests and insert at the angles of the ribs located more cephalad.

Of associated interest are the trapezius and latissiumus dorsi muscles because they can be independently elevated and advanced in conjunction with paraspinous muscle flaps, depending on the demands of the clinical situation.[2,6]

The paraspinous muscles themselves have a Mathes and Nahai type IV segmental blood supply.[7] There are two parallel lines of perforators that run in tandem from a cephalad to caudal direction: one set of perforators is medial and the other is situated laterally.[8] These perforators are branches of the **dorsal branch of the intercostal vessels** from the aorta. Medial and lateral perforators branch off the intercostal vessels at the upper half of the paraspinous muscle complex and from lumbar and sacral vessels at the lower half.[7] When mobilized as a pedicled paraspinous muscle flap, the mobilized paraspinous muscle flap complex is based on the lateral row of intercostal perforators after the sacrifice and division of the medial row of intercostal perforators as needed for flap dissection and mobilization (▶ **Fig. 13.1**).[2,8]

13.4 Variations

- Bilateral paraspinous muscle flaps with trapezius muscle flaps.
- Paired paraspinous with latissimus dorsi (LD) muscle flaps.[2]
- Paired paraspinous with LD flaps and gluteus maximus.[2]

13.5 Preoperative Considerations

Evaluation of the patient should begin with patient history and physical examination, paying attention to the indications for the proposed spine surgery,

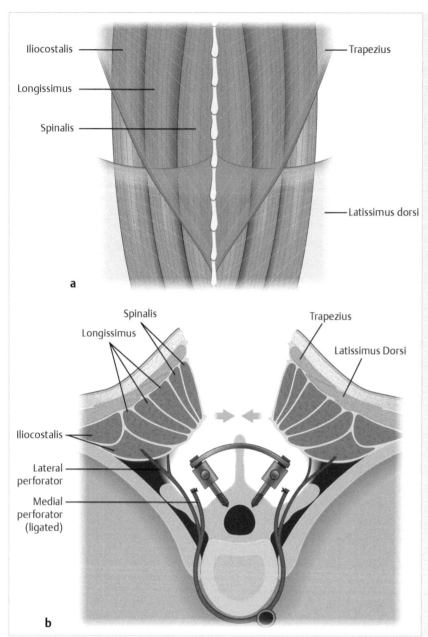

Fig. 13.1 (a) Pertinent anatomy for reconstruction of the typical spine defect. SP, spinous process; S, spinalis; L, longissimus; I, iliocostalis; T, trapezius; LD, latissimus dorsi. The paraspinous muscle is made up of paired spinalis, longissimus, and iliocostalis muscles. These muscle complexes can be mobilized based on the lateral row perforators and can be advanced medially for ablation of empty space and reconstruction of spinal wounds. Superficial to this are the trapezius muscle cephalad and the latissimus dorsi muscle cadual. These can be mobilized to provide an additional layer of reconstruction. (b) Schematic representing the paraspinous muscle flap mobilization on both sides in preparation for reconstruction of both the spine and the coverage of the spinal hardware. At the deepest part of the defect is the spinal cord with spinal hardware adjacent. The paraspinous muscle complexes have been mobilized off the midline. The tripartate nature of the paraspinous muscle complex (spinalis, longissimus, and iliocostalis components) from medial to lateral can be noted. The two rows of perforators that provide blood supply to the paraspinous muscle complex muscles are displayed (medial row and lateral row).

prior surgery to the spine and posterior thorax, and comorbid medical conditions that may impact healing. Previous infections should be taken into consideration. Ideally, the wound bed should definitively be debrided in a meticulous manner and washed out to the point of pristine total eradication of infection prior to flap reconstruction. Basically, certain cases of spinal instability and critical hardware exposure may require coordination with the spine surgeon for simultaneous debridement, washout, and reconstruction in a single-surgical setting due to prohibitive risks to the patient's neurological well-being posed by repeat surgery for debridement and washout prior to reconstruction (▶ Fig. 13.2).

13.6 Positioning and Skin Markings

Positioning is usually prone. Adequate mobilization of the paraspinous muscle flaps can be accomplished with any variation of standard prone positioning that may be required by the spine surgeon.

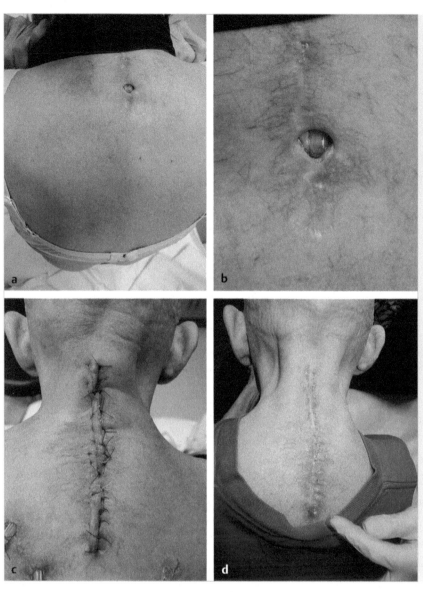

Fig. 13.2 (a,b) The patient had been operated on with instrumentation to stabilize the cervical spine in the setting of cervical myelopathy. The patient had healing problems and underwent surgery for repeat closure of a wound 2 months prior to the presentation, but had redevelopment a wound. The image shows the chronic cervical spinal wound. The patient was taken to surgery for aggressive debridement of the wound to include partial removal of instrumentation by the spine surgeon and thorough washout. Reconstruction was performed with paired paraspinous muscle flaps and a second layer of soft-tissue reconstruction utilizing paired trapezius muscle flaps. **(c)** The patient had an uneventful recovery postoperatively; healing is shown at 10 days postoperative. **(d)** Approximately 1 month postoperative.

13.7 Operative Technique

Before handoff of the operation from the spine surgeon to the reconstructive surgeon, a careful anatomic survey should be conducted together taking note of all pertinent features of the defect to include exposure of the spinal column and neural structures, presence and location of hardware, proposed placement of drains, presence or absence of any dural repair, and any other features unique to the case.

The surgeon begins by placing rake retractors in the paraspinous muscle complex on one side first to begin elevation of the flap. With upward traction, a cleavage plane becomes visible with an areolar layer separating from the underlying fascial and muscular attachments to the transverse processes of the vertebrae. The paraspinous muscle complex is mobilized and lifted off the transverse processes. The dissection lifting the flap off the transverse processes is conducted with cautery and is carried lateral taking care to identify and cauterize any medial perforators that may be encountered. These can safely be sacrificed as the flaps are based on the sequential row of relatively larger lateral perforators. In many cases, the dissection that has been conducted by the spine surgeon, particularly when laminectomy was involved in the procedure, has largely taken care of this part of the muscle complex mobilization and minimal or no further dissection on the undersurface of the paraspinous muscle complex is required. Next, rake retractors are placed superficial to the paraspinous muscle complex to help dissect the skin and subcutaneous fat off the paraspinous muscle complex. This dissection can be conducted in one of two manners: either the trapezius and latissimus stratum can be raised with the adipocutaneous envelope in continuity, or these two layers can be dissected separately to allow an additional layer of tissue for advancement to the midline and closure.[2,6] Mobilization of the superficial tissues from the paraspinous muscle complex below allows for further freedom of the paraspinous muscle complex to be medialized. This superficial dissection laterally should be conducted for a width of approximately 5 cm. The overlying layer of skin and fat can be subsequently closed under no tension on conclusion of inset of the muscle flaps at the midline. The superficial surface of the paraspinous muscle complex is covered with investing fascia that can be scored approximately 3 cm lateral to the midline in a line parallel to the spine. This allows for greater unfurling of the mobilized paraspinous muscle flap.

The flaps are brought together in the midline after gently grasping with Allis clamps in order to coapt them and remove tension. A deep drain is usually placed deep to flap inset adjacent to the spine. Further drains are placed in the more superficial planes. At inset, the flaps are coapted in the midline by placement of interrupted large resorbable stitches placed using either a figure-of-eight or Lembert technique. The goal of this step is to facilitate imbrication of the muscle flaps into the depth of the defect, effectively ablating dead space. The muscle flaps can also be inset one on top of the other in a vest-over-pants manner and inset with figure-of-eight sutures.[9] Alternatively, use of the Lembert suture technique with bites taken medial to lateral offset from the midline in the longissimus component of the complex, then to the other side, and lateral back to medial in the longissiumus offset from midline allows for effective dunking of the spinalis medial-most component of the complex into the depth of the wound on tying of sutures. If a trapezius flap or latissiumus flap is utilized, this layer is closed by placement of interrupted figure-of-eight size zero resorbable stitches.

13.8 Donor Site Closure

The superficial fascia is closed, followed by the deep dermis and then the superficial skin. In many cases, the patient can be mobilized out of bed on the postoperative day 1 unless a dural repair has been performed, or because of other circumstances related to the index spine operation that would dictate longer bed rest. Coordination with the nursing staff to ensure frequent position changes with slight tilting is preferred to keep the patient from exerting too much pressure directly on the midline, if determined acceptable and safe by the spine surgeon.[2]

13.9 Pearls and Pitfalls

- Close communication with the spine surgeon will allow optimal setup, identification of key elements of the defect, awareness of vulnerable anatomic sites, and avoidance of neurologic damage.

- Be prepared to utilize the trapezius or latissimus as either additional layers of coverage or as the primary flaps in cases where the paraspinous muscle complex itself is not sufficient.
- Maneuvers that can enhance the reach of the paraspinous pedicled muscle flaps include scoring of the surface of the paraspinous muscle flap complex in parallel to its long axis and additional mobilization of the myocutaneous or cutaneous element from the underlying paraspinous muscle complex.

References

[1] Cohen LE, Fullerton N, Mundy LR, et al. Optimizing successful outcomes in complex spine reconstruction using local muscle flaps. Plast Reconstr Surg 2016;137(1):295–301

[2] Garvey PB, Rhines LD, Dong W, Chang DW. Immediate soft-tissue reconstruction for complex defects of the spine following surgery for spinal neoplasms. Plast Reconstr Surg 2010;125(5):1460–1466

[3] Manstein ME, Manstein CH, Manstein G. Paraspinous muscle flaps. Ann Plast Surg 1998;40(5):458–462

[4] Mericli AF, Tarola NA, Moore JH Jr, Copit SE, Fox JW IV, Tuma GA. Paraspinous muscle flap reconstruction of complex midline back wounds: Risk factors and postreconstruction complications. Ann Plast Surg 2010;65(2):219–224

[5] Hultman CS, Jones GE, Losken A, et al. Salvage of infected spinal hardware with paraspinous muscle flaps: anatomic considerations with clinical correlation. Ann Plast Surg 2006;57(5):521–528

[6] Casas LA, Lewis VL Jr. A reliable approach to the closure of large acquired midline defects of the back. Plast Reconstr Surg 1989;84(4):632–641

[7] Balogh B, Piza-Katzer H, Ritschl P, Winkelbauer F, Firbas W. Modifications of the paraspinous muscle flap: anatomy and clinical application. Plast Reconstr Surg 1996;97(1):202–206

[8] Wilhelmi BJ, Snyder N, Colquhoun T, Hadjipavlou A, Phillips LG. Bipedicle paraspinous muscle flaps for spinal wound closure: an anatomic and clinical study. Plast Reconstr Surg 2000;106(6):1305–1311

[9] Saint-Cyr M, Nikolis A, Moumdjian R, et al. Paraspinous muscle flaps for the treatment and prevention of cerebrospinal fluid fistulas in neurosurgery. Spine 2003;28(5):E86–E92

14 Latissimus Dorsi Muscle/Myocutaneous Free/Pedicled Flap

Geoffrey L. Robb

Abstract

For over a century, the latissimus dorsi myocutaneous flap has been used in reconstructive surgery. It became popular for breast reconstruction in the mid-1970s, but its popularity waned with the development of the transverse rectus abdominis myocutaneous flap in the early 1980s. The latissimus dorsi myocutaneous and muscle flaps, however, are still popular not only for pedicled flap reconstruction of breast and thoracic defects but also for a variety of microsurgical reconstructive applications in virtually every location of the body. This is due to its large flat shape, ease of flap harvest, and relatively long pedicle with large diameter vessels for microsurgical anastomoses. This chapter covers every salient angle in using the latissimus dorsi muscle as a myocutaneous free or pedicled flap, beginning with indications suggesting its use, to the relevant anatomy, to the preoperative considerations, to surgical techniques. Five variations involving the flap are also cited.

Keywords: intercostal artery, lumbar artery, thoracodorsal nerve, Poland's syndrome

14.1 Introduction

The latissimus dorsi myocutaneous flap was first introduced as a pedicled flap for coverage of mastectomy wounds by Tansini in 1906. This reconstructive approach was a common practice in Europe at the time for radical mastectomy defects, but was eschewed in the United States for many years. Little is known of the further reconstruction history of the latissimus flap until reintroduced by Olivari in 1976. Multiple reports of the flap's application to breast reconstruction then surfaced in the late 1970s, including its use as a free tissue transfer in the United States by Maxwell in 1979.[1] Notably, the popularity of the latissimus dorsi myocutaneous flap waned with the new development of the transverse rectus abdominis myocutaneous (TRAM) flap by Hartramf in 1982.

The latissimus dorsi myocutaneous and muscle flaps still enjoy extensive popularity not only for pedicled flap reconstruction of breast and thoracic defects but also for a variety of microsurgical reconstructive applications in virtually every location of the body because of its large flat shape, ease of flap harvest, and relatively long pedicle with large diameter vessels for microsurgical anastomoses.

14.2 Typical Indications

14.2.1 Pedicled

- Immediate breast reconstruction with or without breast implant, especially in cases with extended skin loss.
- Breast reconstruction in breast conservation (lumpectomy) for larger defects.
- Breast reconstruction with or without breast implant after postmastectomy radiation therapy.

- Breast reconstruction salvage after partial autologous flap loss.
- Delayed repair of mastectomy or lumpectomy defects.
- Contouring a chest wall defect in Poland's syndrome.
- Upper extremity shoulder and arm defects.
- Chest wall and thoracic cavity defects.
- Caudal head and neck defects.

14.2.2 Free Flap

- Head and neck reconstruction, especially for large scalp.
- Extremity coverage for larger surface area or larger dead space defect such as over prosthetic joint, distal third of the lower extremity, or large foot defect.[2]
- Functional transfer upper/lower extremity reconstruction.

14.3 Anatomy

The latissimus dorsi muscle is a large, flat, triangular-shaped superficial muscle in the posterior thorax with a wide origin from the spine and posterior ilium and insertion into the intertubercular grove of the humerus via a flat thickened tendon. The muscle has a large anterior and posterior arc of rotation, with large skin perforator territories often useful for reconstructive applications as a pedicled flap (▶ Fig. 14.1).

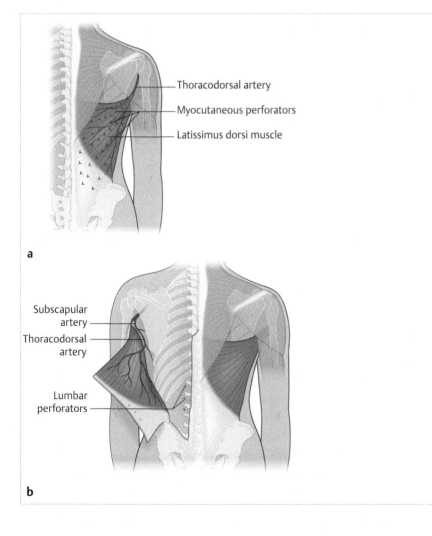

Thoracodorsal artery

Myocutaneous perforators

Latissimus dorsi muscle

a

Subscapular artery

Thoracodorsal artery

Lumbar perforators

b

Fig. 14.1 **(a)** Myocutaneous perforators paralleling the muscle fibers from the thoracodorsal pedicle branches. **(b)** Anatomy of the latissimus dorsi muscle origin and inserting muscle fiber direction with primary blood supply from the thoracodorsal artery and location of lumbar perforators.

The muscle originates from the spine of the lower six thoracic vertebrae through the posterior thoracolumbar fascia, from the spine of the lumbar and sacral vertebrae and the posterior crest of the ilium. There are also small muscle slips from the lower four ribs as well as a slip of muscle from the external oblique muscle of the abdomen. The upper and anterolateral muscle borders are primarily free. The muscle fibers spiral into a tendon that forms the posterior fold of the axilla and inserts into the humeral groove. The major pedicle to the muscle is the **thoracodorsal artery**, which is a terminal branch of the **subscapular artery**. The vessel enters the muscle on the deep surface approximately 10 cm from the origin, essentially where the muscle forms the posterior axillary fold. The thoracodorsal artery follows the border of the subscapularis muscle and sends a branch medially to the serratus anterior muscle, then further divides into several branches that enter the latissimus muscle directly. Segmental minor pedicles, perforating branches from the **intercostal and lumbar arteries**, enter posteriorly and form the vascular basis of a transverse as well as medially based latissimus muscle or myocutaneous flap.

The nerve supply is from the **thoracodorsal nerve**, a branch of the posterior cord of the brachial plexus, which runs along the subscapular and thoracodorsal artery to penetrate the muscle, as the main pedicle is about 10 cm from the insertion. The nerve is frequently divided in breast reconstruction to avoid muscle animation; otherwise the nerve is preserved for functional transfer or for preservation of muscle mass. The flap is usually not harvested as a sensate flap.

14.4 Variations

- Cutaneous thoracodorsal artery perforator flap based on lateral muscle perforators of the thoracodorsal pedicle.[3]
- Split myocutaneous or muscle flap on either the transverse or lateral thoracodorsal branch.
- Chimeric flap with serratus muscle with or without rib segment(s) and/ or scapular cutaneous or osteocutaneous flap with lateral, tip, or medial scapular bone.
- Myocutaneous or muscle flap as posterior transposition or turnover flap based on medial lumbar perforators arising from the posterior intercostal arteries.
- Extended myocutaneous flap with inclusion of regional fat.

14.5 Perioperative Considerations

For patients with small- to medium-sized breasts, the extended latissimus dorsi myocutaneous flap can include as much of the surrounding subcutaneous and submuscular fat as well as overlying skin as practical to provide a larger volume of tissue for breast reconstruction, especially if also missing external breast skin and patients wishing to avoid using an implant.

As a free flap, the muscle flap is commonly used with skin graft coverage for large surface area defects of the extremities that may also require bulk or dead space fill, such as the thigh, the distal lower one-third of the extremity or the foot. The myocutaneous flap can also be very useful for torso as well as head and neck reconstruction. The ideal application for the muscle flap in the head and neck is the large scalp defect coverage covered with a skin graft.

Typically, little to no functional disability is seen from sacrifice of the latissimus dorsi muscle.

14.6 Positioning and Skin Markings

The decubitus position is ideal for positioning and skin markings, although the patient could alternatively be marked preoperatively in the standing position denoting the orientation of the latissimus skin island particularly for breast and arm reconstruction. (▶ Fig. 14.2) The marking of the correct orientation and size of the skin island over the latissimus muscle is important for breast, chest wall, and arm transfer. Moreover, adequate marking of the axillary tunnel transfer size is also important to avoid flap compression as well as limitation of rotation of the muscle flap into a desired defect. The borders of the latissimus muscle are commonly drawn anteriorly along the posterior axillary line, superomedially in relation to the scapular tip, and medially along the perispinal origins of the muscle. Due to the posterior torso's robust thoracodorsal fascia vascular profusion in general, the skin island can be usually placed anywhere on the muscle distribution but should be located appropriately for the desired rotation position for the breast, torso, or arm defect. The width of the skin island is often limited to 8 to 10 cm and the length to 20 cm, so the rotation of the skin island can be tested initially in the decubitus position with a laparotomy sponge held securely in the upper posterior axilla and then using the sponge to simulate the rotated muscle so the orientation and positioning of the skin island markings can then be drawn on the back with the desired angle of rotation and inset in the torso or breast area as needed.

The course of the thoracodorsal neurovascular pedicle will travel centrally within the marked outline of the muscle from the axilla branching into the lateral and transverse branches. If the muscle alone is being harvested, a centrally or laterally located incision of 8 to 10 cm in length can suffice for adequate exposure in muscle elevation. A myocutaneous flap is commonly elevated through the marked skin paddle margin incisions. Endoscopic, or robotically assisted, muscle harvest can be done through an axillary incision or small incisions in the chest.

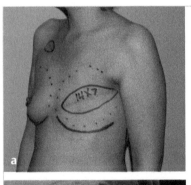
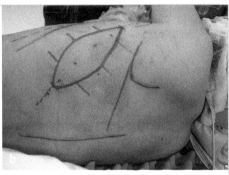
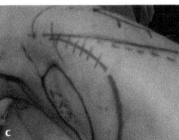

Fig. 14.2 (a) Oblique view preoperatively. **(b)** Decubitus position marking for muscle flap boundaries and skin island, axillary tunnel location. **(c)** Dissection boundary marking the back and the breast with axillary tunnel.

14.7 Operative Technique

Refer to ▶Video 14.1 for an example of the operative technique for the latissimus dorsi muscle flap. After the necessary skin incision for muscle exposure or localization of the skin island, the superficial dissection is beveled slightly to avoid undercutting the skin flap edges and to capture more local perforators. Once Scarpa's fascia is opened, the muscle fascia is easily identified as a satisfactory plane for dissection over the muscle. Typically, all the muscle boundaries are initially defined and identified in the subcutaneous dissection process (▶Fig. 14.3). The undersurface of the muscle can then be dissected from virtually any angle but perhaps the easiest dissection is from the anterior border of the muscle, initially separating the latissimus muscle from the underlying serratus muscle, which immediately establishes the correct plane of dissection.[4]

The dissection progresses inferomedially separating the fibers of origin from the posterior ilium and from the paravertebral fascial layers. The muscle is then elevated superiorly toward the axilla over the serratus anterior muscle. The serratus vascular branch is easily visualized on the superficial surface of the serratus muscle and can be traced superiorly directly to the thoracodorsal pedicle. As the elevation of the flap continues superomedially, the muscle border is freed from the trapezius and teres muscles and the thoracodorsal pedicle can be identified on the undersurface of the latissimus muscle, followed proximally toward the axilla. At this juncture, dissection should meticulously expose and release the thoracodorsal pedicle from the surrounding soft tissues on the chest

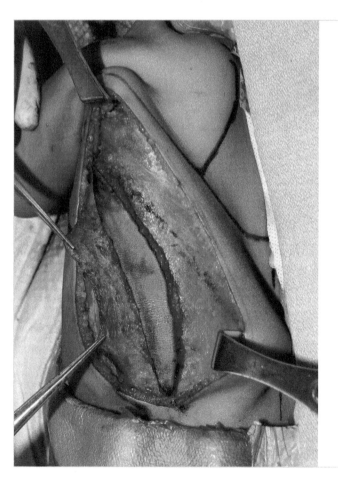

Fig. 14.3 Exposure of the latissimus dorsi muscle after making incisions around the planned skin paddle.

wall. If the transfer of the muscle, anteriorly, is impeded by restricted rotation of the thoracodorsal pedicle, the serratus branch can be divided for greater length of the pedicle arc.

Typically, the insertion of the muscle into the humerus is not disturbed, but the muscle tendon can be partially or completely transected as necessary for rotation and transfer of the flap.[5] In the radiated chest wall and axilla, a slower, more deliberate dissection technique is necessary to avoid damaging the pedicle vessels that may have become more fibrotic and scarred down, following radiation therapy.

For harvesting the muscle or myocutaneous flap for free tissue transfer, the thoracodorsal pedicle can be dissected more proximally to the subscapular vessels for increased length and caliber, facilitating vessel anastomoses (▶ Fig. 14.4). This requires ligation of the serratus anterior branch of the thoracodorsal artery, angular (scapular tip) branch of the thoracodorsal artery, and circumflex scapular artery. By doing so, a pedicle of 8 to 10 cm can be harvested with the flap.

The latissimus dorsi muscle or myocutaneous flap can be split longitudinally, basing the flap on either the descending (lateral) or transverse (medial) branch of the thoracodorsal artery (▶ Fig. 14.5). The branch point usually occurs

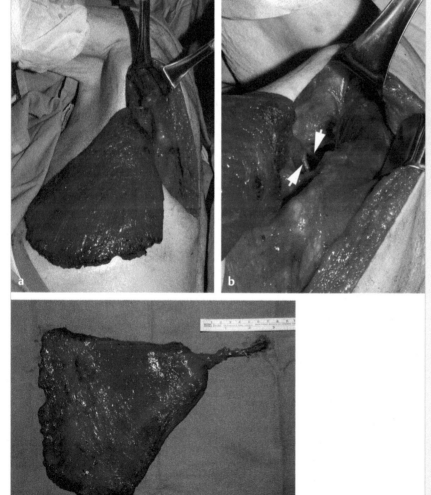

Fig. 14.4 (a) Completed dissection of a latissimus dorsi muscle free flap. (b) Close up of the axillary area showing the pedicle dissected to include the subscapular artery and vein (arrows). (c) Completed flap harvest demonstrating flap pedicle length.

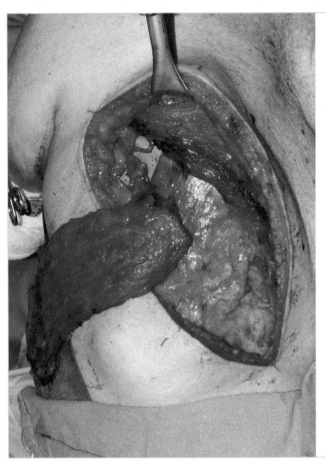

Fig. 14.5 The latissimus dorsi muscle flap has been split to include the descending branch of the thoracodorsal artery. The thoracodorsal nerve still innervates the medial muscle, which now gets its blood supply solely from the lumbar perforators.

1 to 2 cm before entering the muscle. The blood vessel supplying portion of the muscle that will be used for flap reconstruction is preserved while the other branch is ligated. The remaining muscle is supplied by the lumbar perforators. Conversely, the branch of the thoracodorsal nerve, which also branches 1 to 2 cm before entering the muscle, that supplies the portion of the muscle used for flap reconstruction is divided while the other branch is preserved.

14.8 Donor Site Closure

The undermining of the back skin necessary to harvest the muscle or myocutaneous flap allows relative tension-free closure unless a wider skin island beyond 10 to 12 cm is used or the length of the flap is in excess of 20 cm. Rarely will skin grafting of the donor site be necessary. Performing quilting of the back skin to the posterior chest wall and use of closed suction drainage catheters are felt to help minimize the incidence of postoperative back sarcoma. A multilayer closure of the donor site skin margins is important for reliable healing, considering the necessity of progressive early postoperative arm and shoulder movement.

14.9 Pearls and Pitfalls

- Special attention should be paid to the proper plane of muscle flap elevation just inferior to the scapular tip, which should be over the serratus anterior muscle to avoid including the deeper back musculature in the flap harvest.

- Recognition of good latissimus contraction preoperatively is important, since latissimus muscle atrophy can occur in breast cancer patients postmastectomy, possibly reflecting compromise of the vascular pedicle of the latissimus muscle.
- Subcutaneous and intermuscular fat can be added to the margins of the harvested muscle to increase overall flap volume in the extended flap.[4]
- Use of the latissimus dorsi myocutaneous flap based on retrograde flow from the serratus anterior branch has been described in cases where the proximal pedicle has been transected during an axillary dissection or other prior surgery.

References

[1] Maxwell GP, Stueber K, Hoopes JE. A free latissimus dorsi myocutaneous flap: case report. Plast Reconstr Surg 1978;62(3):462–466

[2] Watson JS, Craig RD, Orton CI. The free latissimus dorsi myocutaneous flap. Plast Reconstr Surg 1979;64(3):299–305

[3] Angrigiani C, Grilli D, Siebert J. Latissimus dorsi musculocutaneous flap without muscle. Plast Reconstr Surg 1995;96(7):1608–1614

[4] Maves MD, Panje WR, Shagets FW. Extended latissimus dorsi myocutaneous flap reconstruction of major head and neck defects. Otolaryngol Head Neck Surg 1984;92(5):551–558

[5] Bostwick J III, Nahai F, Wallace JG, Vasconez LO. Sixty latissimus dorsi flaps. Plast Reconstr Surg 1979;63(1):31–41

15 Thoracodorsal Artery Perforator Flap

David S. Cabiling and Roman J. Skoracki

Abstract

The thoracodorsal artery perforator flap is a variant of the workhorse latissimus dorsi myocutaneous flap, which is harvested as an adipocutaneous flap sparing the underlying Latissimus dorsi muscle. It is supplied by thoracodorsal artery perforators that course through the latissimus dorsi muscle. The flap is useful in the reconstruction of axillary, shoulder, chest wall, and breast defects. As a free flap, it can provide a relatively thin and pliable cutaneous flap useful for the reconstruction of shallow defects as well as extremity and head and neck resurfacing. Its donor site can be concealed in the midaxillary line and make it an attractive alternative to the anterolateral thigh and lateral arm flaps. Every critical consideration in the utilization of the thoracodorsal artery perforator flap is covered in this chapter, from indications for its use, to anatomy, to preoperative considerations, to the operative technique. Two paragraphs in the chapter are devoted to a mention of the variations to the standard flap procedure.

Keywords: descending/vertical branch, transverse/horizontal branch, posterior rami of the lateral cutaneous branches of the intercostal nerves

15.1 Introduction

The thoracodorsal artery perforator (TDAP) flap is a variant of the workhorse latissimus dorsi (LD) myocutaneous flap, which is harvested as an adipocutaneous flap sparing the underlying LD muscle. It is supplied by TDAPs that course through the LD muscle. The TDAP flap was first described by Angrigiani et al in 1995.[1] As a pedicled flap, it is useful in the reconstruction of axillary, shoulder, chest wall, and breast defects. As a free flap, it can provide a relatively thin and pliable cutaneous flap useful for the reconstruction of shallow defects as well as extremity and head and neck resurfacing. Its donor site can be concealed in the midaxillary line and make it an attractive alternative to the anterolateral thigh and lateral arm flaps.

15.2 Typical Indications

- Axillary, chest wall, and shoulder defects.
- Extremity defects when a thin pliable reconstruction is desired.
- Correction of breast defects such as post lumpectomy asymmetry, breast skin envelope deficits, or congenital breast deformities.

15.3 Anatomy

The thoracodorsal vascular pedicle originates at the subscapular branch of the axillary vessels. It courses toward the LD muscle and enters its deep surface about 2 to 3 cm medial to its edge and approximately 4 cm inferior to the tip of the scapula (or 8–10 cm inferior to the posterior axillary fold). Here, the thoracodorsal pedicle splits into two main branches: the **descending (or vertical) and transverse (or horizontal) branches** (▶Fig. 15.1a). The TDAP flap can be designed around either branch, although the descending branch is more

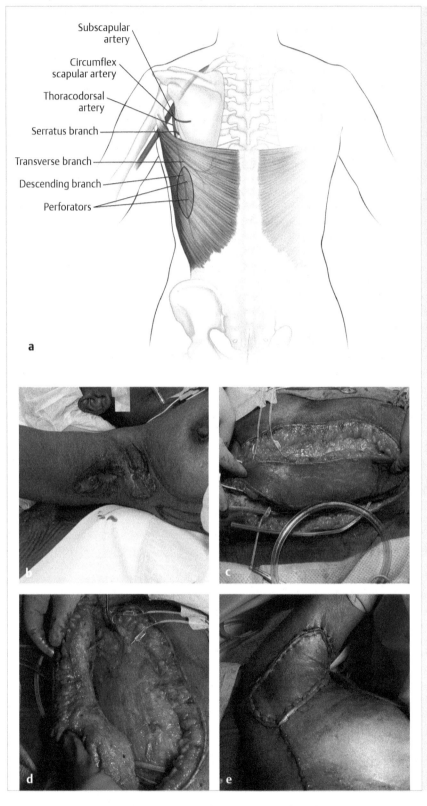

Fig. 15.1 (a) Vascular anatomy of the thoracodorsal artery. (b–e) Patient with long-standing axillary hidradenitis reconstructed with a pedicled single perforator TDAP flap. The flap was designed over the descending branch of the thoracodorsal pedicle. The undersurface of the flap demonstrates the perforator dissection through the latissimus dorsi muscle fibers. In this case, dissection beyond the thoracodorsal pedicle bifurcation was unnecessary to cover the defect. (Adapted from Zenn MR, Glyn J. Reconstructive Surgery: Anatomy, Technique, and Clinical Applications. New York: Thieme Medical Publishers; 2012.)

commonly utilized because it supplies a larger number of perforators. The descending branch of the thoracodorsal pedicle courses about 2 cm medial to the lateral border of the LD muscle. Along this course, the first perforator is typically about 6 cm inferior to the tip of the scapula. Additional perforators may be found in 2 to 4 cm intervals inferior to this first perforator. The descending branch artery has a diameter of 0.8 to 1.5 mm. The transverse branch runs about 3 cm inferior to the superior border of the LD muscle and has a similar caliber. Both branches reliably supply one to three perforators to the overlying skin. The perforators have a variable intramuscular course of about 3 to 5 cm before reaching their source vessels (▶ **Fig. 15.1b-e**). Of note, more distal perforators occasionally originate from intercostal vessels rather than the thoracodorsal pedicle. Additionally, in 55 to 75% of patients a direct cutaneous branch arises from the thoracodorsal pedicle and wraps around the anterior border of the LD muscle.[2]

Sensation to the TDAP skin paddle is provided by **the posterior rami of the lateral cutaneous branches of intercostal nerves**. These originate more anteriorly between serratus anterior and external oblique muscles. The motor supply to the LD muscle is the thoracodorsal nerve, which runs in close proximity to the vascular pedicle and should be preserved.

15.4 Variations

Both transversely and vertically oriented flaps can be designed depending on patient and surgeon preference as well as indication. Transversely oriented flaps are best suited in breast reconstruction where the skin pattern is oriented in a similar fashion to an LD flap for breast reconstruction. Additionally, a pedicled bilobed flap can be designed with a larger vertical limb and a smaller secondary horizontal limb, which can facilitate the closure of the vertical limb donor site after a 90-degree rotation of the flap.

Being based on the thoracodorsal pedicle, the TDAP can also be incorporated into any of the many tissue components based on this pedicle including LD muscle, serratus anterior muscle, thoracodorsal fascia, and scapular bone and rib.

15.5 Preoperative Considerations

In obese patients, the adipose component of the flap can be substantial. It is possible to delaminate the deeper layer of fat to thin the flap, but consideration should be given to other flaps if a thin reconstruction is required. In females, closure of a large flap can lead to lateral distortion of the breast.

15.6 Positioning and Skin Markings

The TDAP flap is typically harvested in the lateral decubitus position in a similar fashion to an LD flap. The ipsilateral arm can be secured to the operating table with a lateral position arm board or prepped into the field and left free on a padded Mayo stand. A position change may be necessary for free TDAP flaps intended for recipient sites not easily accessed in the lateral position, but this is usually unnecessary for regional defects. Pedicled flaps are best inset and positioned for breast indications after the donor site is closed and the patient has been repositioned supine.

The anterior border of the LD muscle as well as the tip of the scapula are palpated and marked. The flap is designed as an ellipse over the descending branch of the thoracodorsal pedicle. The anterior edge of the flap should be marked more anterior to the anterior border of the latissimus muscle to ensure

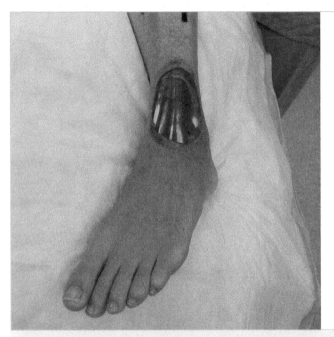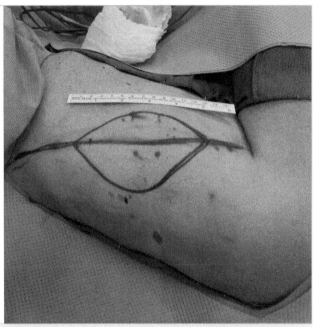

Fig. 15.2 Patient with a radiated sarcoma defect of the distal leg reconstructed with a free TDAP flap. The markings demonstrate the anterior border of the latissimus dorsi muscle as well as the dominant perforators identified on the Doppler examination. In addition, the anterior border of the flap extends anteriorly to the anterior border of the latissimus dorsi muscle.

perforator capture (▶Fig. 15.2). A skin pinch test will assist in determining the maximum width of flap that can be primarily closed.

Surface Doppler examination can be helpful to identify the location of the TDAP perforators but one must be aware that this is not as reliable in perforator location identification as it is in other perforator flaps (e.g., DIEP or ALT flaps). This is because the TDAP perforators can run a variable distance on top of the LD fascia before entering the skin and due to the presence of intercostal perforators.[3]

One of the advantages of the TDAP flap is that the perforator does not need to be centered on the skin paddle and can be distal or proximal in the flap. The maximal size of skin paddle supplied by a single perforator has not been determined but flaps as large as 14 × 25 cm have been described. The desire for a primary closure of the donor site may be a limiting factor for flap width.

15.7 Operative Technique

Typically, the anterior incision is made first and the dissection begins posteriorly in the loose areolar plane between the LD muscle fascia and the subcutaneous fat. This allows for identification and selection of the perforator(s). A single perforator will reliably supply most flaps. Care should be taken to look for direct cutaneous perforators wrapping around the anterior border of the LD muscle as these are present in more than half of the patients. Perforator selection will depend on the size of the flap, the size of perforator(s), and the pedicle length required. More distal perforators require longer intramuscular dissection but provide longer pedicle length.

Once a suitable perforator has been identified, the flap can be completely islandized and the perforator(s) can be dissected through its intramuscular course, carefully ligating any muscular branches. The descending branch is then dissected free from the posterior surface of the LD muscle, carefully sparing the motor nerve branches. One can stop the dissection at the thoracodorsal vessel bifurcation if a short pedicle is suitable and the pedicle vessel caliber is adequate, thereby preserving the thoracodorsal vessels and the remaining branch to the LD muscle. If a longer pedicle is needed or a larger caliber vessel is desired for microsurgery, the dissection can be carried further to the origin of the thoracodorsal vessels at the subscapular system (▶ Fig. 15.3).

The flap can then be divided and transferred as a free flap or tunneled to reach local defects as a pedicled flap. Transferring the flap through the spit latissimus fibers rather than around the edge of the muscle helps to increase the reach of the pedicled TDAP.

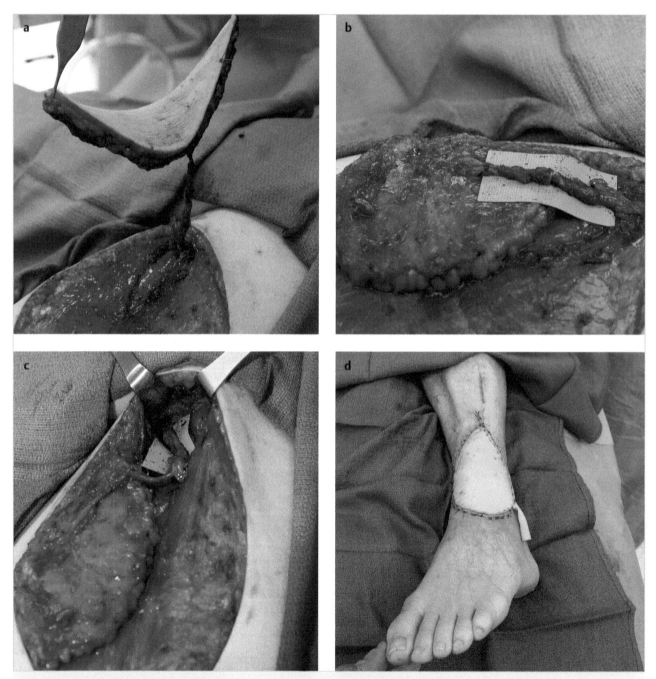

Fig. 15.3 (a-d) Elevated free TDAP flap. Here the transverse branch was ligated and the flap was harvested on the thoracodorsal vessels. Flap inset to the distal leg demonstrating good contour.

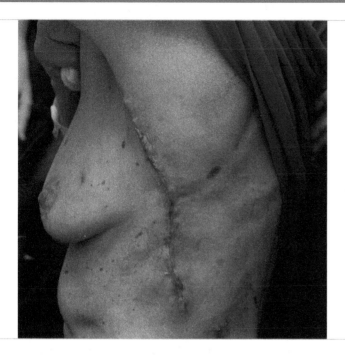

Fig. 15.4 Donor site following free TDAP flap 2 weeks postoperatively. Drains have been removed as seroma formation is less with complete latissimus dorsi (LD) muscle sparing in comparison to traditional LD flaps.

15.8 Donor Site Closure

Primary donor site closure can be ensured by skin pinch testing the donor site while designing the flap. Wide undermining and progressive tension sutures assist in cases when the closure is under tension. Closed suction drains are utilized and standard layered skin closure is performed. As no muscle is taken with the flap, arm motion is unrestricted postoperatively (▶ **Fig. 15.4**).

15.9 Pearls and Pitfalls

- Surface Doppler identification of TDAP perforators can be useful but should be taken with an ounce of caution as the perforators may travel several centimeters on the muscle fascia before entering the skin. Additionally, it is possible to have a false positive surface Doppler signal in thin patients as the descending branch itself can easily be audible.
- The perforators can be located proximally or distally. Proximal perforators require the shortest and quickest dissection. Distal perforators allow for longer pedicle length but require a longer dissection and may be supplied by intercostal vessels.
- The majority of patient will have a direct cutaneous branch.
- The donor scar from transversely oriented flaps can be hidden in a bra or bathing suit and may be preferable in female patients.

References

[1] Angrigiani C, Grilli D, Siebert J. Latissimus dorsi musculocutaneous flap without muscle. Plast Reconstr Surg 1995;96(7):1608–1614

[2] Heitmann C, Guerra A, Metzinger SW, Levin LS, Allen RJ. The thoracodorsal artery perforator flap: anatomic basis and clinical application. Ann Plast Surg 2003;51(1):23–29

[3] Kim JT. Latissimus dorsi perforator flap. Clin Plast Surg 2003;30(3):403–431

16 Serratus Anterior Muscle/Muscle with Rib Flap

Noopur Gangopadhyay and Roman J. Skoracki

Abstract

The serratus anterior muscle pedicled flap has use in many plastic surgery applications. Because of its robust vascular supply, it is a useful flap for a wide variety of composite defects. The muscle or fascia can be harvested by themselves, but it can also be designed with a skin paddle, with rib, or with the tip of the scapula. The steps involved in the operation are logically laid out, beginning with typical indications, to anatomy, to preoperative considerations, to surgical technique. Four variations involving the flap are also covered.

Keywords: lateral thoracic artery, serratus branches of the thoracodorsal artery, long thoracic nerve, segmental intercostal nerves

16.1 Introduction

The serratus anterior muscle pedicled flap has been in use for over 100 years for plastic surgery applications. Microsurgical applications of this muscle flap were first described by Takayanagi and Tsukie in 1982, and were further popularized by Buncke in the mid-to-late 1980s.[1] Because of its robust vascular supply, vascular pedicle that is exposed before the flap is elevated, and variability from the subscapular system, it is a useful flap for a wide variety of composite defects. The muscle or fascia can be harvested by themselves, but it can also be designed with a skin paddle, with rib, or with the tip of the scapula.[2,3] Chimeric flaps incorporating the latissimus dorsi muscle and even the scapular or parascapular skin islands have also been described.

16.2 Typical Indications

- Intrathoracic defects after tumor resection, tracheoesophageal fistula repair, or for bronchopleural fistula coverage.[4]
- Breast reconstruction for partial defects and chest wall defects.
- Axillary defects.
- Oromandibular, maxillary, and orbital floor defects, as an alternative to free fibula reconstruction.[3]
- Lower extremity and upper extremity wounds requiring thin pliable coverage for small to medium defects.
- Free functional muscle transfer, as in facial reanimation.

16.3 Anatomy

The serratus anterior muscle is a thin, broad muscle on the lateral chest wall that originates from the first eight or nine ribs and inserts on the scapula (▶ Fig. 16.1a). The area that is harvested for flap reconstruction is between the anterior border of the latissimus dorsi muscle and the lateral border of

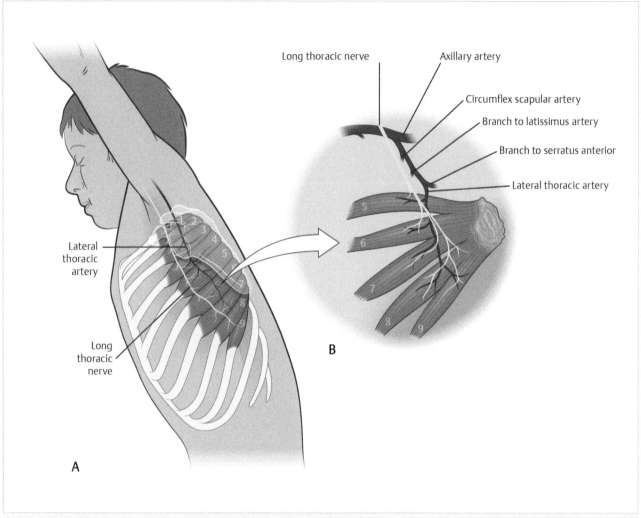

Fig. 16.1 (a) Relevant anatomy. (b) Vascular anatomy of the flap.

the pectoralis major muscle (▶ **Fig. 16.1b**).[1,2] Each leaflet of the serratus anterior arises from a separate rib (first nine ribs), running obliquely posteriorly to blend into a wider muscle belly. The insertion is the medial border of the scapula. Functionally, the serratus anterior stabilizes the scapula against the chest during elevation and abduction of the arm.

This is a Mathes and Nahai type III muscle. The two dominant pedicles are the **lateral thoracic artery** for the superior portion of the muscle and the **serratus branches of the thoracodorsal artery** for the inferior portion of the muscle (▶ **Fig. 16.2**). The lateral thoracic artery comes directly from the axillary artery, and runs along the anterolateral surface of the muscle. The thoracodorsal artery arises from the subscapular trunk, and gives rise to a single serratus branch that divides into two to five smaller branches, supplying the five lower slips of the muscle, before entering the latissimus dorsi muscle.[5] The thoracodorsal pedicle branches are posterior on the thorax in relation to the lateral thoracic pedicle. Each artery is accompanied by a single vein. The motor innervation is the **long thoracic nerve**, from the C5 to C7 nerve roots. Sensory supply to the overlying skin is from the **T2 to T4 segmental intercostal nerves**.

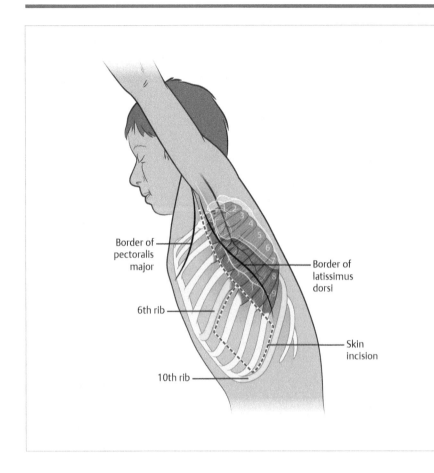

Fig. 16.2 Incision markings.

16.4 Variations

- Serratus anterior fascia-only flap based on the serratus anterior branches with preservation of the long thoracic nerve.
- Myocutaneous flap in rare instances.
- Myo-osseous flap including the fifth or sixth rib or the inferolateral border of the scapula (based on the angular branch).
- Composite serratus anterior–latissimus dorsi muscle flap (chimeric flap) based on the thoracodorsal vessels with preservation of the serratus anterior branches.

16.5 Preoperative Considerations

A skin paddle is challenging to design with this flap. In obese patients and in women due to the lateral breast, the skin paddle may be bulky or the harvest may distort the breast shape. If a skin paddle is needed, consideration should be given to other flaps first. This flap is an elegant solution for small defects requiring thin pliable coverage, as fascia-only or muscle-only flaps can be harvested. The serratus anterior flap with rib or with scapular tip can be an alternative to free fibula flap reconstruction of head and neck defects, and is useful in patients who have extensive peripheral vascular disease that may preclude harvest from an extremity.[2,3,4]

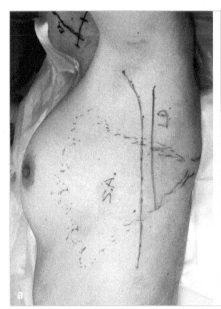
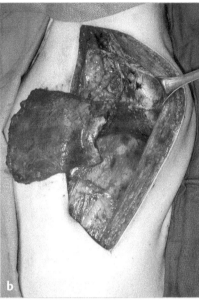

Fig. 16.3 Skin markings for **(a)** serratus anterior flap and **(b)** flap elevation. (Image courtesy of Matthew M. Hanasono.)

16.6 Positioning and Skin Markings

This flap is harvested best in the lateral decubitus position, either complete or in a "sloppy lateral" approach.[1] The patient should be placed on a beanbag with an axillary roll placed in the axilla that is facing downward. The entire upper extremity on the side of flap harvest should be prepped into the field to allow for intraoperative position changes during flap elevation. If the patient is supine and the arm is abducted at the shoulder, only the anterior portion of this flap can be elevated.

The serratus anterior muscle is usually not harvested with a skin paddle. If a skin paddle is desired, hand-held Doppler is useful to mark perforating blood vessels in the region of interest.[5] More often than not, these vessels will arise from intercostal branches that do not communicate with the serratus branch. An oblique lateral chest wall incision or a vertical incision in the lateral chest wall can be made for harvest (▶ **Fig. 16.3**). If the patient is muscular, with little body fat, sometimes slips of the serratus muscle can be seen on the lateral chest wall. This is hidden in women by the lateral breast.

Landmarks for the surrounding musculature can be more easily identified preoperatively. The latissimus dorsi muscle can be forcefully contracted, such that the anterior border is visible or palpable in the posterior axillary line. Similarly, the pectoralis major muscle can be forcefully contracted, such that the lateral border is visible or palpable in the anterior axillary line.[1] Part of the serratus anterior muscle, its blood supply, and its potential skin island will lie in this space. The tip of the scapula should also be marked, as this denotes the posterior border of the muscle.

16.7 Operative Technique

A vertical or oblique skin incision is made in the lateral chest wall between the borders of the latissimus dorsi and pectoralis major muscles. Dissection is deepened through the subcutaneous tissues until the thin fascia overlying the serratus anterior muscle is exposed. It is useful to expose the latissimus dorsi muscle and elevate the latissimus partially to identify the superficial surface of the serratus anterior. One should be careful during this dissection, as the long thoracic nerve, lateral thoracic artery, and thoracodorsal pedicle lie on the superficial surface of the muscle.[5] The upper slips of the serratus anterior muscle are best harvested on the lateral thoracic artery while the lower slips are best harvested on the thoracodorsal pedicle.

The lower three to five slips of muscle are typically harvested with the flap, based on the thoracodorsal pedicle. These can be harvested as a pedicled flap for regional applications, or as a free flap for distant microvascular applications. Once the pedicle is identified, the deep surface of each muscle leaflet is dissected free from their corresponding rib origin in an anterior to posterior approach, unless rib is to be included in which case the muscle attachment is carefully preserved as it is the blood supply to the underlying bone.[2] Dissection continues posteriorly toward to the scapula, where the muscle can be divided and the rest of the flap is elevated from caudad to cephalad. Care should be taken to preserve the long thoracic nerve above the slips to be harvested, which joins the thoracodorsal pedicle at the level of the fifth or sixth rib. After the nerve is identified, it can be separated from the vessels circumferentially. The nerve is divided at the superior most edge of the flap that is harvested, maintaining the innervation to the slips above the flap intact. To avoid scapula winging, at least three to four slips including their innervation should be preserved.

The flap can be used as a pedicled flap or as a free flap. As a pedicled flap, it can reach the chest wall, shoulder, axilla, and central back. It is also useful for intrathoracic defects.[4] One to two ribs are often removed completely or partially to allow an appropriate window for pedicled serratus muscle flaps to reach intrathoracic defects and avoid compression of the pedicle.[4] When using the serratus muscle flap intrathoracically, it is important to take into consideration the anatomic relationship of the rib cage, the vascular pedicle, and the lung in its inflated state, as the inset will likely be performed with the lung collapsed on the affected side. Reinflation of the lung may cause vascular compression or stretch if this is not taken into consideration during the surgery.

A flap of 20 × 15 cm (more commonly a flap the size of the palm of the patient's hand) can be harvested as a free flap, with a maximal pedicle length of 6 to 8 cm, unless the thoracodorsal and subscapular vessels are included, in which case a much greater (15 cm) pedicle length can be achieved.

If thin pliable coverage is desired, as in dorsal hand or dorsal foot coverage, the serratus fascia can be harvested as a free flap. The standard approach is the same for elevation of the serratus muscle. The lateral edge of the latissimus dorsi is identified and elevated to expose the deeper serratus anterior fascia and muscle. Both the main thoracodorsal artery and the serratus branches must be identified and protected within the boundaries of the proposed flap. The fascia and vessel are then dissected off the underlying serratus anterior muscle, from distal to proximal. The thoracodorsal branch to the latissimus muscle will be ligated during the dissection and the long thoracic nerve should be preserved.

For composite defects, harvesting rib or scapula with the flap is useful (▶ **Fig. 16.4**). The superficial dissection is similar to serratus anterior muscle-only elevation.[2] The fifth or sixth rib is usually included in a myo-osseous serratus flap.[2] The muscle slip is left attached to the fifth or sixth rib, such that the selected rib is on the deep surface of the flap. Care should be taken to avoid injury to the parietal pleura. A single rib defect in the chest wall will not lead to any significant donor site morbidity.[2] Of note, the portion of the rib that lies posterior to the serratus insertion will not be covered by the flap when it is transferred to the recipient bed.[3] This may be important, depending on

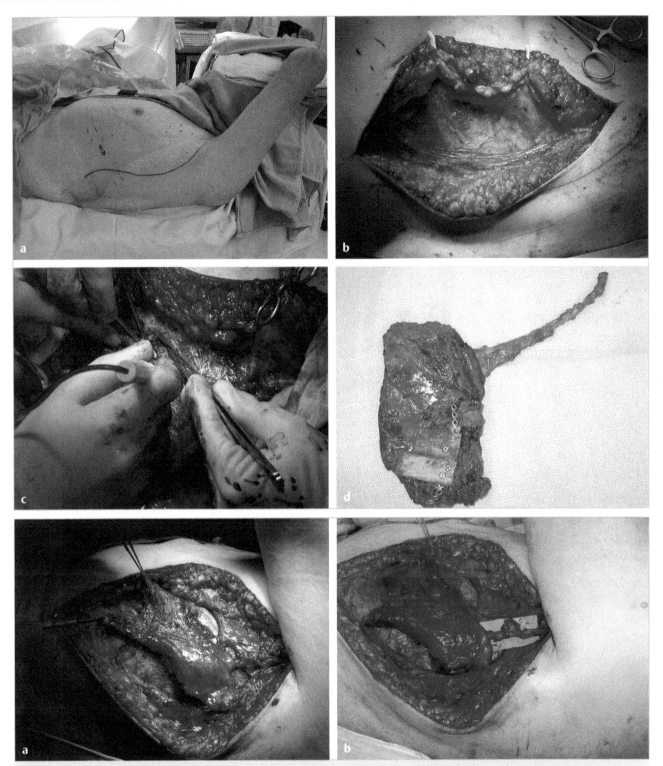

Fig. 16.4 (a–d) Harvest of serratus–rib myo-osseous flap. The standard skin markings are the same. The rib was harvested with the serratus anterior muscle as a composite flap and plated prior to reconstruction of a maxillary defect. **(e,f)** It is useful to expose the latissimus dorsi muscle and elevate the latissimus partially to identify the superficial surface of the serratus anterior. In this case, the lower slips of serratus were harvested with a single rib, based on the thoracodorsal pedicle.

the indication for the myo-osseous flap harvest. The scapular tip can also be harvested with the serratus muscle, as the scapular tip has an independent blood supply.[3,5] The angular branch that originates from the thoracodorsal artery directly or from a serratus branch of the thoracodorsal artery is accompanied by venae comitantes, and must be captured with the flap to vascularize the bone.[3,5]

The serratus anterior muscle can be harvested with the latissimus dorsi muscle based on the thoracodorsal vessels.[5] The serratus branches are preserved during the dissection. Skin islands in the scapular or parascapular territories can be harvested by incorporating the circumflex scapular branches.

The flap can be neurotized with the addition of the long thoracic nerve, as is useful in facial reanimation.[1,5] Given its minimal bulk, it is suitable for transplantation into the paralyzed side of the face. It can be anchored to multiple points of the facial mimetic muscles due to the separate nature of each leaflet harvested. Each slip can be further spilt into superficial and deep bellies if necessary. Anastomosis of the facial nerve to the long thoracic nerve is performed using standard nerve coaptation techniques.

16.8 Donor Site Closure

As this flap is usually harvested without a skin paddle, the donor site is able to be closed primarily in the standard fashion. Even in scenarios where a small skin paddle is harvested, the donor site can be closed without tension and without need for significant undermining. Surgical drains should be placed for adequate drainage of dead space.

16.9 Pearls and Pitfalls

- The codominant pedicles—thoracodorsal and lateral thoracic—should be identified early in the dissection, as they lie on the superficial surface of the muscle.
- The long thoracic nerve to the muscle slips that are not included with the flap should be identified and protected during the dissection to prevent functional deficits, including scapular winging.
- The flap can be harvested with bone, with the best choices being the fifth or sixth ribs, or the scapular tip, which has an independent blood supply.

References

[1] Whitney TM, Buncke HJ, Alpert BS, Buncke GM, Lineaweaver WC. The serratus anterior free-muscle flap: experience with 100 consecutive cases. Plast Reconstr Surg 1990;86(3):481–490, discussion 491

[2] Chang DW, Miller MJ. A subperiosteal approach to harvesting the free serratus anterior and rib myo-osseous composite flap. Plast Reconstr Surg 2001;108(5):1300–1304

[3] Kim PD, Blackwell KE. Latissimus-serratus-rib free flap for oromandibular and maxillary reconstruction. Arch Otolaryngol Head Neck Surg 2007;133(8):791–795

[4] Meyer AJ, Krueger T, Lepori D, et al. Closure of large intrathoracic airway defects using extrathoracic muscle flaps. Ann Thorac Surg 2004;77(2):397–404, discussion 405

[5] Takeishi M, Ishida K, Makino Y. The thoracodorsal vascular tree-based combined fascial flaps. Microsurgery 2009;29(2):95–100

17 Scapular and Parascapular Flaps

Sydney Ch'ng

Abstract

Scapular and parascapular flaps are made up of various combinations of skin (scapular/parascapular), muscle (latissimus dorsi/serratus anterior), and bone (lateral segment/ scapular tip). They can be harvested to fulfill the reconstructive requirements for a variety of defects, particularly of the head and neck. This chapter covers the procedure, from start to finish, involved in the use of the scapular and parascapular flaps, starting with indications for use, anatomy, preoperative considerations, and operative technique. Three variations to the standard procedure are listed.

Keywords: circumflex scapular artery, triangular space, cutaneous scapular branch, parascapular branch, subscapular artery, axillary artery, circumflex scapular artery, thoracodorsal artery

17.1 Introduction

In 1980, dos Santos published the first anatomical study of the scapular fasciocutaneous flap in cadavers.[1] Gilbert and Teot published the first clinical series of scapular flap for resurfacing of ankle and lower leg defects in 1982.[2] In 1986, Swartz et al popularized the flap with inclusion of the lateral segment of the scapular bone in head and neck reconstruction.[3] In 1991, Coleman and Sultan demonstrated that the angular branch of the thoracodorsal artery was consistently the blood supply to the scapular tip, and its inclusion allowed two separate segments of scapular bone to be raised reliably.[4]

Various combinations of skin (scapular/parascapular), muscle (latissimus dorsi/serratus anterior), and bone (lateral segment/scapular tip) can be harvested to fulfill the reconstructive requirements of a variety of defects, particularly of the head and neck.[5]

17.2 Typical Indications

- Pedicled cutaneous flap for resurfacing of the shoulder and axilla.
- Free flap:
  - Fasciocutaneous flap for skin and soft-tissue defects.
  - Osteocutaneous flap for maxillary or mandibular reconstruction, especially when the fibular free flap is not an option.
  - Osteocutnaeous flap for composite scalp reconstruction.

17.3 Anatomy

17.3.1 Landmarks

The fasciocutaneous flap can be oriented transversely (scapular flap), or obliquely (parascapular flap), or a boomerang-shaped skin paddle can be elevated based on the parent vessels (▶**Fig. 17.1**).

The **circumflex scapular artery** (external diameter: 2.5–3.5 mm) traverses the **triangular space** before dividing into its terminal **cutaneous scapular and parascapular branches**. The triangular space, bounded by the long head of triceps laterally, the teres minor and subscapularis superiorly, and the teres major inferiorly, is situated two-fifths of the distance from the scapular spine to the

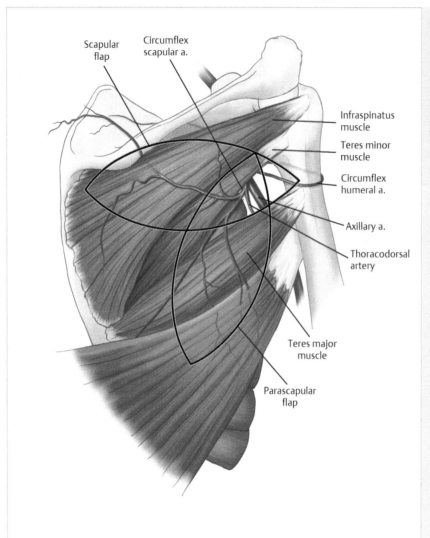

Scapular flap

Circumflex scapular a.

Infraspinatus muscle

Teres minor muscle

Circumflex humeral a.

Axillary a.

Thoracodorsal artery

Teres major muscle

Parascapular flap

Fig. 17.1 The circumflex scapular artery and vein traverse the triangular space and divide into the scapular cutaneous branch, on which the horizontal scapular flap is based, and the parascapular cutaneous branch, on which the vertical parascapular flap is based.

scapular tip along the lateral border. The axis of the scapular flap therefore extends from the triangular space to the midline, with the superior boundary being the scapular spine and the inferior boundary being the scapular tip. The axis of the parascapular flap extends from the triangular space along the lateral border of the scapula to the posterior superior iliac spine. The width of the flap is determined by ease of primary closure, usually 5 to 7 cm.

17.3.2 Vascular Anatomy

The **subscapular artery** originates from the **axillary artery**, and after an average course of 2.2 cm, divides into the **circumflex scapular artery** and **thoracodorsal artery** (▶ Fig. 17.2). The circumflex scapular artery is about 3 to 4 cm long, and passes through the triangular space. In the triangular space, it gives off the subscapular, infrascapular, and direct muscular branches to the teres major and minor muscles. Beyond the triangular space, it becomes known as the descending branch of the circumflex scapular artery, which eventually bifurcates into the terminal cutaneous scapular and parascapular branches.

The lateral border of the scapula receives vascular supply from the musculoperiosteal branches of the circumflex scapular artery at the triangular space. The scapular tip is supplied by the angular branch of the thoracodorsal artery and can be used as an alternate blood supply for the scapular bone.

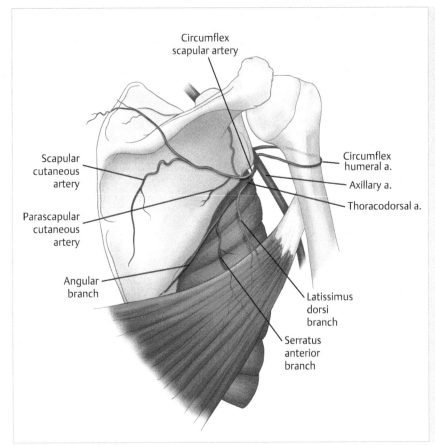

Fig. 17.2 The subscapular system supplies the scapula, scapular and parascapular skin flaps, and latissimus dorsi and serratus anterior muscles.

The thoracodorsal artery travels an average of 8.4 cm before diving into branches to serratus anterior and latissimus dorsi. The angular branch arises most commonly from the latissimus dorsi branch (51%), but can arise from the serratus anterior branch (25%), as the third branch of a trifurcation of the thoracodorsal vessel (20%), or as a branch of thoracodorsal proximal to its bifurcation (4%). It travels just deep to the superior border of latissimus dorsi, and at around the scapular tip, it divides into its terminal branches.

17.3.3 Variations

- Fasciocutaneous flap: parascapular and/or scapular skin paddle.
- Osteocutaneous flap: parascapular (usually) or scapular skin paddle and the lateral border of the scapula (based on the circumflex scapular artery) or the tip of the scapula (based on the angular artery).
- Myo-osseous flap: the lateral border and/or tip of the scapula and latissimus dorsi muscle and/or the superior four slips of serratus anterior can be included.

17.4 Preoperative Considerations

Generally, the ipsilateral scapula is used for convenience of patient positioning except in situations where one arm is involved in the use of a walking stick or cane, there has been previous axillary dissection or irradiation, or there is lymphedema of the upper limb, in which case the contralateral scapula is preferred.

Loss of shoulder abduction has been reported for up to 6 months postoperatively, after which the range of movement should return to normal.

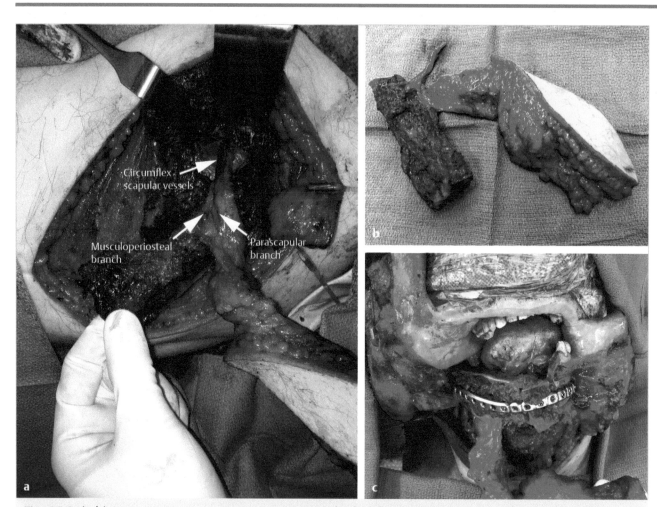

Fig. 17.3 **(a,b)** A composite osseocutaneous–parascapular free flap with the lateral border of the scapula based on the circumflex scapular vessels, and **(c)** following a single osteotomy for reconstruction of the anterior and right lateral mandible.

17.4.1 Mandible

The lateral border of the scapula is harvested with the medial scapular osteotomy placed such that the width of the bony segment matches the height of the native mandible to be reconstructed. The thicker cortical bone along the lateral edge can be placed along the inferior margin of the mandible so that the resultant tapering neoalveolus is well suited for retention of a conventional denture (but poor for osseointegrated dental implants due to inadequate bone thickness). If the lateral edge is placed superiorly, the opposite is true (▶ **Fig. 17.3**).

When bilateral mandibulectomy is performed, especially if combined with total glossectomy, the scapula bone can be oriented transversely where the angular tip is used to reconstruct the mentum, and the dorsal surface of the scapula oriented cephalad. Grooves of 1.0 to 1.5 cm deep are cut into the remaining body of the mandible to allow slotting of the scapula bony segment in a tongue-in-groove manner.[6]

17.4.2 Maxilla

The angular tip of the scapula is preferred for reconstruction of the maxilla.

For an infrastructure maxillectomy defect, the scapular tip is uniquely shaped, and can reconstruct the entire palatoalveolar complex without the need for contouring osteotomies when placed horizontally (▶ **Fig. 17.4**). The thin bone of the scapular tip where the serratus anterior muscle attaches is not ideal for osseointegration, but can accommodate a non–implant-retained denture.

For the hemimaxillectomy defect, the scapular tip is usually oriented vertically with its natural convexity facing anteriorly, and with the broader lateral edge placed inferiorly along the alveolar arch to allow osseointegration if desired. The ipsilateral scapula is used generally with the thoracodorsal vessels entering posteriorly at the tip. The oral surface of the reconstructed alveolar process is usually left to mucosalize with the periosteum or a cuff of teres major muscle, thereby providing an immobile sturdy base for denture retention. For a more extensive defect, a single osteotomy is possible for further refinement of the curvature if the angular and teres major branches of the thoracodorsal artery are maintained (▶ **Fig. 17.5**). The latissimus dorsi or teres major muscle can be harvested with the angular tip and used for soft-tissue reconstruction of the palate the way the internal oblique muscle is used in conjunction with the iliac crest.

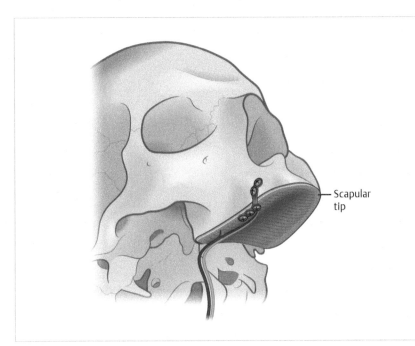

Fig. 17.4 The scapular tip can be placed transversely for reconstruction of an infrastructure palatoalveoler defect without contouring osteotomies.

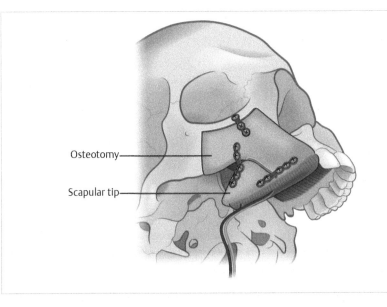

Fig. 17.5 The scapular tip can be oriented vertically for reconstruction of a hemimaxillectomy defect with an osteotomy fashioned for zygomaticonasal contouring. In this configuration, the palate is often reconstructed with the latissimus dorsi or teres major muscle.

17.4.3 Calvaria

The scapula is well suited to reconstruct the calvaria with the latissimus dorsi muscle (and skin grafting) used for scalp reconstruction. The long thoracodorsal vessels mean that vein grafting to the superficial temporal vessels is seldom required.

17.5 Positioning and Skin Marking

The patient is placed on a suction bean bag at 45 degrees to the operating table, and strapped at the pelvis. The table is rotated 45 degrees, thus making the patient horizontal during ablation, and rotated back 60 degrees during flap harvesting to avoid the need to reposition the patient intraoperatively. Alternatively, the patient can be repositioned in a lateral decubitus position following completion of ablation. The entire ipsilateral upper limb (prepared to the elbow) is kept in the operating field to allow flexion and abduction of the shoulder as required. For access to the flap, the scapular angle needs to be readily palpable. More extensive medial dissection toward the midline is usually not required unless the scapular (transverse) skin paddle is required in addition to the parascapular (vertical) skin paddle.

An anastomotic network from branches of the circumflex scapular and thoracodorsal arteries is found within teres major. Some of these branches should be preserved in cases where an osteotomy is planned, or a large cuff of teres major is required. Up to 14 cm of bone, extending 1 cm from the glenoid fossa, can be harvested based on a single osseous branch from either the circumflex scapular or the thoracodorsal artery alone.

The triangular space, bounded by the teres minor muscle superiorly, the teres major muscle inferiorly, and the long head of the triceps laterally, corresponds to a point two-fifths of the distance between the scapular spine and the scapular angle along the lateral border of the scapula. The axis of the parascapular flap extends from the triangular space along the lateral border of the scapula to the posterior superior iliac spine—that of the scapular flap extends from the triangular space horizontally to the posterior midline. The skin territory of the parascapular flap extends from the scapular spine superiorly to midpoint between the scapular angle and the posterior superior iliac spine inferiorly—that of the scapular flap from the posterior axillary line laterally to the posterior midline medially. The width of the flap, however, is in practice limited to that which can be closed primarily.

17.6 Operative Technique

17.6.1 Parascapular Skin Paddle

The skin paddle is centered along the flap axis (i.e., the lateral border of the scapular bone), and can be designed to be as long as 30 to 35 cm. Dissection usually commences superolaterally where the incision is taken down to the muscular aponeurosis covering the infraspinatus, the teres minor and major, and the long head of triceps. Immediately superficial to the muscular aponeurosis is a loose subfascial areolar plane that allows for a bloodless dissection. Dissection is carried out medially until the descending branch of the circumflex scapular vessel emerging from the triangular space is identified. The inferolateral and medial incisions are then made, and the flap is islanded with the dissection converging onto the triangular space. The muscles are retracted to facilitate dissection of the vascular pedicle. Numerous muscular and periosteal branches are ligated, and once the infrascapular branch is ligated, the circumflex scapular vessels are reached.

Shoulder abduction and flexion will facilitate dissection of the most proximal segment of the circumflex scapular vessels, or a counterincision can be made in the axilla. If additional length is required, the thoracodorsal branch can be ligated thereby including the subscapular vessels, which originate from the axillary vessels, in the flap pedicle.

17.6.2 Scapular Skin Paddle

The skin paddle is centered on transversely along the cutaneous scapular branch axis, and the superolateral incision is made first. The circumflex scapular artery branching into its terminal cutaneous branches are observed emerging at the triangular space. The superomedial and inferior incisions are then made, and dissection continues as described above converging toward the triangular space where the muscular and periosteal branches are ligated. The remainder of the dissection is as described earlier.

17.6.3 Lateral Scapular Bone Flap

The lateral scapular bone can be harvested with a parascapular/scapular skin paddle. Following exposure of the triangular space and the circumflex scapular vessels, muscular and musculoperiosteal branches that enter the muscles that originate and insert along the lateral border are identified and preserved. The desired segment of bone is outlined by retracting infraspinatus laterally, and dividing the muscle fibers of teres minor superiorly and teres major inferiorly, down to the periosteum, which is scored with diathermy. Osteotomies are then carried out along the outline, ending at least 1 cm from the glenoid fossa to prevent inadvertent entry into the shoulder joint, and stopping short of the scapular tip. The bone segment is then retracted laterally to reveal the underlying subscapular muscle, which is divided, leaving a thin stippling of fibers on the ventral surface of the scapula to avoid injury to the periosteal blood supply. The vascular dissection continues proximally until the desired length of vascular pedicle is achieved.

17.6.4 Scapular Tip Bone Flap

The scapular tip can be accessed through a parascapular fasciocutaneous or latissimus dorsi myocutaneous free flap incisions if a chimeric flap is required. If only an osseous flap is required, an incision is made along the lateral border of the scapula. The angular branch originates from the thoracodorsal vessels, and is identified by retracting the latissimus dorsi muscle inferiorly, or tracing it from the thoracodorsal vessels by reflecting the latissimus dorsi muscle superiorly if the muscle is to be harvested as well (▶ **Fig. 17.6**). The teres major muscle is partially released from the lateral border of the scapula, and the rhomboid major muscle from the medial border. The infraspinatus is released from the dorsal surface of the scapula for the amount of bone required. On completion of osteotomy, the subscapularis muscle fibers are divided on the ventral surface.

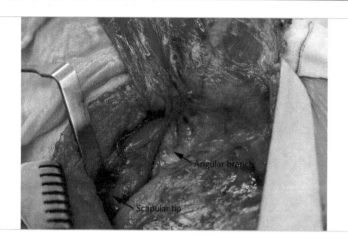

Fig. 17.6 The latissimus dorsi muscle is reflected superiorly to reveal the angular branch of the thoracodorsal vessels coursing towards the scapular tip.

17.7 Donor Site Closure

The width of the skin flaps is designed so that the incision can be closed primarily. Skin grafting on the back is best avoided due to poor graft take.

To minimize flap ischemia, as much of the donor site is closed as possible when the flap is still connected at the pedicle. Musculature divided or detached from the scapula in the harvest of an osseous component needs to be repaired. Drill holes may facilitate this if suturing is not possible to the muscular remnants or through the scapula bone by direct piercing with a heavy suture needle. Closed suction drains are used. Range of movement exercises are started within several days after surgery, and should normalize by 1 month postoperatively.

17.8 Pearls and Pitfalls

- The scapular flap is useful as a second-line option for mandibular and maxillary reconstruction when the fibular flap is not available. Combined with the latissimus dorsi, it has also been used as a chimeric flap for scalp and calvarial reconstruction.
- The scapular (transverse) or parascapular (oblique) skin paddle is based on the circumflex scapular artery, which also supplies the lateral scapular bone. The scapular tip is based on the angular branch of the thoracodorsal artery.
- The circumflex scapular artery is located at the triangular space formed by teres minor superiorly, teres major inferiorly, and the long head of triceps laterally, about two-fifths of the distance from the scapular spine to the scapular tip. The angular branch of thoracodorsal artery is found beneath the latissimus dorsi muscle within a pad of fat, extending from the thoracodorsal artery to the angular tip of the scapular bone.
- The scapular tip oriented transversely is well suited for reconstruction of the infrastructure maxillectomy palatoalveolar defect or the bilateral (anterior) mandibulectomy defect. The lateral border of the scapula oriented vertically is used to reconstruct an ipsilateral hemimaxillectomy or lateral mandibulectomy defect.
- Detached or divided muscles, such as teres major laterally and rhomboid major medially, should be reattached to the remaining scapula during closure of the donor site.

References

[1] Dos Santos LF. The scapular flap: a new microsurgical free flap. Rev Bras Cir 1980;70:133–144

[2] Gilbert A, Teot L. The free scapular flap. Plast Reconstr Surg 1982;69(4):601–604

[3] Swartz WM, Banis JC, Newton ED, Ramasastry SS, Jones NF, Acland R. The osteocutaneous scapular flap for mandibular and maxillary reconstruction. Plast Reconstr Surg 1986;77(4):530–545

[4] Coleman JJ III, Sultan MR. The bipedicled osteocutaneous scapula flap: a new subscapular system free flap. Plast Reconstr Surg 1991;87(4):682–692

[5] Hasan Z, Gore SM, Ch'ng S, Ashford B, Clark JR. Options for configuring the scapular free flap in maxillary, mandibular, and calvarial reconstruction. Plast Reconstr Surg 2013;132(3):645–655

[6] Hanasono MM, Skoracki RJ. The scapular tip osseous free flap as an alternative for anterior mandibular reconstruction. Plast Reconstr Surg 2010;125(4):164e–166e

18 Scapular and Parascapular Cutaneous Free Tissue Transfer

Michelle Lee and Samuel Lin

Abstract

The scapular and parascapular cutaneous flaps are derived from the skin and subcutaneous tissue of the back based on branches of the circumflex scapular artery. The versatility and reliability of the scapular and parascapular flaps make them workhorse flaps for head and neck reconstruction. The advantages of the back skin for head and neck reconstruction are as follows: (1) it is similar to facial skin in texture and color, (2) it can be hairless, and (3) it has a relatively small amount of subcutaneous fat in thin individuals. Furthermore, the subscapular vascular system is unique because multiple types of flaps (skin, muscle, bone) can be raised based on branches of the same subscapular vascular tree. These flaps can be inset independently while sharing the same source vessel—thus simplifying the microsurgery to only one set of anastomoses. The scapular/parascapular flaps can be used to reconstruct a wide range of composite craniofacial defects where different combinations of flaps are necessary to resurface complex, three-dimensional defects. In addition, cutaneous scapular and parascapular flaps can provide large amounts of soft tissue with minimal donor-site morbidity. This chapter puts before the surgeon, in logical sequence, the steps involved in the use of scapular and parascapular cutaneous flap transfer. Beginning with typical indications, anatomy, preoperative considerations are discussed, and operative techniques are detailed. Three variations to the standard procedure are also listed.

Keywords: axillary artery, circumflex scapular artery, deep branch, superficial branch, triangular space

18.1 Introduction

The scapular and parascapular cutaneous flaps are derived from the skin and subcutaneous tissue of the back based on branches of the circumflex scapular artery. In 1978, Sajjo first recognized the potential to transfer the fascia and soft tissue of the scapular region by injecting dye into the circumflex scapular artery.[1] Clinically, Dos Santos was the first to perform a free scapular flap in 1980. Nassif was credited with describing the parascapular flap in 1982 when he designed a vertically based skin paddle based on the descending branch of the circumflex scapular artery.[2,3] The versatility and reliability of the scapular and parascapular flaps make them workhorse flaps for head and neck reconstruction. The advantages of the back skin for head and neck reconstruction are as follows: (1) it is similar to facial skin in texture and color, (2) it can be hairless, and (3) it has a relatively small amount of subcutaneous fat in thin individuals. Furthermore, the subscapular vascular system is unique because multiple different types of flaps (skin, muscle, bone) can be raised based on branches of the same subscapular vascular tree. Those flaps can be inset independently while sharing the same source vessel—thus simplifying the microsurgery to only one set of anastomoses. The scapular/parascapular flaps can be used to reconstruct a wide range of composite craniofacial defects where different combinations of flaps are necessary to resurface complex three-dimensional defects. In addition, cutaneous scapular and parascapular flaps can provide large amounts of soft tissue with minimal donor site morbidity.

18.2 Typical Indications

- Volume reconstruction in hemifacial macrosomia.
- Large skin and subcutaneous defects of the head and neck.
- When taken as a composite flap, it can reconstruct a wide spectrum of head and neck defects ranging from cutaneous and contour defects to complex three-dimensional composite tissue defects of the skull base, orbit, midface, and mandible. The various flaps supplied by a single subscapular vascular system can simultaneously resurface areas such as intraoral lining, extraoral lining, and bone.
- Axillary defects.
- Large skin and subcutaneous defects of the upper and lower extremity.

18.3 Anatomy

The scapular and parascapular cutaneous flaps are based on the circumflex scapular artery, which is a branch of the subscapular artery. The **subscapular artery** originates from the distal third of the **axillary artery**. It branches into the **thoracodorsal artery** and the **circumflex scapular artery**. The thoracodorsal artery supplies the latissimus dorsi muscle and gives off the serratus artery branch, which supplies the serratus muscle. The circumflex scapular artery divides into a **deep and superficial branch**. The deep branch of the circumflex scapular artery supplies the periosteum of the lateral border of the scapular bone. The superficial branch of the circumflex scapular artery travels through the **triangular space** in the fascial septum between the teres major and teres minor muscle. The triangular space that the superficial circumflex scapular artery exits from is an important anatomical landmark. The space is bordered by teres major muscle, teres minor muscle, and the long head of the triceps muscle. After exiting the triangular space, the circumflex scapular artery divides into a transverse and descending branch. The scapular flap is based on the transverse branch of the superficial circumflex scapular artery and the parascapular flap is based on the descending or vertical branch of the superficial circumflex scapular artery (▶ **Fig. 18.1**).

The circumflex scapular artery is accompanied by two venae comitantes, which drain into the thoracodorsal vein. The diameter of the circumflex scapular artery at the origin from the subscapular artery ranges from 2 to 6 mm. The diameter of the subscapular artery at the origin of the axillary artery ranges from 4 to 8 mm. The length of the vascular pedicle varies between 7 and 14 cm based on the level of proximal dissection: at the level of cutaneous circumflex scapular artery (4–6 cm), at the level of subscapular artery (7–10 cm), at the level of axillary artery (11–14 cm).

The vascular pedicle for the scapular/parascapular flap is extremely reliable. The circumflex scapular artery is consistently found in the triangular space nearly 100% of the time. Infrequent (< 5%) anatomical variations of the subscapular vascular tree include the descending branch of the circumflex scapular artery, which travels deep to the teres major muscle; the circumflex scapular artery, which arises directly from the axillary artery; duplicate

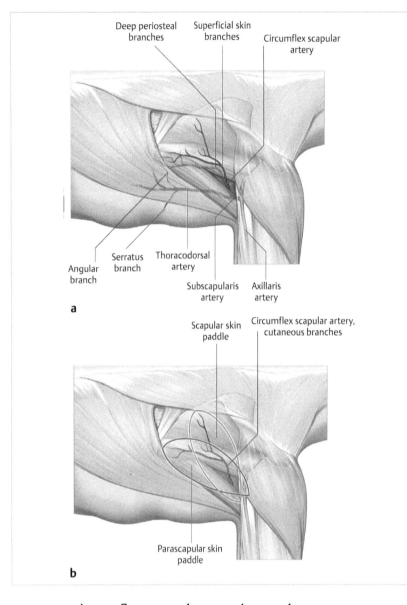

Deep periosteal branches
Superficial skin branches
Circumflex scapular artery

Angular branch
Serratus branch
Thoracodorsal artery
Subscapularis artery
Axillaris artery

a

Scapular skin paddle
Circumflex scapular artery, cutaneous branches

Parascapular skin paddle

b

Fig. 18.1 (a) Vascular anatomy of the subscapular vasculature. (b) Cutaneous design of the scapular and parascapular flaps.

circumflex scapular arteries; and separate venous drainage of the circumflex scapular vein into the axillary vein instead of the thoracodorsal vein.

The dorsal rami of the spinal nerves provide cutaneous sensation to the back. The scapular and parascapular flap is not transferred as a sensate flap.

18.4 Variations of Flap Configuration

- Osteocutaneous flap by including the lateral or medial border of the scapula bone through osseous branches of the deep circumflex scapular artery. Of note, the tip of the scapula is supplied by the angular artery, which is a branch of the thoracodorsal artery.
- Myocutaneous flap by including any of the following muscles: latissimus, teres minor, infraspinatus, and subscapularis via the subscapular vascular tree.

- Chimeric flap variations for the scapular or parascapular flap: it can be harvested with the scapular flap, scapular bone, latissimus muscle, serratus muscle, and serratus with rib based on a single vascular pedicle (the subscapular vessel system).

18.5 Preoperative Considerations

No preoperative imaging is usually necessary. The triangular space is palpated and the vascular pedicle is traced with a handheld Doppler preoperatively. In obese patients, the triangular space may be difficult to palpate. The flap may also be excessively bulky due to the thick subcutaneous tissue. The flap can be thinned by removing the fat underneath the superficial fascia; however, this technique is rarely used given that thinning of the fat may compromise the flap's vascularity. In patients with previous surgeries in areas near the circumflex subscapular artery, vascular studies can be obtained preoperatively to ensure the patency of the pedicle.

18.6 Positioning and Skin Markings

Lateral decubitus position is the preferred position in most scenarios. The patient's ipsilateral arm should be prepped into the operative field with full range of motion. This ability to move the arm in multiple directions facilitates maximum exposure during the dissection. The following landmarks are palpated and marked preoperatively: posterior midline, the scapular angle, the scapular spine, the scapular lateral border, the posterior iliac spine, and the triangular space (▶Fig. 18.2). The superficial circumflex scapular artery emerges from the triangular space. The triangular space is bordered by the teres minor, teres major, and the long head of the triceps muscles.

18.6.1 Scapular Flap

The scapular flap skin paddle is centered along the axis of the horizontal branch of the superficial circumflex scapular artery. The flap axis runs parallel to the

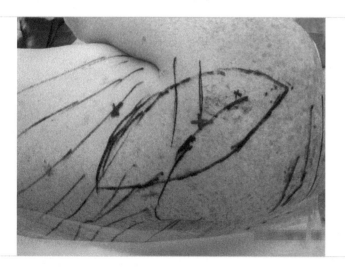

Fig. 18.2 Preoperative design of a parascapular flap centered over the vertical branch of the superficial circumflex scapular artery.

spine of the scapula transversely across the scapula. The course of the horizontal branch of the superficial circumflex scapular artery is marked and confirmed by a hand-held Doppler preoperatively. An elliptical-shaped skin flap is then designed around this line. The extent of the skin paddle should be approximately 2 cm below the scapular spine, 2 cm above the scapular angle, and 2 cm lateral to the midline.[4] However, most flaps with a width of 10 cm can be closed primarily and flap length can be extended to the medial border of the contralateral scapula if necessary. It is critical to mark the lateral or proximal part of the skin paddle over the triangular space to ensure the pedicle enters within the boundaries of the flap.

18.6.2 Parascapular Flap

The parascapular flap skin paddle is centered along the vertical branch of the superficial circumflex scapular artery. Similar to the scapular flap, the triangular space is palpated preoperatively and the Doppler confirms the superficial circumflex scapular artery emerging from the triangular space. A line drawn from the triangular space to the posterior iliac spine approximates the course of the vertical branch of the artery. An elliptical skin flap is then designed around this line. The flap dimensions can be up to 15 cm in width by 25 cm in length. The distal portion of the flap can extend to the posterior iliac spine or the 12th rib. The lateral or proximal part of the skin paddle should be outlined over the triangular space (▶ **Fig. 18.2**).

18.7 Operative Technique

18.7.1 Scapular Flap

Starting medially, incision is made around the skin island down to the deep fascia. Dissection proceeds from distal to proximal in a suprafascial plane toward the triangular space. The descending branch of the circumflex scapular artery is clipped if the scapular flap is taken in isolation. The pedicle emerges superior to the superior border of the teres major muscle. Once the pedicle has been identified, the lateral skin incision of the flap is then completed. The deep fascia is incised and dissection continues around the pedicle in a subfascial plane. Dissection around the pedicle continues until sufficient caliber and length is achieved. It can be taken to the origin of the thoracodorsal artery as well as the axillary artery if additional length or vessel size is necessary. Branches to the teres minor muscle, lateral border of the scapula, and the deep branch of the circumflex scapular artery as it courses under the scapula can be divided if the flap is not taken as a composite flap.

18.7.2 Parascapular Flap

Dissection of the parascapular flap is similar to the scapular flap. Starting distally, incision is made around the skin island down to the deep fascia. Dissection proceeds from distal to proximal in a suprafascial plane toward the vascular pedicle exiting from the triangular space. The transverse or horizontal branch of the circumflex scapular artery is clipped if the parascapular flap is taken in isolation. Once the pedicle has been identified, the lateral skin incision of the flap is then completed. The deep fascia is incised and dissection continues around the pedicle in a subfascial plane. Dissection around the pedicle continues until sufficient caliber and length is achieved. It can be taken to the origin of the thoracodorsal artery as well as the axillary artery if additional length or vessel size is necessary. Branches to the teres minor muscle, lateral border of the scapula, and the deep branch of the circumflex scapular artery as they course under the scapula can be divided if the flap is not taken as a composite flap.

Alternatively, the dissection can also be completed by identifying the circumflex scapular artery first as it exits the triangular space and proceed in a proximal to distal fashion for both the scapular and parascapular flaps. The skin incisions surrounding the pedicle entrance into the skin/subcutaneous tissue are made first and the pedicle is identified first, followed by making incisions distally. Identifying the pedicle proximally early in the flap dissection can be fairly expedient followed by determining the remainder of the flap given the vascular anatomy is very consistent.

18.8 Donor Site Closure

Flaps less than 8 to 9 cm can be closed primarily. There should be no tension on defects being closed primarily. Defects unable to be closed primarily may be either skin grafted or allowed to heal secondarily. Preoperative tissue expansion of the back tissue can also be performed to allow ease of closure of the donor site. It is important not to violate the normal anatomy and place the expanders away from the triangular space and the area of the proposed flap elevation. ▶ Fig. 18.3a–c illustrates skin markings and proximal to distal pedicle elevation. ▶ Fig. 18.3d–h demonstrates a patient after oncological resection of a postauricular tumor resulting in loss of skin and subcutaneous tissue. A free parascapular flap was used to cover the defect.

18.9 Pearls and Pitfalls

- The parascapular and scapular cutaneous territory can be harvested together on a single vascular pedicle.
- The parascapular flap vascular pedicle is within the substance of the cutaneous tissue and not directly above the muscular fascia.
- The descending branch of the circumflex scapular artery (parascapular flap) is usually the dominant artery in comparison to the transverse circumflex scapular artery (scapular flap).
- When elevating the scapular or parascapular flaps from distal to proximal, it is important to stay in the areolar plane just above the back fascia. Once the pedicle has been identified in the triangular space, the dissection proceeds deep to the fascia. This minimizes confusion and facilitates ease of dissection.
- A proximal to distal dissection is an expedient means of flap elevation in most cases. Secondary to a relatively short vascular pedicle, flap pedicle length is increased by increasing the length of the cutaneous portion of the flap.

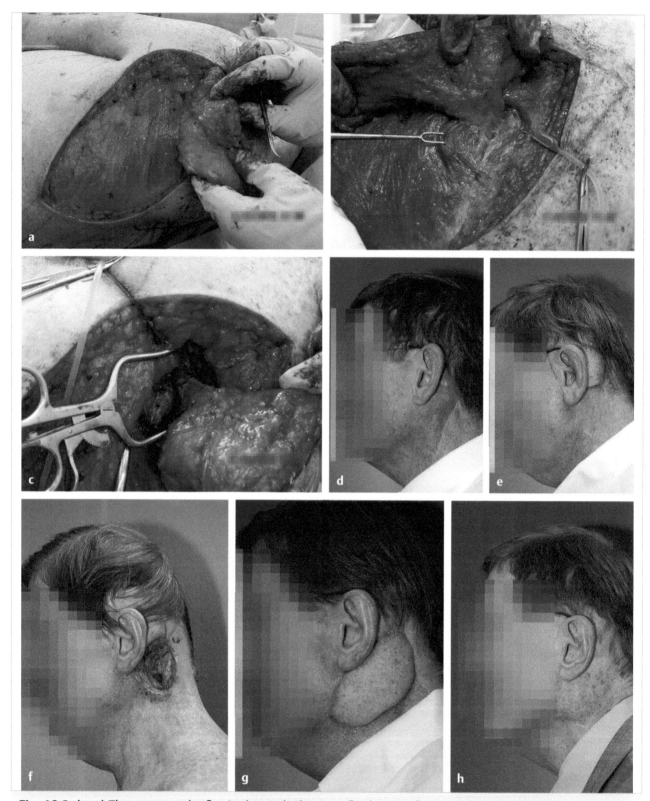

Fig. 18.3 (a–c) The parascapular flap is elevated. The superficial circumflex scapular artery is demonstrated as it exits the triangular space. **(d–h)** Preoperative and postoperative photos of a patient after a free parascapular flap was used to resurface a postauricular defect.

References

[1] Saijo M. The vascular territories of the dorsal trunk: a reappraisal for potential flap donor sites. Br J Plast Surg 1978;31(3):200–204

[2] Dos Santos LF. The scapular flap: a new microsurgical free flap. Bol Chir Plast 1980;70:133

[3] Nassif TM, Vidal L, Bovet JL, Baudet J. The parascapular flap: a new cutaneous microsurgical free flap. Plast Reconstr Surg 1982;69(4):591–600

[4] Urbaniak JR, Koman LA, Goldner RD, Armstrong NB, Nunley JA. The vascularized cutaneous scapular flap. Plast Reconstr Surg 1982;69(5):772–778

19 Keystone Flap

Michel Saint-Cyr

Abstract

The keystone perforator island flap is a versatile, multiperforator fasciocutaneous advancement flap useful in closing skin defects following excision of skin cancers. It can be used for reconstruction of small, moderate, and extensive soft-tissue defects utilizing well-vascularized adjacent tissue based on known vascular perforator clusters, which help to avoid the need of a free flap for many complex reconstructions. The keystone perforator island flap can also be used as a primary or adjunct flap and, with additional modifications, can be individualized to reconstructive needs. The salient elements in the surgical use of this flap are described in this chapter, from typical indications, to anatomy, to preoperative considerations, to operative technique. A listing of four variations to the standard procedure is also included.

Keywords: keystone perforator island flap, perforasome, linking vessels

19.1 Introduction

The **keystone perforator island flap** (KPIF) is a multiperforator fasciocutaneous advancement flap first described by Behan in 2003 for closure of skin defects following excision of skin cancers.[1] This flap can be used for reconstruction of small, moderate, and extensive soft-tissue defects utilizing well-vascularized adjacent tissue based on known vascular perforator clusters, successfully avoiding the need of a free flap for many complex reconstructions. The KPIF is a versatile flap, which can be used as a primary or adjunct flap and, with additional modifications, can be individualized to reconstructive needs.

19.2 Typical Indications

- Defects secondary to tumor extirpation (commonly soft-tissue sarcoma and skin cancers) or trauma.
- Coverage of exposed hardware, enterocutaneous fistulae, or chronic wounds.
- Upper and lower extremity soft-tissue defects.
- Defects of trunk, perineum, hip, and buttocks.

19.3 Anatomy

The keystone flap is a multiperforator island advancement flap. It is based on perfusion through musculocutaneous and/or fasciocutaneous perforators.[2]

A **perforasome** describes the arterial network surrounding a single perforator.[3] Direct and indirect **linking vessels** connect multiple perforators and allow perfusion of a larger surface area (▶ **Fig. 19.1**).

The orientation of linking vessels corresponds to the maximal blood flow to the overlying tissue. This is generally axially oriented in the extremities (along the underlying main axial vessels) and perpendicular to the midline in the trunk (in line with muscle fibers and ribs). Perforator blood flow tends to be

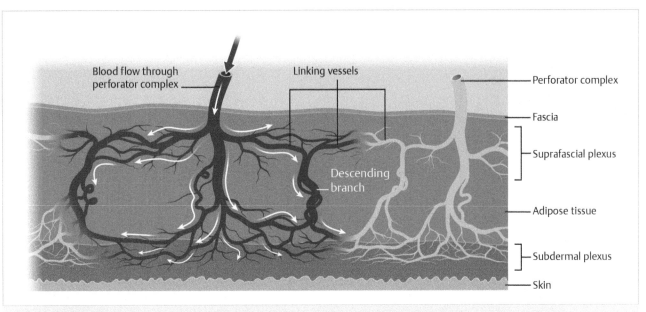

Fig. 19.1 Vascular basis of extended ALT flap demonstrating interperforator flow.

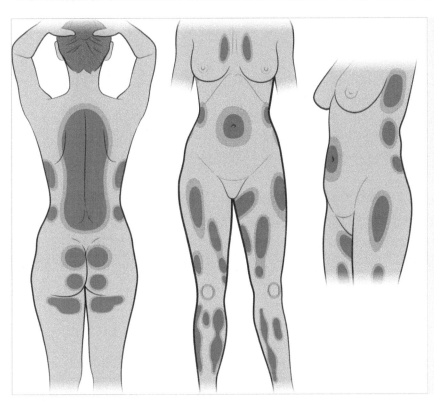

Fig. 19.2 Perforator "hotspots" around which a keystone perforator flap is ideally designed.

unidirectional, away from articulations, and bidirectional, if midway between the two articulations.[3]

Understanding the perforator anatomy allows identification of perforator hotspots. This is where there is maximal blood flow, thus better flap perfusion.[3] One should also be aware of areas with a paucity of perforators, particularly the scalp where the use of keystone flaps is discouraged.[3] Flaps are often centered over known hotspots, although they can be centered over random perforators detected via Doppler ultrasound examination.

Flap design should be guided by knowledge of this perforator anatomy (▶ Fig. 19.2).

19.4 Variations

- Flap to defect ratio may be extended to 2:1, 3:1, 4:1, or greater depending on laxity of the tissue.[2] Flaps created over an underlying muscle belly allow for large flap design and more mobility.
- Asymmetrically designed limbs at varying angles may be used[2] in order to prevent crossing joint lines, expose critical structures, and violate lymphatic basins.
- Complete circumferential versus partial incision of the deep fascia. Fascia may not need to be incised at all, depending on tissue mobility. Progressive release of the deep fascia as needed to provide necessary movement.[2]
- Double opposing keystone flaps.

19.5 Preoperative Considerations

Evaluate the planned flap site for prior trauma, prior surgery, and radiation changes as they might compromise blood flow or mobilization of the flap. Flap size should be increased to incorporate more perforators, decrease tension on closure, and to increase flap viability in cases where significant undermining, radiation treatment, or other forms of soft-tissue injury have occurred. Ensure laxity of tissue in region of the planned KPIF to allow adequate advancement and tension-free closure. The central portion of the flap should ideally involve highest density of perforators for maximal vascularity. The flap axis is designed parallel to long axis of extremities and perpendicular to the trunk. Limbs of the KPIF should respect aesthetic lines. Avoid crossing joints to reduce scar and joint contracture. Care should be taken to avoid lymph node basins to minimize risk of lymphedema.

19.6 Positioning and Skin Markings

Patient positioning is dependent on the location of the defect and area of planned KPIF. This requires exposure of the areas with perforators. This may be supine, prone, or lateral decubitus position based on availability and laxity of adjacent soft tissue.

The flap was historically designed with a 1:1 flap to defect ratio, but can be modified, depending on the adjacent tissue laxity, up to a ratio of 5:1 or greater.[2] The ratio is dependent on the size of the defect, with smaller defects amenable to a greater ratio to ensure capture of perforators.

KPIF design is dependent on the adjacent tissue dominant perforators, concentrated in hotspots that are further localized with the use of a handheld Doppler ultrasound. Perforators are marked with a marking pen. This aids in flap design and decreases the risk of injury to the vascular supply during surgical dissection. Maximize perforator concentration along the central portion of the flap to allow fascial undermining and greater mobility and flexibility (▶ Fig. 19.3).

Traditionally, a 90-degree angle was employed for designs of symmetric flap limbs with a 1:1 flap to defect width ratio. However, the angle of the limbs can be asymmetric and should be modified to meet the individual needs of the defects.[2]

Care must be taken to plan the incisions to avoid injury to underlying critical structures, particularly neurovascular bundles and lymphatic basins. Scar

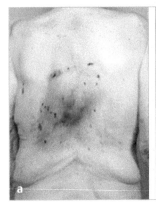
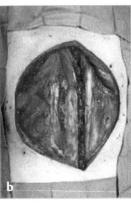
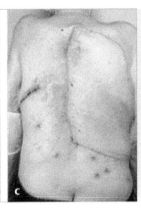

Fig. 19.3 (a) Patient with a large soft-tissue tumor of the back, centered to the right of the patient's midline. **(b)** Sugical defect. **(c)** Wound closed with left back keystone perforator island flap.

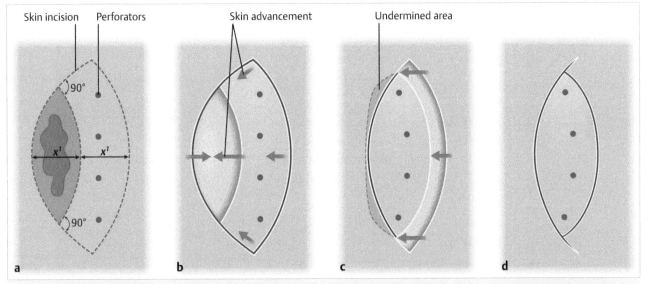

Fig. 19.4 (a-d) Schematic illustration of a keystone perforator island flap. The red dots indicate hypothetical perforators. Arrows indicate direction of skin advancement. The shaded area in the third figure indicates the area undermined to help with closure.

placement must avoid crossing of joint lines, in an attempt to reduce postoperative morbidity and ideally planned along the aesthetic lines of the body to decrease scar visibility.[2] When necessary, use hand surgery principles with zigzag limbs across flexion creases.

Preoperative planning should also evaluate the need for a second keystone flap if the defect is too large for closure by a single flap. The second KPIF is planned on the contralateral side of the defect.

19.7 Operative Technique

Position the patient to allow for easy access of the wound and donor site. This will vary depending on the wound location. Perform addition excision of the defect if necessary to make an ellipse (▶Fig. 19.4). Design flap adjacent to the defect, over known perforator hotspots when possible. Confirm perforator capture via hand-held Doppler ultrasound.

Sharply incise through skin and fat straight down to the underlying deep fascia. Care should be taken to avoid any superficial vital structures in the area. Assess flap mobility and determine if fascia incision is necessary. Perform progressive fascial incisions until enough flap mobility is achieved to allow for

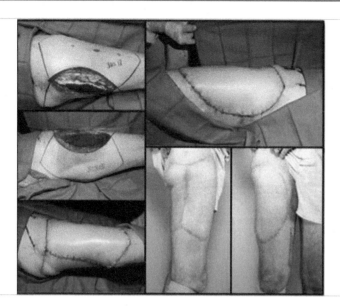

Fig. 19.5 Flap mobilization and final appearance of a keystone perforator island flap used of right thigh wound closure.

tension-free closure of the wound. Care should be taken when incising fascia to protect perforators that may traverse directly under these fascial openings. Assess the need for undermining of adjacent tissue or fascial undermining of the flap itself. Undermine only as needed for flap mobilization, taking care not to injure any perforators supplying the skin. Close the donor area using a V–Y technique at the lateral apices of the donor site.

After sufficient flap mobilization, close in layers (▶ **Fig. 19.5**). For large defects, use progressive tension sutures, and closed suction drains are used to prevent seromas. Reapproximate the superficial fascia. Complete the skin closure in a typical layered fashion.

19.8 Donor Site Closure

Closure/flap inset is performed in layers (i.e., superficial fascia, dermis, and epidermis). Reapproximate the superficial fascia, but avoid undue tension with these stitches near perforators since this can occlude those vessels.

For large defects, or if there has been significant undermining, it is necessary to use progressive tension three-point sutures to close off dead space, and/ or bulb-suction drains, as mentioned earlier. Avoid positioning drain tubing in close proximity to perforating vessels to prevent vessel occlusion or rupture. Use the progressive tension sutures to advance the donor defect leading edge toward the flap in the same vector as flap advancement.

19.9 Pearls and Pitfalls

- Design over known perforator "hotspots." Avoid "coldspots" with a paucity of perforators (e.g., scalp).
- Design the flap on healthy native skin, away from traumatized and/or irradiated tissue.
- If bilateral flap donor site options exist, choose the side with greater laxity and perforator density.
- Increase the flap to defect size ratio, if necessary, to improve tissue mobility, increase potential for undermining, and increase perforator capture.

- Design flaps over areas of relative mobility/laxity to decrease tension. Incise fascia as needed and consider progressive tension sutures for closure.
- Modify incisions to respect aesthetic units, to avoid joints lines, and to prevent exposure of critical structures and violation of lymph basins.

References

[1] Behan FC. The keystone design perforator island flap in reconstructive surgery ANZ J Surg 2003;73(3):112–120

[2] Mohan AT, Rammos CK, Akhavan AA, et al. Evolving concepts of keystone perforator island flaps (KPIF): principles of perforator anatomy, design modifications, and extended clinical applications. Plast Reconstr Surg 2016;137(6):1909–1920

[3] Saint-Cyr M, Wong C, Schaverien M, Mojallal A, Rohrich RJ. The perforasome theory: vascular anatomy and clinical implications. Plast Reconstr Surg 2009;124(5):1529–1544

20 Transverse Rectus Abdominis Myocutaneous Free Flap

Amanda K. Silva and David W. Chang

Abstract

The transverse rectus abdominis myocutaneous free flap for breast reconstruction procedure (and its variations) has been developed to help minimize donor site morbidity—from the free muscle-sparing and deep inferior epigastric perforator, which spare more muscle and fascia, to the free superficial inferior epigastric artery flap, which is based off the superficial system—thus avoiding fascia and muscle dissection. This chapter examines the crucial considerations in this procedure, starting with indications and contraindications, anatomy, the blood supply, innervation, preoperative considerations, and the operative technique. The discussion of the technique goes into detail on the preparation of the recipient vessels, flap dissection, inset, and shaping, and donor site closure. Five variations to the standard procedure are listed.

Keywords: deep superior epigastric artery, deep inferior epigastric artery, intercostal vessels, linea semilunaris, semicircular line, arc of Douglas

The transverse rectus abdominis myocutaneous (TRAM) free flap for breast reconstruction was first described in 1979 by Holmström.[1] Over the years, variations have been developed to help minimize donor site morbidity, from the free muscle-sparing (MS-TRAM) and deep inferior epigastric perforator (DIEP), which spare more muscle and fascia, to the free superficial inferior epigastric artery (SIEA) flap, which is based off the superficial system, thus avoiding fascia and muscle dissection altogether.

20.1 Typical Indications

Breast reconstruction in a healthy patient with abdominal skin laxity and excess fat.

20.2 Contraindications

Patient unwilling to accept donor site scars and potential donor morbidities.

Patient unwilling to undergo a long, complex procedure with prolonged postoperative recovery.

Medical comorbidities such as hypercoagulability that significantly increases risk of free flap.

20.3 Anatomy

20.3.1 Rectus Abdominis Muscle and Sheath

The rectus abdominis muscles are a pair of long, straight muscles that arise from the symphysis pubis and insert on the fifth, sixth, and seventh ribs. The rectus sheath is formed by the aponeurotic extensions of the laterally located external oblique, internal oblique, and transversus abdomnius muscles. The midline fusion of these aponeuroses between the rectus abdomini is the linea alba. The lateral border of the rectus sheath is referred to as the **linea semilunaris**. Each

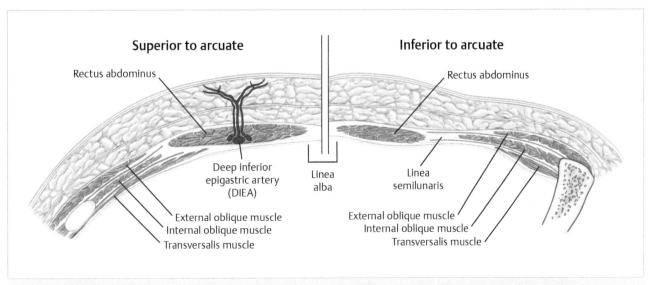

Fig. 20.1 Axial view of anterior abdominal wall superior and inferior to the arcuate line. DIEA, deep inferior epigastric artery. (Adapted from Jones GE. Bostwick's Plastic and Reconstructive Breast Surgery, Third Edition. New York: Thieme Medical Publishers; 2010.)

rectus abdominis muscle is subdivided by two to five tendinous inscriptions that are adherent to the overlying anterior rectus sheath. An important transition in the posterior sheath is the arcuate line (**semicircular line** or **arc of Douglas**), which is generally located halfway between the umbilicus and symphysis pubis. Inferior to this point the internal oblique aponeurosis ceases to split around the rectus abdomini and instead the aponeuroses of all three muscles pass anterior. The transversalis fascia is the only layer deep to the rectus abdomini and therefore this is an area of weakness postoperatively (▶ **Fig. 20.1**).

20.3.2 Blood Supply

The rectus abdominis muscle has two major vascular pedicles: **deep superior epigastric artery** (DSEA) and **deep inferior epigastric artery** (DIEA), and minor blood supply from the **intercostal vessels**. The DSEA arises from the internal mammary artery at the level of the sixth intercostal space. The DIEA usually originates 1 cm above the inguinal ligament from the external iliac artery and pierces the transversalis fascia to enter the rectus sheath just below the arcuate line where it runs on the deep surface of the rectus abdominis muscle. It usually divides into two branches below the level of the umbilicus to form the medial and lateral rows; however, variations include no or multiple branching. The DIEA has two venae comitantes, which usually join to form a single vein prior to their junction with the external iliac vein (▶ **Fig. 20.2**).

The deep arteries supply the overlying abdominal skin by perforators that travel through the muscle. The highest concentration of perforators is in the periumbilical area. These perforators communicate with other regional superficial vessels through a system of choke vessels. One key superficial vessel is the **SIEA**, which if large enough in caliber can be used for reconstruction. This vessel is usually found just deep to Scarpa's fascia, two-thirds the distance from the midline symphysis pubis to the anterior superior iliac spine. The veins of the superficial system travel above Scarpa's fascia and communicate extensively across the midline. The superficial veins drain into the deep venous system by way of the veins accompanying the arterial perforators.

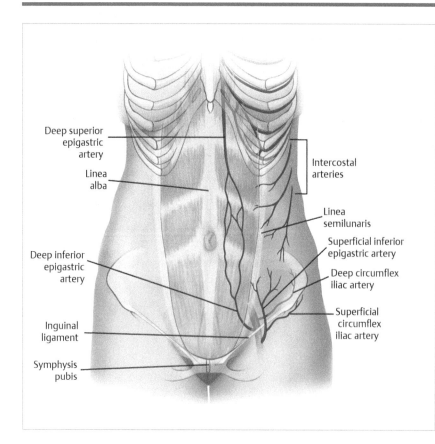

Fig. 20.2 Blood supply to the abdominal wall. DSEA, deep superior epigastric artery; DIEA, deep inferior epigastric artery; SIEA, superficial inferior epigastric artery; DCIA, deep circumflex iliac artery; SCIA; superficial circumflex iliac artery. (Adapted from Jones GE. Bostwick's Plastic and Reconstructive Breast Surgery, Third Edition. New York: Thieme Medical Publishers; 2010.)

The transverse abdominal skin overlying the rectus abdomini can be divided into zones representing levels of perfusion from the DIEA, referred to as Hartrampf zones. The robustness of the blood supply diminishes as the zone numbers go higher. Zone I refers to the skin overlying the rectus abdominis muscle on the side ipsilateral to the vessel used. Zone II is the skin overlying the contralateral rectus abdominis muscle. The skin lateral to **linea semilunaris** on the ipsilateral side is referred to as zone III, and the skin lateral to the contralateral linea semilunaris is zone IV. Some studies suggest that medial row perforators supply zone IV more reliably than lateral row perforators. The SIEA reliably perfuses the hemiabdomen.[2]

20.3.3 Innervation

The motor and sensory innervation comes from the T7 to T12 intercostal nerves, which traverse the plane between the transversus abdominis and the internal oblique muscles. The nerves enter the midportion of the rectus muscles at the posterior surface. Although the majority of the nerves may need to be sacrificed to harvest the flap, efforts should be made to preserve the inferior-most larger nerve near the arcuate line as this nerve has been shown to provide motor innervation to the entire muscle.[3]

20.4 Variations

- Pedicled TRAM: pedicle flap based on the deep superior epigastric vessels, all or most muscle taken.
- Free TRAM: free flap based on the deep inferior epigastric vessels, all muscle taken.

- MS-TRAM: free flap based on the deep inferior epigastric vessels, some muscle taken, pedicle not completely skeletonized.
- DIEP: free flap based on the deep inferior epigastric vessels, rectus abdominis muscle, and majority of anterior rectus sheath spared.
- SIEA: free flap based on the superficial inferior epigastric vessels, rectus abdominis muscle, and anterior rectus sheath completely spared and not dissected.

20.5 Preoperative Considerations

Preoperatively, the patient's abdomen should be evaluated to make sure that she is a good candidate for a TRAM flap. The patient should have enough excess abdominal skin and fat to reconstruct an adequately sized breast and be able to close the abdominal donor site. Additionally, if the patient has had previous surgery on abdomen one should consider whether a TRAM flap is feasible. Although concerning for soft-tissue vascularity, successful TRAM/DIEP flap reconstruction following abdominoplasty and liposuction have been reported.[4,5] Some advocate use of preoperative imaging in these patients to help guide flap design and flap delay procedures.

20.6 Positioning and Skin Markings

The flap is designed on the lower abdomen with a transverse ellipse shape. The upper marking is usually just at or above the umbilicus, and the lower marking is just above the pubis. The blood supply is more robust as the flap is placed more superior, however the scar is then placed higher as well. The design of the flap is tapered lateral (▶ Fig. 20.3).

For positioning, the patient is supine and her waist is at the proper bend of the table so that she can be placed in a sitting position during flap inset and to aid with donor site closure. The patient's arms can be out or tucked depending on the surgeon's preference.

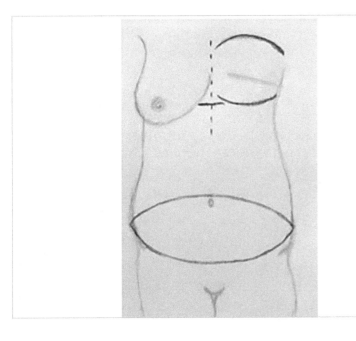

Fig. 20.3 Markings for a TRAM/DIEP flap. The patient's midline is marked, as well as both inframammary folds and the breast footprint in delayed reconstructions. The height of the flap at the midline should be roughly equal to the desired breast base width.

20.7 Operative Technique

20.7.1 Preparation of the Recipient Vessels

Currently, the author uses the internal mammary vessels as the primary recipients of choice; however, the thoracodorsal vessels may be used as well. The intercostal spaces are palpated to find an optimal space that is wide and readily accessible for comfortable microvascular anastomoses. This is usually at the second or third intercostal space. Next, the pectoralis muscle is split in the direction of its fibers to expose the intercostal space. The intercostal muscle fibers are carefully divided layer by layer with a bipolar. Dissection starts laterally to avoid injury to the internal mammary vessels, which are usually within 1 to 3 cm from the edge of the sternum. If there is a single vein, it is usually medial to the artery. If there are two veins, then the artery is usually between the veins.

Adjacent cartilage does not need to be removed routinely; however, if the intercostal space is narrow or deep, thus making anastomoses difficult, cartilage should be removed for better exposure. Some surgeons prefer to remove a 2 to 4 cm segment of rib cartilage routinely to access the internal mammary vessels. To accomplish this, the perichondrium is incised and dissected off, the cartilage is then removed directly over the internal mammary vessels using a rib dissector or rongeur. The perichondrium is then carefully dissected off the internal mammary vessels. Final preparation of the recipient vessels is best performed under a microscope.

20.7.2 Flap Dissection

The inferior skin incision is made first and the superficial inferior epigastric vein (SIEV) is identified. If there is a good SIEV, it is dissected out and clipped long in case it is needed later for additional or alternative venous drainage. Next the SIEA is identified. This usually lies lateral to the SIEV and deep to Scarpa's fascia. If there is a SIEA present with large enough caliber and the patient is a good candidate, this flap maybe chosen.

If there is no adequate SIEA, the incision on the hemiabdomen is completed down to the abdominal wall fascia inferior and superior. Extra sub-Scarpa's fat is included in the superior portion of the flap to improve the closure of the abdomen and add extra flap bulk if necessary. Next the umbilicus is dissected out. It helps to make four small stab incisions with a number 11 blade at the 12-, 3-, 6-, and 9-o'clock positions. Single prong skin hooks are then placed into the adjacent incisions to provide tension while incisions are made to connect the stab incisions. A tenotomy scissors is then used to dissect the umbilical stalk down to its base.

Dissection next proceeds from lateral to medial, raising the flap off the abdominal wall in the loose areolar plane. Dissection can be rapid at this point as there are no important perforators in this area. Once the linea semilunaris is approached, dissection slows as perforators will start to be encountered (▶ Fig. 20.4).

20.7.3 Tram

If a full-muscle TRAM is planned, careful dissection is performed up to the major perforators on the preferred side. Once these perforators are encountered, a fascia-sparing technique is used to open the rectus sheath fascia, incorporating

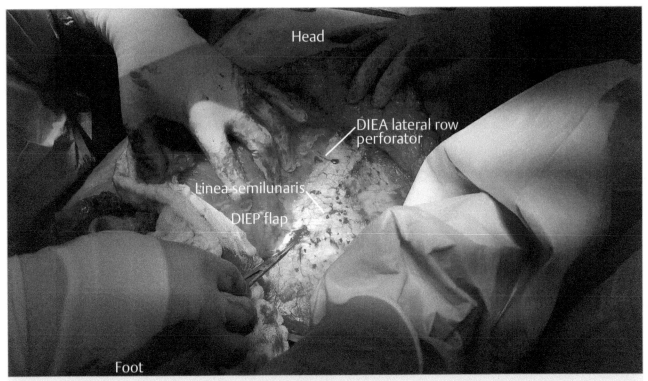

Fig. 20.4 Lateral flap dissection. DIEA, deep inferior epigastric artery; DIEP, deep inferior epigastric perforator.

only a small cuff of fascia around the perforators. The rectus sheath incision is extended inferiorly and laterally to expose the underlying rectus abdominis muscle.

The anterior rectus sheath is dissected off the underlying rectus abdominis. Several intercostal nerves and vessels will be seen on the surface of the posterior rectus sheath, which are ligated. The lateral border of the muscle is identified and dissected inferiorly, where the DIEA pedicle is found. The rectus abdominis muscle is separated from the posterior sheath.

The rectus abdominis muscle is then gently retracted to expose the deep inferior epigastric vessels. Once the vascular pedicle has been isolated and protected, the inferior muscle attachment at the symphysis pubis is detached. The pedicle is then traced toward its origin at the external iliac vessels. The superior muscle attachment is divided, and the superior epigastric artery and vein are ligated. Superiorly, the muscle can be divided at any level above the perforators to the flap. The deep inferior epigastric pedicle is left intact until the recipient site is prepared.

20.7.4 MS-TRAM and DIEP

If a muscle-sparing TRAM is planned, dissection continues with elevation of the skin and subcutaneous tissues off the anterior rectus sheath from lateral to medial until the lateral perforators are seen. Large perforators are preserved. Next the medial flap incision is made, whether that be at the midline in the case of a hemiabdominal flap or slightly past midline in the event of the need for a slightly larger flap. Dissection proceeds in the same plane from medial to lateral to identify the medial row perforators. Once all potential perforators are identified, the perforators are chosen for inclusion in the flap.

Medial perforators provide longer pedicles and their harvest results in less functional damage to the remaining rectus muscle, as the muscle is innervated

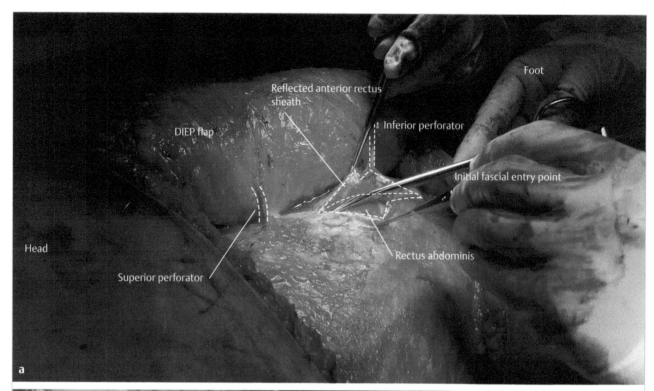

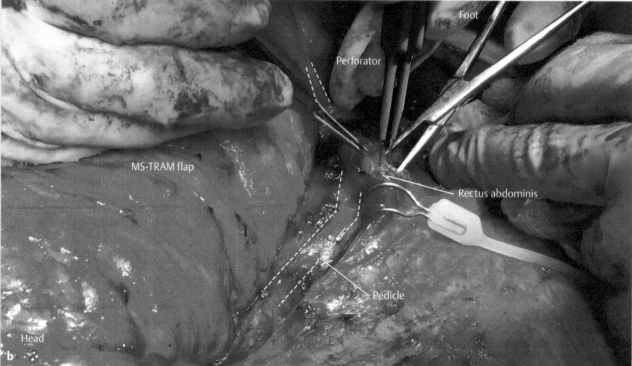

Fig. 20.5 **(a)** Anterior rectus sheath incision. Note minimal amount of fascia sacrificed, leaving a small fascial cuff around the perforator. DIEP, deep inferior epigastric perforator. **(b)** Muscle sparing TRAM showing division of rectus abdominis muscle to include a small cuff of muscle with the flap.

from lateral to medial. Also, compared to the laterally located perforators, more medially located perforators may provide better perfusion to the tissues across the midline of the flap. Generally, two or three moderate to large perforators will provide sufficient circulation to the flap.

Next, an incision is made in the anterior rectus sheath inferior to and connecting the perforators taking a small cuff of fascia (▶ **Fig. 20.5a**). The anterior sheath is dissected off the underlying rectus abdominis muscle. The decision to perform an MS-TRAM or a DIEP flap is based on the number, caliber, and location of perforators as well as their orientation and course within the rectus muscle. A DIEP flap is selected when there is a single large perforator, or when two or more perforators are located within the same intramuscular septum. If the perforators are located in different intramuscular layers, the muscle fibers between them would need to be divided for a DIEP flap; under these circumstances, a small cuff of muscle between and around the perforators is incorporated (▶ **Fig. 20.5b**).

Once the extent of the muscle that needs to be taken with the flap is decided, the muscle is carefully divided taking care to avoid injury to the perforators or pedicle. Once the inferior portion of the muscle is divided, the main pedicle should be exposed. The rectus muscle fibers are then split inferiorly to further expose and dissect out the main pedicle.

20.7.5 Flap Inset and Shaping

The flap can be inset vertically or horizontally. The authors prefer to place the flap vertically for breast reconstruction with zones I and II inferomedial, to form the majority of the new breast and zone III superolateral. When a flap based off the DIEA is used, this is best done with a flap from the contralateral side of the abdomen rotated approximately 90 degrees counterclockwise, resulting in the vascular pedicle lying medial, in an anatomically natural position, toward the internal mammary recipient vessels (▶ **Fig. 20.6**).

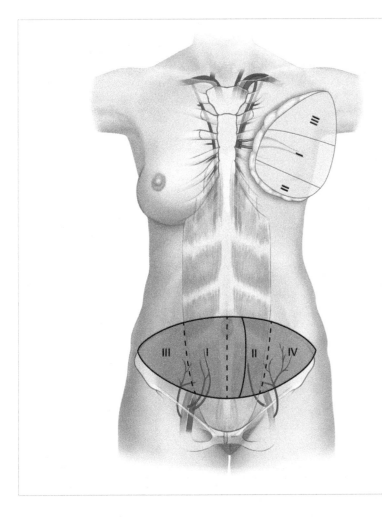

Fig. 20.6 Flap in situ and showing inset with the Hartrampf zones denoted. (Adapted from Jones GE. Bostwick's Plastic and Reconstructive Breast Surgery, Third Edition. New York: Thieme Medical Publishers; 2010.)

After microvascular anastomosis, the flap is inset. Usually, the mastectomy skin flap alone will provide good support, however, when the flap is significantly smaller than the mastectomy defect, it needs to be secured medially and superiorly so that it does not fall within the pocket. The corner of the flap from zones III and IV are trimmed away as necessary. It is better to make the initial breast mound volume slightly larger than the contralateral breast and allow for revision if necessary. Attention also needs to be paid to make sure the inframammary fold is placed in the correct location, as it is very difficult to adjust this later on. Once the optimal size and shape have been achieved compared to the contralateral breast, the skin paddle is marked. The patient is then placed back in a supine position, and the buried portion of the skin is deepithelialized.

In delayed breast reconstruction, the surgeon must decide how to manage the inferior portion of the mastectomy skin flap. If the skin flap is abundant and soft, the author prefers to preserve it and use it for the breast reconstruction, as this allows for more "natural"-appearing shape. If the skin flap is fibrotic due to irradiation, it may be better to discard it and replace that area with flap skin.

20.8 Donor Site Closure

Proper closure of the donor site defect is essential to prevent abdominal bulge or hernia. If a fascia-sparing technique was used, it should be able to be closed primarily. It is important to ensure the aponeuroses of the external and internal obliques are included in the fascial closure. If the fascia integrity is poor or a significant amount of fascia was harvested thus making a tension-free primary closure difficult, mesh is used to reinforce the closure. Closed-suction drains are placed above the fascia closure in the subcutaneous tissue.

After the abdomen is closed, the umbilicus is brought out through an incision made in the midline of the abdominal flap and secured with sutures. There are many different ways to inset the umbilicus. The author prefers to make an upside-down U incision and to resect a small wedge from the inferior portion of the umbilicus to inset the U.

20.9 Pearls and Pitfalls

- Fat necrosis and partial flap loss result from inadequate perfusion. In almost all cases zone IV should be discarded. Usually, a small portion from the corner of zone III is also discarded.
- As many perforators as necessary should be included to provide optimal perfusion to the flap. In many cases only two or three perforators, and occasionally even a single large perforator, will provide sufficient perfusion. However, in higher-risk patients, such as smokers or the obese, the surgeon should consider including more perforators to reduce the risk of significant fat necrosis or partial flap loss.
- Consider previous abdominal scars with placement of incisions and amount of undermining needed for abdominal closure.

References

[1] Holmström H. The free abdominoplasty flap and its use in breast reconstruction. An experimental study and clinical case report. Scand J Plast Reconstr Surg 1979;13(3):423–427

[2] Schaverien M, Saint-Cyr M, Arbique G, Brown SA. Arterial and venous anatomies of the deep inferior epigastric perforator and superficial inferior epigastric artery flaps. Plast Reconstr Surg 2008;121(6):1909–1919

[3] Rozen WM, Ashton MW, Kiil BJ, et al. Avoiding denervation of rectus abdominis in DIEP flap harvest II: an intraoperative assessment of the nerves to rectus. Plast Reconstr Surg 2008;122(5):1321–1325

[4] Kim JY, Chang DW, Temple C, Beahm EK, Robb GL. Free transverse rectus abdominis musculocutaneous flap breast reconstruction in patients with prior abdominal suction-assisted lipectomy. Plast Reconstr Surg 2004;113(3):28e–31e

[5] Ribuffo D, Marcellino M, Barnett GR, Houseman ND, Scuderi N. Breast reconstruction with abdominal flaps after abdominoplasties. Plast Reconstr Surg 2001;108(6):1604–1608

21 Transverse Rectus Abdominis Myocutaneous Pedicled Flap

Amanda Murphy and Jason G. Williams

Abstract

The transverse rectus abdominis myocutaneous pedicled flap was a truly important innovation in plastic surgery, as it was the first completely autologous, single-stage option for breast reconstruction. Despite advances in microsurgical free tissue transfer, the pedicled transverse rectus abdominis myocutaneous flap remains the most widely utilized flap for breast reconstruction among North American surgeons. This chapter fully covers the sequential steps in implementation of this procedure, from typical indications, to anatomy, to preoperative considerations, to the operative technique itself. Five variations to the standard procedure are also listed.

Keywords: deep inferior epigastric vessels, deep inferior epigastric artery, internal mammary artery, musculophrenic epigastric artery, superior epigastric artery, 8th to 12th intercostal vessels

21.1 Introduction

The transverse rectus abdominis myocutaneous (TRAM) pedicled flap, described by Dr. Carl Hartrampf in 1982, was a truly important innovation in plastic surgery as it was the first completely autologous, single-stage option for breast reconstruction.[1] His description of a pedicled myocutaneous flap based on the superior epigastric vessels marked the advent of a new era in breast reconstruction. Despite advances in microsurgical free tissue transfer, the pedicled TRAM remains the most widely utilized flap for breast reconstruction among North American surgeons.

21.2 Typical Indications

- Breast reconstruction.
- Chest wall reconstruction:
  - Tumor excision.
  - Poland syndrome.

21.3 Anatomy

The pedicled transverse rectus abdominis myocutaneous (pTRAM) flap is composed of a lower abdominal skin island elevated on one of the paired rectus muscles, with perfusion from the superior epigastric vessels.

The rectus muscles originate from the anterior aspect of the xyphoid process and sixth, seventh, and eighth costal cartilages. They run the length of the anterior abdomen encased in the rectus sheath, and insert on the pubic symphysis. The rectus sheath is formed by the aponeuroses of the external oblique, internal oblique, and transverse abdominal muscles. The external oblique and transversus abdominis muscles form the outer and innermost layers, respectively. Above the arcuate line, the internal oblique aponeurosis splits contributing to both anterior and posterior rectus sheath. Below the arcuate line, the leaflets converge and contribute only to the anterior sheath. The muscles are divided by three tendinous intersections that attach only to the anterior rectus sheath.

The anterior abdominal wall is perfused by two main sources, the superior and **deep inferior epigastric vessels** (DIEVs). The **deep inferior epigastric artery** (DIEA) and its accompanying veins are the dominant source of blood flow to the lower abdominal tissue, meaning that the skin island transferred with the pTRAM is perfused by the nondominant superior epigastric pedicle, which arises from the **internal mammary artery** (IMA) (▶ **Fig. 21.1**).

Deep to the sixth interspace, the IMA divides into **musculophrenic** and **superior epigastric arteries** (SEAs). The superior epigastric vessels travel inferiorly

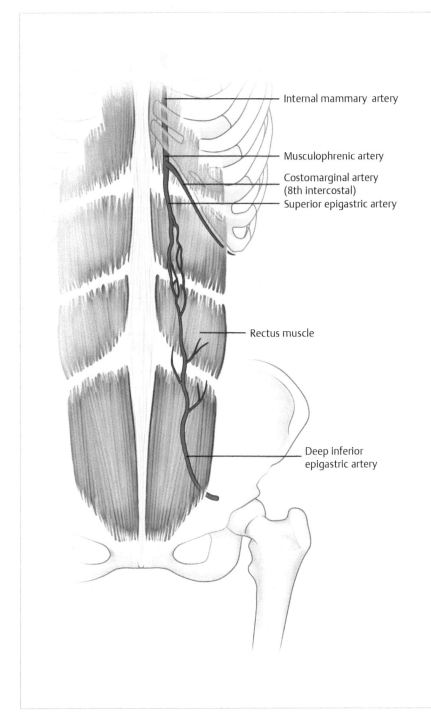

Internal mammary artery

Musculophrenic artery

Costomarginal artery
(8th intercostal)

Superior epigastric artery

Rectus muscle

Deep inferior
epigastric artery

Fig. 21.1 Vascular anatomy of the rectus muscle and anterior abdominal wall. (Adapted from Jones GE. Bostwick's Plastic and Reconstructive Breast Surgery, Third Edition. New York: Thieme Medical Publishers; 2010.)

either within or on the deep surface of the rectus muscle, at a distance of approximately 2.5 to 4 cm from the midline. Just above the umbilicus, the superior epigastric vessels combine with the deep inferior epigastric system in a web of choke anastomoses.

In addition to the epigastrics, the rectus muscles receive minor segmental blood flow from the **8th to 12th intercostal vessels**. These vessels form anastomotic connections with the epigastrics on the deep surface of the muscle. The eighth intercostal artery is the largest of these, anastomosing with the SEA at the midportion of the rectus muscle. In situations where the IMA has been divided, such as with coronary bypass or previous harvest for flap recipients, preservation of this minor pedicle can maintain flow through the SEA in a retrograde fashion.

Moon and Taylor describe three patterns of flap perfusion based on the DIEA.[2] In type I, the SEA descends to anastomose with a single DIEA. In type II, the most commonly encountered variant, the DIEA branches into two vessels at the arcuate line, communicating with the superior system in a complex network of choke vessels. In type III, the DIEA branches into three vessels at the arcuate line, with a greater number of anastomoses with the superficial system. The epigastric vessels send perforating vessels through the muscle in two rows, medial and lateral, to the overlying skin. These perforating vessels are of greatest density at the level of the umbilicus, and should therefore be included in the skin island of the pTRAM.

The blood supply to cutaneous portion of the TRAM from either rectus muscle is divided into four zones in order of decreasing perfusion. Zone I lies directly over top of the ipsilateral rectus muscle. Originally it was felt that zone II constituted the tissue directly across the midline, overlying the contralateral rectus muscle, with zone III lateral to the ipsilateral rectus, and zone IV in the same position contralaterally. It is now widely recognized that the tissue lateral to the ipsilateral rectus (traditionally zone III) has superior perfusion than the tissue directly across midline (zone II). As such, the ipsilateral hemiabdomen now is composed of zones I and II as well as the contralateral hemiabdomen zones III and IV (►**Fig. 21.2**).

Motor innervation to the rectus muscles is supplied segmentally by the lower six **intercostal nerves** that travel between internal oblique and transversus abdominis accompanied by their vascular pedicles. Cutaneous sensation is provided by T7, T8, and T9 above the umbilicus; T10 at the umbilicus; and T11, T12, and L1 below the umbilicus.

21.4 Variations

- Double/bipedicle TRAM:
  - Both rectus muscles used for one skin island.
  - Improves vascularity and allows more tissue to be transferred.
  - Consider if large volume is needed, or consider with risk factors (e.g., smokers, chest radiation, and abdominal scars impairing distal flow).
  - Additional donor site morbidity with potential for loss of abdominal wall strength and stability if both rectus mucles are harvested.
- Vascular delay (►**Fig. 21.3**):
  - Mechanism described by Taylor to recruit additional tissue that would otherwise undergo hypoxic injury.[3]
  - Hartrampf advocated use of delay in his original description of pTRAM as a means to improve reliability.

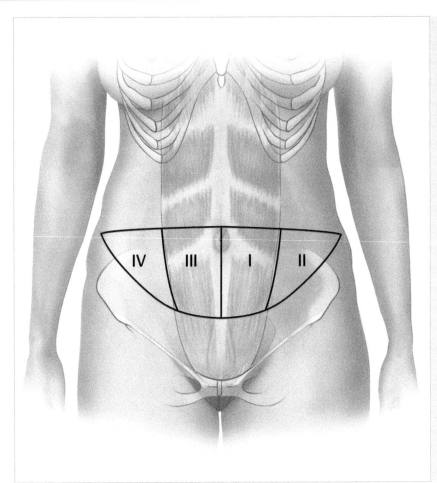

Fig. 21.2 Vascular zones of the pedicled myocutanious TRAM flap. (Adapted from Jones GE. Bostwick's Plastic and Reconstructive Breast Surgery, Third Edition. New York: Thieme Medical Publishers; 2010.)

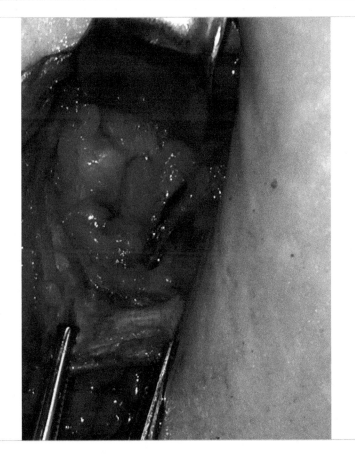

Fig. 21.3 Exposure of the deep inferior epigastric pedicle through a 5cm lower abdominal incision prior to ligation during flap delay procedure.

- Mustoe demonstrated that delay procedure improves tissue survival across a midline scar.[4]
- Performed 7 to 14 days prior to flap elevation.
- The DIEA/V is ligated through a small incision along the lower border of the planned skin island.
- Midabdominal TRAM:[5]
  - Inferior incision positioned at or just below umbilicus so that the skin transferred is supplied primarily by SEA with potential improved vascularity.
  - Theoretical improvement in abdominal wall integrity as the fascia below arcuate line not violated.
  - Consider in morbidly obese patients.
- Muscle-sparing TRAM.
- Free TRAM.

21.5 Preoperative Considerations

The optimal patients for pedicle TRAM breast reconstruction are nonsmokers with mild/moderate abdominal tissue requiring less than 1,000 g tissue. For a unipedicled TRAM, about 50% of the lower abdominal tissue can be harvested reliably. Patients requiring more tissue should be considered for one of the variations listed earlier to enhance flap viability.

Obesity, smoking, and prior chest radiation are associated with significantly increased risk of complications following pedicled TRAM. Abdominal obesity or pannus compromises blood flow to the flap and carries increased risk of partial flap loss. Also, because the pedicled TRAM is elevated on the nondominant system this procedure is not as reliable in smokers. Patients with significant cardiovascular or obstructive lung disease are not good candidates for pTRAM. Other considerations include history of lumbosacral disease, as sacrificing the rectus muscle is thought to exacerbate these conditions. In addition, because the abdominal site can only be used once, the risk of future disease in the opposite breast must be taken into consideration and discussed with the patient.

Abdominal scars that should raise concern for pedicle viability include subcostal scars from open cholecystectomy and paramedian scars. Vertical midline scars traditionally prevent use of tissue across the scar without the use of a bilateral pedicle. Interestingly, Mustoe demonstrated that some tissue across the scar can be harvested with the use of a delay procedure.[4] Suprapubic or Pfannenstiel incisions are inconsequential in terms of blood flow to the pedicled TRAM. All abdominal scars, however, should alert the surgeon to the possibility of scarring between the rectus muscle and peritoneal cavity that can complicate dissection.

21.6 Positioning and Skin Markings

Similar to planning a free TRAM or DIEP flap, the abdominal incisions are marked with the patient standing. The amount of redundant tissue and abdominal skin stretch is estimated. A transverse elliptical skin island is marked over the lower abdomen, extending from 2 cm above the umbilicus to the suprapubic crease in the midline and tapering to each ASIS laterally. The inferior incision should lie above the hair-bearing region of the pubis to avoid wound healing complications. The midline is marked both above the umbilicus and on the pubis to facilitate closure. The flap height should equal to the desired breast width.

In the operating room, the patient is positioned supine on a table that can be flexed to facilitate abdominal closure. Midline marks can be reinforced with staples.

21.7 Operative Technique

The superior incision is made first, beveling through subcutaneous fat to the abdominal wall fascia. The dissection then proceeds elevating the skin and fat over the abdominal wall fascia and muscles to the level of the xyphoid and costal margins. If desired, the patient can then be flexed to confirm the position of the suprapubic incision, avoiding excessive tension on abdominal skin closure. The inferior dissection proceeds straight down to the abdominal wall fascia and the skin flaps are elevated off the external oblique muscle and fascia from lateral to medial. This dissection proceeds rapidly using electrocautery until the lateral edge of the rectus muscle is encountered, and continued carefully until the lateral row of perforators are visualized. The umbilicus is then incised and dissected free on its stalk. Then, corresponding to the required flap dimensions, the skin island is divided and elevated on the contralateral side to expose the medial row of perforators (▶ Fig. 21.4).

The anterior rectus sheath is then incised medially and laterally along its length preserving a 1 to 2 cm cuff of fascia on either side. This leaves a 2 to 4 cm strip of anterior sheath attached to the rectus cranial to the skin paddle. The muscle is then exposed and dissected from the posterior rectus fascia. The DIEVs are identified at the lateral edge of the rectus muscle, two-thirds of the way inferior between the umbilicus and pubic symphysis. If the patient did not undergo a delay procedure, these vessels are then ligated as proximally

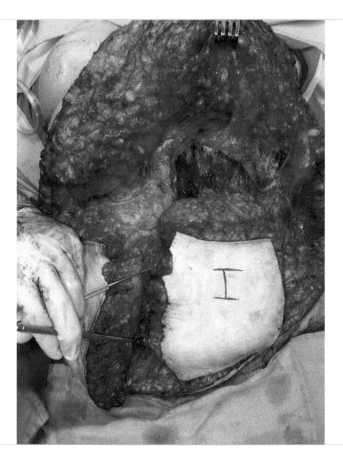

Fig. 21.4 Intraoperative image of lower abdominal skin and adipose tissue island isolated on rectus muscle.

as possible to preserve length for possible microanastamosis (supercharge) in case of vascular compromise. Intercostal neurovascular bundles are cauterized or ligated (▶ **Fig. 21.5**).

Using electrocautery, the muscle is divided distally and the skin paddle secured to the underlying muscle using a sutures to avoid avulsion. The musculocutaneous unit is then elevated to the costal margin. For breast reconstruction, the musculocutaneous unit is most commonly contralateral to the mastectomy defect, but may also be ipsilateral. Ipsilateral design may lead to decreased epigastric bulging. A subcutaneous tunnel approximately four fingerbreadths in width is made, and the flap is carefully fed through into the mastectomy defect. Passage of a large flap can be aided by placing the entire unit in a sterile plastic bag for transfer (▶ **Fig. 21.6**). A right flap is rotated counterclockwise approximately 180 degrees through the tunnel so that the lateral edge of zone II lies in the lateral aspect of the defect. Similarly, a left flap is rotated clockwise.

The muscular pedicle is then inspected for any kinking (▶ **Fig. 21.7**). It may be necessary to incise rectus fascia and release lateral rectus fibers over the costal margin to relieve potential compromise to the pedicle from rotation. The flap is then circumferentially deepithelialized and inset to match the contralateral breast mound.

21.8 Donor Site Closure

The fascial defect is repaired using the surgeon's preferred suture, such as a looped 0 permanent or long-term resorbable monofilament suture in a running locking fashion, ensuring at least 1 cm bites of fascia are taken. If there

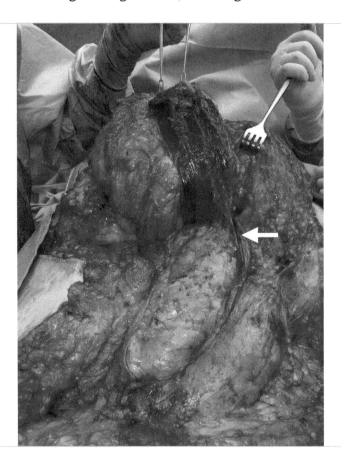

Fig. 21.5 Elevated pTRAM flap showing the eighth intercostal artery *(white arrow)* entering the rectus muscle. In situations where the IMA has been divided, this minor pedicle can provide retrograde flow to the pTRAM via anastamoses with the SEA.

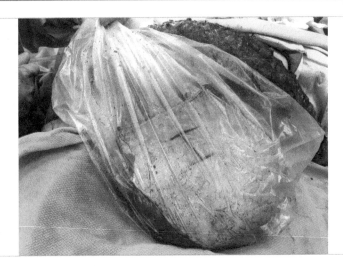

Fig. 21.6 Once elevated, large flaps can be placed in a sterile bag for passage into the mastectomy defect. This facilitates transport through the subcutaneous tunnel and protects the skin paddle from avulsion.

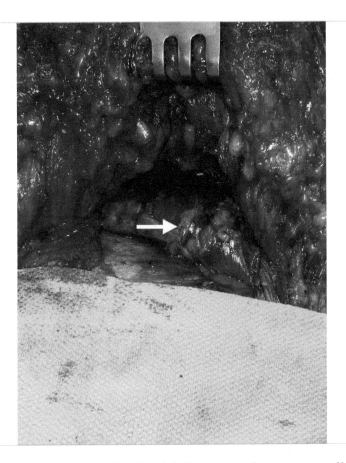

Fig. 21.7 The superior epigastric artery pedicle *(white arrow)* can be visualized on the deep surface of the rectus after the flap has been rotated into the mastectomy defect.

is tension on the fascial closure or the suture pulls through, then use of mesh is indicated. Some surgeons routinely choose to reinforce the donor defects with mesh. Two closed suction drains are placed exiting through the lateral corners of the incision or separate stab incisions, and the abdominal wall closed in layers in the surgeon's preferred method. The authors use 2–0 resoluble suture in Scarpa's fascia, followed by 3–0 absorbable suture inverted dermal sutures and a final layer of 4–0 resoluble sutures running subcuticular sutures if required.

An incision is made in the position of the neoumbilicus through which the umbilical stalk is retrieved and inset with 4–0 absorbable buried sutures and interrupted 5–0 permanent monofilament skin sutures.

21.9 Pearls and Pitfalls

- Consider delay procedure in patients with comorbidities, or where more than 50% of lower abdominal tissue required. Ensure division of the DIEA as proximal to take off from iliac as possible to preserve DIEA pedicle length for potential supercharging.
- Some degree of venous congestion occurs in many pedicled flaps initially but typically resolves over 24 hours.
- In cases where the IMA has been divided, the flap can survive via retrograde flow through the eighth intercostal artery.
- There is low risk of total flap loss, but higher risk of fat necrosis or partial flap loss as compared to free TRAM or DIEP flaps.
- In flaps that appear vascularly compromised, supercharging of the DIEA/V to the thoracodorsal vessels can be a salvage option.

References

[1] Hartrampf CR, Scheflan M, Black PW. Breast reconstruction with a transverse abdominal island flap. Plast Reconstr Surg 1982;69(2):216–225

[2] Moon HK, Taylor GI. The vascular anatomy of rectus abdominis musculocutaneous flaps based on the deep superior epigastric system. Plast Reconstr Surg 1988;82(5):815–832

[3] Taylor GI, Corlett RJ, Caddy CM, Zelt RG; Clinical Applications. An anatomic review of the delay phenomenon: II. Clinical applications. Plast Reconstr Surg 1992;89(3):408–416, discussion 417–418

[4] O'Shaughnessy KD, Mustoe TA. The surgical TRAM flap delay: reliability of zone III using a simplified technique under local anesthesia. Plast Reconstr Surg 2008;122(6):1627–1630

[5] Slavin SA, Goldwyn RM. The midabdominal rectus abdominis myocutaneous flap: review of 236 flaps. Plast Reconstr Surg 1988;81(2):189–199

22 Deep Inferior Epigastric Perforator Flap

Liza C. Wu

Abstract

The deep inferior epigastric perforator flap is a viable option for breast reconstruction and is a skin and subcutaneous tissue free flap over the lower abdomen. It was designed to spare the rectus muscle and fascia entirely, thus decreasing the abdominal donor site morbidity encountered with the transverse rectus abdominus myocutaneous flap. Because of its reliable anatomy, preferred donor site, and low donor site morbidity, the deep inferior epigastric perforator flap has become the preferred method for autologous breast reconstruction. This chapter takes the surgeon through the sequential and logical steps involved in the procedure, from initial indications, to anatomy, to preoperative considerations, to operative technique, to donor site closure. Four variations also come in for discussion.

Keywords: Adipocutaneous, deep inferior epigastric artery, stacked flaps

22.1 Introduction

The deep inferior epigastric perforator (DIEP) flap was first described by Koshima and Soeda in 1989 and further popularized by Allen for breast reconstruction.[1,2] The DIEP flap is a skin and subcutaneous tissue free flap over the lower abdomen. It was designed to spare the rectus muscle and fascia entirely, decreasing the abdominal donor site morbidity encountered with the transverse rectus abdominus myocutaneous (TRAM) flap. Because of the reliable anatomy, preferred donor site, and low donor site morbidity, the DIEP flap has become the preferred method for autologous breast reconstruction.

22.2 Typical Indications

- Breast reconstruction.
- Soft-tissue defects of the head and neck, trunk, and extremities.

22.3 Anatomy

The DIEP flap is an adipocutaneous flap supplied by the deep inferior epigastric artery perforators, which are usually located within a 5-cm radius from the umbilicus.

The **deep inferior epigastric artery** originates from the medial aspect of the external iliac artery just proximal to the inguinal ligament. It courses anterior to the peritoneum below the arcuate line and enters the rectus muscle compartment from the posterolateral border of the rectus muscle. The deep inferior epigastric artery then most commonly divides into two branches that give off perforating vessels to the muscle and skin via a medial and lateral row (►Fig. 22.1).

The perforators may assume a musculocutaneous or an extramuscular course. After entering the rectus abdominis muscle, musculocutaneous perforators may follow a short transverse course, a long transverse course, or a directly perpendicular course. Lateral row perforators are more frequently perpendicular, whereas

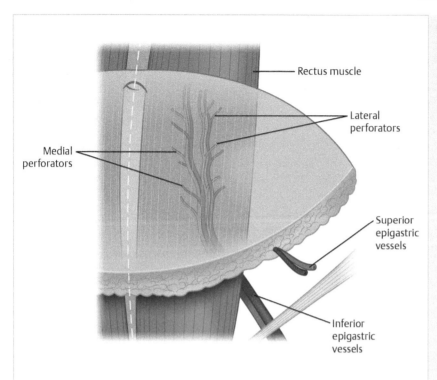

Fig. 22.1 Deep inferior epigastric artery then most commonly divides into two branches that give off perforating vessels to the muscle and skin via a medial and lateral row.

medial row perforators tend to exhibit a longer intramuscular course. Less muscle dissection will be necessary the shorter the intramuscular course of the perforator. Extramuscular perforators may follow a paramedian or a tendinous course, allowing for a faster dissection and little muscle disruption.[3]

It is important to note that the medial and lateral rows form a substantial vascular network in the subdermal plexus with medial row perforators branching medially to form anastomoses across the midline and lateral row perforators rarely extending across the midline.

The venous drainage occurs through perforator venae comitantes that drain into two inferior epigastric veins that unite and drain into the external iliac vein. It's important to note, however, that the dominant venous drainage of the anterior abdominal wall can be through the superficial epigastric venous system can be disrupted during DIEP flap harvest.

A sensory branch arising from the intercostal nerves may be isolated as it joins the perforating vessels where they perforate the anterior rectus fascia. This may be dissected distally along with the perforator dissection and elevated with the flap for sensory innervation.

22.4 Variations

- For cases where large volume is needed, a double-pedicle DIEP flap may be harvested in continuity or as "stacked" flaps.
- Inguinal lymph nodes based on the superficial circumflex iliac vessels may be harvested with the DIEP flap for treatment of upper extremity lymphedema.
- In thin patients, DIEP flaps may be used together with breast implants for increased volume.
- The DIEP flap may be designed in a vertical fashion and based on single perforators to cover small soft-tissue defects.

22.5 Preoperative Considerations

Preoperative imaging may be obtained, although not advocated by all, by way of computed tomography angiography (CTA) or magnetic resonance angiography (MRA) to aid in information concerning the location, course, caliber, and flow of the perforating vessels. The data can then be brought together in a surgical road map that will determine an intraoperative strategy in terms of choosing and dissecting the perforators and vascular pedicle.[4]

In patients with previous abdominal surgeries, the DIEP flap may be precluded due to potential injury to perforating vessels and/or the pedicle. In these cases, imaging is warranted to ensure presence of inferior epigastric perforators.

22.6 Positioning and Skin Markings

The markings are made with the patient in a standing position following standard TRAM guidelines. Superiorly, the markings extend just above the umbilicus centrally and join the lateral markings lateral to the anterior superior iliac spine (ASIS). The inferior marking extends from the pubic crease centrally tapering in an elliptical fashion laterally to end over the iliac crest lateral to the ASIS.

The patient is positioned in the supine position with appropriate padding for pressure points, sequential compression devices are applied. The arms may be kept out or in a tucked position. If preoperative imaging was obtained, the perforators may be marked on the skin with a marking pen. Before prepping and draping the operating table should be tested to ensure that it flexes at the waist, this will be necessary at the time of closure to decrease the tension on the incision line.

22.7 Operative Technique

Refer to Video 22.1 for an example of the operative technique for the deep inferior epigastric perforator flap. The upper abdominal incision is made following the surgical markings. The superior abdominal skin flap is raised to ensure closure prior to making the inferior incision. The inferior incision is made and special care is taken to identify and preserve 5 cm of length of any superficial inferior epigastric vein in case the venous drainage of the DIEP is inadequate through the deep system.

The flap is raised from lateral to medial and medial to lateral in the suprafascial plane until the perforators are encountered overlying the rectus muscle. It is important to identify the perforator topography of the lower abdomen to determine the best perforator to base the DIEP flap (▶ Fig. 22.2a). Once the perforators are defined, careful consideration is given to choose the best perforator or perforators to support the amount of tissue to be transferred. Guidelines to choose a single perforator flap are loosely based on the 1.5 mm palpable artery and a 2 mm vein unless multiple perforators are included in the flap. When the best perforator(s) is chosen, the anterior rectus sheath is incised along the trajectory from the inferolateral border of the rectus muscle toward the particular neurovascular bundle. If more than one perforator will be taken with the flap, the anterior rectus sheath is opened in line with the perforators to be dissected. The pedicle is dissected out to the origin from the external iliac vessels. The perforator dissection is performed by releasing the fascia surrounding the perforator and then dissecting the muscle and branches from the perforator retrograde toward the pedicle. The vessels are followed within the muscle and the muscle is carefully split in

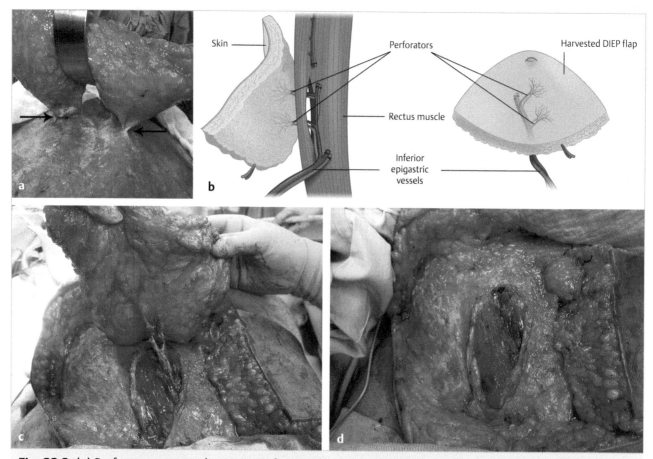

Fig. 22.2 **(a)** Perforator topography. Main perforators have been dissected (*black arrows*). One medial perforator on the right side of the patient and one medial and one lateral perforator on the left. **(b)** Diagram of perforator dissection and DIEP flap based on two perforators in same line, facilitating the dissection and minimizing injury to the muscle. **(c)** DIEP flap based on two perforators, form lateral and medial rows. **(d)** Donor site following DIEP flap harvest. Note the defect on the anterior rectus sheath on both sides. Muscles are preserved. A polypropelene mesh may or may not be used to reinforce closure, either as an underlay or onlay mesh of the anterior rectus sheath.

the direction of its fibers to expose the deep inferior epigastric pedicle. Small side branches of the pedicle are ligated with vascular clips or carefully coagulated with electrocautery to avoid any bleeding into the operating field. Once the pedicle is fully exposed and the desired length is achieved, the vessels are ligated proximally and then distally with vascular clips and the flap is harvested (▶ **Fig. 22.2b–d**).

Branches of the intercostal nerves that pass anterior to the pedicle should be left intact to avoid denervating the muscle medially, thus optimizing muscle function postoperatively.

Pure sensory nerves running with the perforators can often be dissected for several centimeters for innervation of the skin island.

22.8 Donor Site Closure

The anterior rectus fascia is closed primarily with nonabsorbable sutures. A polypropelene mesh may or may not be used to reinforce closure, either as an underlay or onlay mesh of the anterior rectus sheath. A bridged mesh repair may be needed in some cases depending on the amount of muscle sacrificed, amount of fascia taken, or the number of nerves divided.

The abdominal wound is closed in layers, with absorbable suture, and the umbilicus is reinset in its proper position, much like an abdominoplasty procedure.

22.9 Pearls and Pitfalls

- The superficial epigastric vein should be dissected for 3 to 7 cm and saved. This vein can be anastomosed to the deep inferior epigastric vein or to an additional recipient vein to augment venous drainage when necessary.[5]
- If the patient has had previous abdominal surgeries, there is a risk that the inferior epigastric vessels or its perforators may have been injured. In this case, imaging studies such as CTA or MRA should be obtained. Previous Pfannenstiel incisions will generally not cause injury to the inferior epigastric vessels.
- Branches of the intercostal nerves should be left intact to avoid denervating the rectus muscle.

References

[1] Koshima I, Soeda S. Inferior epigastric artery skin flaps without rectus abdominis muscle. Br J Plast Surg 1989;42(6):645–648

[2] Allen RJ, Treece P. Deep inferior epigastric perforator flap for breast reconstruction. Ann Plast Surg 1994;32(1):32–38

[3] Ireton JE, Lakhiani C, Saint-Cyr M. Vascular anatomy of the deep inferior epigastric artery perforator flap: a systematic review. Plast Reconstr Surg 2014;134(5):810e–821e

[4] Selber JC, Serletti JM. The deep inferior epigastric perforator flap: myth and reality. Plast Reconstr Surg 2010;125(1):50–58

[5] Sbitany H, Mirzabeigi MN, Kovach SJ, Wu LC, Serletti JM. Strategies for recognizing and managing intraoperative venous congestion in abdominally based autologous breast reconstruction. Plast Reconstr Surg 2012;129(4):809–815

23 Superficial Inferior Epigastric Artery Flap

Gordon K. Lee and Laurence S. Paek

Abstract

The superficial inferior epigastric artery flap is a lower abdominal wall flap used as a free flap for facial reconstruction. It can provide the same results as the transverse rectus abdominis myocutaneous, muscle-sparing transverse rectus abdominis myocutaneous, and deep inferior epigastric perforator flaps, but involves less extensive dissection. The superficial inferior epigastric artery flap does not require opening the rectus sheath or dissection of the rectus abdominis muscles, thereby completely preserving the strength and integrity of the abdominal wall. In autologous free flap breast reconstruction, this flap is applied less frequently than other abdominal-based free flaps, mainly due to the variable presence and caliber of the superficial inferior epigastric artery. While this flap is largely used as a free flap most commonly for breast reconstruction, it can also be used as a pedicled flap for reconstruction of local defects around the thigh, pubic region, and abdominal wall. In this chapter, the authors walk the surgeon through each critical step in the procedure, beginning with initial indications and followed by anatomy, preoperative considerations, and operative technique. Augmenting the discussion is the listing of three variations to the standard procedure.

Keywords: deep inferior epigastric artery, superficial circumflex iliac artery, deep circumflex iliac artery, superior epigastric artery, intercostal arteries, anterior superior iliac spine, superficial inferior epigastric vein, 10th to 12th intercostal nerves

23.1 Introduction

The **superficial inferior epigastric artery** (SIEA) flap is a lower abdominal wall flap, first described in 1971 by Antia and Buch as a free flap for facial reconstruction. In 1979, Holmström performed the first breast reconstruction using a SIEA free flap. The SIEA flap can provide the same results as the transverse rectus abdominis myocutaneous (TRAM), muscle-sparing TRAM (MS-TRAM), and deep inferior epigastric perforator (DIEP) flaps, but involves less extensive dissection. The SIEA does not require opening of the rectus sheath or dissection of the rectus abdominis muscles, thereby completely preserving the strength and integrity of the abdominal wall.[1] In autologous free flap breast reconstruction, this flap is applied less frequently than the TRAM, MS-TRAM, and DIEP flaps, mostly due to the variable presence and caliber of the SIEA.[2,3,4] While the SIEA flap is largely used as a free flap, most commonly for breast reconstruction, it can also be raised as a pedicled flap for reconstruction of local defects around the thigh, pubic region, and abdominal wall.

23.2 Typical Indications

- Autologous breast reconstruction.
- Penile or vaginal reconstruction.
- Head and neck reconstruction.
- Coverage (usually as a pedicled flap) of
  - Upper and lower extremity defects.
  - Contralateral abdominal defects.
  - Groin and perineum defects.

23.3 Anatomy

The blood supply of the lower abdominal wall is a network of arteries and veins originating from the SIEA, **deep inferior epigastric artery** (DIEA), **superficial and deep circumflex iliac arteries**, the **superior epigastric artery**, and the **intercostal arteries** (▶Fig. 23.1). While the DIEP and TRAM flap tissue is vascularized by the musculocutaneous perforators of the DIEA, the SIEA is an adipocutaneous flap vascularized by a pedicle with a subcutaneous course.

The difficulty in using the SIEA flap lies in the unpredictable anatomy of the vessels first documented by Taylor and Daniel in 1975.[2] Several variations of the SIEA vessels have been described in anatomical studies.[3,4,5,6] Overall, the SIEA has been shown to be present in approximately 58% of clinical dissections; on computed tomographic angiography (CTA), it may be detected up to 94% of the time.[2,3,4] The diameter of the SIEA ranges from 0.3 to 3.1 mm.[2,3,4,5] It is estimated that the SIEA can suitably support a flap in 24 and 31% of patients; many surgeons seek a SIEA diameter of 1.5 mm or greater when considering harvesting this flap.[3,4]

The SIEA most often originates from the common femoral artery, approximately 2 to 3 cm below the inguinal ligament.[1,2,3,4] It most often arises from a common trunk with the superficial circumflex artery. Less commonly, it may arise as a side branch of the deep femoral artery or pudendal artery. After piercing the deep fascia at its origin, the SIEA crosses the inguinal ligament and lies deep to Scarpa's fascia. As it courses toward the umbilicus, the SIEA eventually pierces Scarpa's fascia and is located subcutaneously. The SIEA crosses the inguinal ligament at the midpoint between the **anterior superior iliac spine** (ASIS) and pubic symphysis.[5] Venous drainage of the SIEA flap is usually provided by the **superficial inferior epigastric vein** (SIEV) or the associated venae comitantes.[2,3,4,5] The SIEV is located superficial and medial to the SIEA. The pedicle length of this flap ranges from 4 to 8 cm.[1,5]

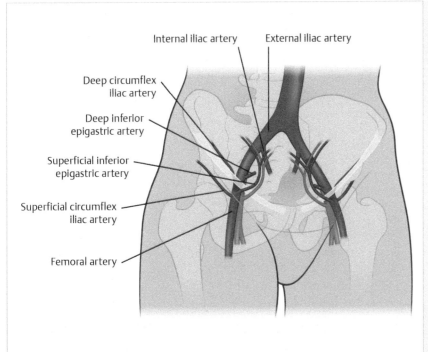

Fig. 23.1 Arterial anatomy of the lower abdominal skin and subcutaneous adipose tissue.

Internal iliac artery

External iliac artery

Deep circumflex iliac artery

Deep inferior epigastric artery

Superficial inferior epigastric artery

Superficial circumflex iliac artery

Femoral artery

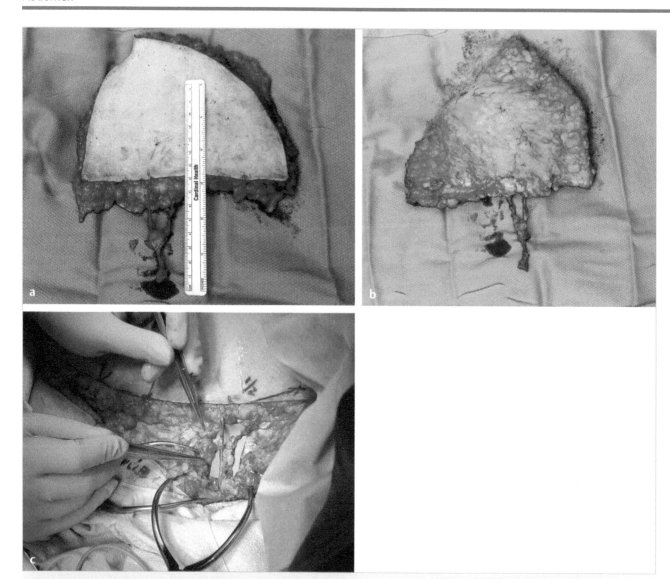

Fig. 23.2 (a, b) A dissected SIEA flap with a pedicle length of approximately 8 cm. Note that this flap includes only ipsilateral abdominal tissue. **(c)** The location of the SIEA is approximately at the midpoint of the ASIS and pubic symphysis and may be superficial (or deep) to Scarpa's fascia. The SIEV is found medial and superficial to the artery.

The SIEA flap may be raised with a sensory component via the **10th to 12th intercostal nerves**. However, the flap is rarely harvested as a sensory flap, since this typically requires an intramuscular dissection (▶ **Fig. 23.2**).[1,2,3,4,5]

23.4 Variations

- Double pedicled using SIEA/SIEA or SIEA/DIEP.
- Unilateral or bilateral.
- The flap can be harvest using the SIEV or the venae comitantes as venous drainage.

23.5 Preoperative Considerations

Contraindications for the SIEA flap include previous abdominoplasty, a long Pfannenstiel scar that transects the SIEA, or any other abdominal scar that would cut across the course of the SIEA. Relative contraindications would include prior abdominal liposuction and/or active smoking, which may lead to a higher incidence of partial flap or fat necrosis.

Vascular imaging (i.e., ultrasound or CTA) can be used preoperatively to assess the size and location of the vessels, but is not routinely used by the senior author. As a consequence of its inherent anatomic variation, the suitability of the SIEA should be evaluated intraoperatively.

Importantly, the SIEA typically only reliably perfuses the ipsilateral hemiabdomen with the possibility of very limited extension across the midline depending on the course and caliber of the SIEA.[3,6] This should be taken into account when assessing the abdominal wall in being able to adequately reconstitute the desired volume for breast reconstruction. When more than the hemiabdomen is needed, either bilateral SIEA flaps or a combination of an SIEA and another abdominal flap, such as a contralateral DIEP flap, is used.

23.6 Positioning and Skin Markings

Preoperative markings are performed with the patient in the upright position. The ASISs and midline are marked. Optionally, the expected locations of the SIEAs, SIEVs, and DIEAs may be delineated on both hemiabdomens. The lower incision marking for the SIEA flap should be as low as possible in order to increase the chance of finding an SIEA of adequate diameter, typically, just above the pubic hairline, at least 5 to 7 cm above the vulvar commissure, and may extend just past the ASIS bilaterally. If abdominal skin laxity permits, the upper abdominal incision line is drawn just above the umbilicus and joins the inferior marking with a gentle curve. The level of the superior marking should be adjusted as necessary in order to avoid excess tension on closure (▶ **Fig. 23.3**).

23.7 Operative Technique

Patients with a SIEA of approximately 1.5 mm or greater diameter should be considered potentially suitable candidates for the SIEA flap. There is a significantly higher chance of thrombosis with SIEAs of smaller diameter.[4] Optimally, two teams can simultaneously perform the surgery: one team operating on the donor site and the other team preparing the recipient site.

The flap elevation starts with the inferior incision. The SIEV on the side(s) of interest is typically encountered first and is located more superficially; caution is advised when dissecting the subcutaneous layer in order to avoid damage to this vessel. Following the identification of the SIEV, the SIEA and its

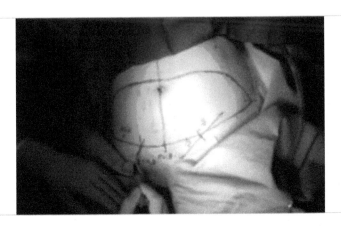

Fig. 23.3 Standard markings for the SIEA flap. The approximate location of the SIEA, which is found halfway between the ASIS and pubic symphysis, is marked on the skin.

two venae comitantes are identified. At the level of the inferior incision, the SIEA is typically located deep and lateral with respect to the SIEV and may be above or below Scarpa's fascia. Subsequently, the vessels are dissected and the diameter is assessed. Complete elevation of the flap tissue from the abdominal wall fascia should not be carried out until adequate caliber of both the SIEV and SIEA is confirmed; in those cases where the SIEA is unsuitable, a DIEP or MS-TRAM flap should be elevated. In cases of sufficient diameter, the SIEA and SIEV may be isolated using vessel loops and dissection performed caudally toward their origins. A Gelpi retractor may facilitate this dissection through the inferior suprapubic fat. The dissection should be done until vessel diameter is satisfactory and sufficient pedicle length is reached, which is typically near its origin from the femoral vessels. Side branches are coagulated or ligated. If lymph nodes from the groin superficial lymphatic system are encountered, they should be left in situ. If the ability of a given SIEA vessel to supply the flap is questionable, DIEA perforators can be left intact and temporarily clamped to observe the perfusion of the flap by the SIEA.[1] This strategy allows conversion to a DIEP flap if necessary.

Next, the upper incision is made down to the abdominal wall. At this time, the upper abdominal flap may be raised up to the xiphoid process with limited lateral dissection in preparation for eventual donor site closure. The umbilicus is also separated from the abdominal flap tissue while making sure to leave a cuff of tissue around its stalk to avoid devascularizing it. If bilateral SIEA flaps are planned, a midline incision between the two hemiabdominal flaps is then performed. The flap(s) are then elevated from the abdominal wall, with meticulous hemostasis, from lateral to medial. Once the recipient site exposure is complete, the SIEA flap pedicle is divided and stabilized at the recipient site in preparation for the requisite microanastomoses. Importantly, in the context of autologous breast reconstruction and internal mammary vessel recipients, the contralateral hemiabdomen is generally preferred due to the favorable orientation of the SIEA/SIEV and internal mammary vessels. Care should be taken when positioning the flap at the recipient site in order to prevent pedicle kinking or tension. The SIEA pedicle is overall shorter, more superficial, and laterally located in comparison to the DIEA, which increases the difficulty of flap inset (▶ **Fig. 23.4**).

23.8 Donor Site Closure

The patient is flexed during closure in order to minimize tension. The elevated upper abdominal flap is then pulled caudally and temporarily fixed to the

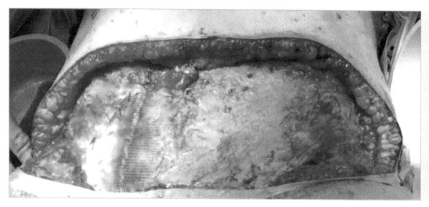

Fig. 23.4 Intraoperative donor site defect following bilateral abdominal-based flap harvest. On the left hemiabdomen, a SIEA flap was harvested with the full integrity of the abdominal wall preserved. On the right side, an MS-TRAM flap was raised. Note that fascial closure and onlay Prolene mesh placement was performed in order to reinforce the donor site on this side.

inferior incision with staples. The eventual location of the umbilicus is then marked and two 19 French Blake drains are placed and brought out through the skin in the suprapubic area. Closure is executed in layers with the Scarpa's layer closed with 2–0 absorbable suture and the dermal layers with 3–0 absorbable suture. Lastly, a 3–0 monfilament absorbable suture is used for subcuticular closure. Notably, the SIEA flap obviates the need for rectus sheath closure since it is not violated during the procedure. The umbilicus is then brought out and secured in place with absorbable sutures.

23.9 Pearls and Pitfalls

- Due to the high variability in anatomy of the SIEA flap pedicle, it is not a viable option in all patients.
- The SIEA unreliably supplies the contralateral hemiabdomen. As such, great caution should be taken and serial intraoperative evaluation should be performed when considering inclusion of flap tissue more than 2 cm lateral to the midline on the contralateral side.
- The inset can be more challenging than other abdominal-based free flaps since the SIEA pedicle is shorter and located more laterally and superficially as compared to the DIEP flap.
- SIEA flap dissection is less extensive and causes substantially less donor site morbidity than the TRAM and DIEP flaps.
- In breast reconstruction, after the microanastomoses are performed, the risk of pedicle traction and avulsion can be reduced by securing the flap with a few absorbable sutures from scarpa's fascia down to the chest wall.

References

[1] Hall-Findlay EJ, Evans GRD, Kim KK. Aesthetic and Reconstructive Surgery of the Breast. 1st ed. Philadelphia, PA: Elsevier; 2010:147–159
[2] Taylor GI, Daniel RK. The anatomy of several free flap donor sites. Plast Reconstr Surg 1975;56(3):243–253
[3] Rozen WM, Chubb D, Grinsell D, Ashton MW. The variability of the Superficial Inferior Epigastric Artery (SIEA) and its angiosome: a clinical anatomical study. Microsurgery 2010;30(5):386–391
[4] Spiegel AJ, Khan FN. An Intraoperative algorithm for use of the SIEA flap for breast reconstruction. Plast Reconstr Surg 2007;120(6):1450–1459
[5] Wei F-C, Mardini S. Flaps and Reconstructive Surgery. 1st ed. Philadelphia, PA: Elsevier; 2009:501–617
[6] Holm C, Mayr M, Höfter E, Ninkovic M. The versatility of the SIEA flap: a clinical assessment of the vascular territory of the superficial epigastric inferior artery. J Plast Reconstr Aesthet Surg 2007;60(8):946–951

24 Vertical Rectus Abdominis Myocutaneous Flap Free/Pedicled Flap

Christopher A. Campbell

Abstract

The vertical rectus abdominis myocutaneous flap is an abdominally based soft-tissue flap with a skin paddle oriented vertically over the epigastric perforators that arborize through the rectus abdominis muscle. Due to its dual blood supply involving the superior and inferior epigastric systems, this flap has been described as a pedicled flap for chest wall and sternal reconstruction and for abdominal, perineal, and vaginal reconstruction, respectively. The vertical rectus abdominis myocutaneous flap has been instrumental in improving outcomes after oncologic pelvic resections due to its significant bulk, which obliterates pelvic dead space and a skin paddle of sufficient size to allow for partial or total vaginal reconstruction. The rectus abdominis muscle's length, combined with an extended skin paddle design, allow the inferiorly based flap to be used in a transpelvic manner to reach sacrectomy defects as well. The vertical rectus abdominis myocutaneous is most commonly used as a pedicled flap, but due to its ease of pedicle dissection and reliable anatomy, it is also used as a free flap for upper extremity, lower extremity, and head and neck reconstruction. In this chapter, the author lays out the considerations surgeons encounter in the use of this flap including typical indications, anatomy, preoperative considerations, and operative technique. Two variations to the common procedure are also mentioned.

Keywords: linea alba, linea semilunaris, arcuate line, deep inferior epigastric artery, superior epigastric artery, eighth intercostal vessels, 7th through 12th intercostal motor and sensory nerves

24.1 Introduction

The vertical rectus abdominis myocutaneous (VRAM) flap is an abdominally based soft-tissue flap with a skin paddle oriented vertically over the epigastric perforators that arborize through the rectus abdominis muscle. Due to its dual blood supply involving the superior and inferior epigastric systems, the VRAM has been described as a pedicled flap for chest wall and sternal reconstruction and for abdominal, perineal, and vaginal reconstruction, respectively.[1,2,3] The VRAM flap has been instrumental in improving outcomes after oncologic pelvic resections due to its significant bulk which obliterates pelvic dead space and a skin paddle of sufficient size to allow for partial or total vaginal reconstruction.[4] The rectus abdominis muscle's length combined with an extended skin paddle design allow the inferiorly based VRAM to be passed in a transpelvic manner to reach sacrectomy defects as well. The VRAM is most commonly used as a pedicled flap, but due to its ease of pedicle dissection and reliable anatomy, it is also used as a free flap for upper extremity, lower extremity, and head and neck reconstruction.[4]

24.2 Typical Indications

- Based on the superior epigastric artery:
  - Sternal and chest wall defects after cardiac surgery requiring muscle to fill the mediastinum and a skin paddle to resurface the chest.
- Based on the deep inferior epigastric artery:
  - Pelvic defects after pelvic exenteration or abdominoperineal resection (APR) requiring significant soft-tissue bulk to fill the pelvic dead space and a skin paddle for resurfacing of the perineum and/or vagina.
  - Sacrectomy defects with transpelvic passage of the skin paddle, often with an extended or oblique skin pattern design.
  - Free flap option for breast/chest wall, extremity, or head and neck reconstruction after oncologic resection or trauma.

24.3 Anatomy

The rectus abdominis muscle is a vertically oriented rectangularly shaped series of four muscle bellies linked together by tendinous inscriptions extending from the costal margin to the pubic bone (▶ Fig. 24.1). The rectus muscle is bordered medially by the **linea alba** at midline and the **linea semilunaris** laterally and is encased within the anterior and posterior rectus fascial sheaths. Above the **arcuate line**, the rectus fascia is composed of tough anterior and posterior sheaths that encase the rectus muscle circumferentially. Below the arcuate line, the anterior sheath is bilaminate—composed of both the anterior and posterior fascial elements, leaving only the transversalis fascia separating the posterior surface of the rectus muscle from the preperitoneal fat. In patients with diastasis recti the rectus muscles will have translated laterally resulting in the fusion of the anterior and posterior rectus fascial sheaths medially.

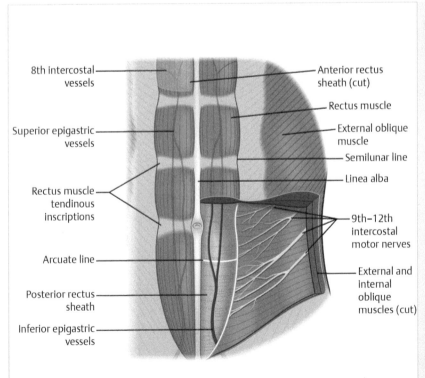

Fig. 24.1 Rectus abdominis muscle fascial and neurovascular anatomy.

8th intercostal vessels

Superior epigastric vessels

Rectus muscle tendinous inscriptions

Arcuate line

Posterior rectus sheath

Inferior epigastric vessels

Anterior rectus sheath (cut)

Rectus muscle

External oblique muscle

Semilunar line

Linea alba

9th–12th intercostal motor nerves

External and internal oblique muscles (cut)

The rectus abdominis muscle has a dual blood supply consisting of the **deep inferior epigastric artery** and its paired venae comitantes entering the posterior surface of the lowest muscle belly of the rectus muscle, and the **superior epigastric artery** (a continuation of the internal mammary artery that emerges from beneath the costal margin) and its paired venae comitantes that enter the substance of the most superior muscle belly. The **eighth intercostal vessels** are a known contributor to the superior epigastric pedicle and provide collateral flow in the event the internal mammary system has been harvested for cardiothoracic indications. The inferior epigastric pedicle is used as the flap's vascular pedicle when the VRAM is rotated inferiorly and for free flap applications, while the superior epigastric system is used as the pedicle when the VRAM is rotated superiorly toward the chest.

The nerve supply of the rectus abdominis consists of the **7th through 12th intercostal motor and sensory nerves** that enter the muscle bellies laterally. The nerves travel beneath the internal oblique muscle on their way to the lateral edge of the rectus abdominis muscle. These nerve branches and minor vascular pedicles that travel with them are divided during flap harvest. The sensory branches of the 7th through 12th intercostal nerves course through the skin paddle of the VRAM from lateral to medial and are also divided during flap harvest.

24.4 Variations

- Extended skin paddle design by extending the skin paddle to the anterior axillary line parallel to the costal orientation.[4]
- Fascial-sparing flap harvesting technique includes only the anterior rectus sheath of the inferior epigastric perforator zone sparing all other medial and lateral fascia to assist with abdominal wall closure.[4]

24.5 Preoperative Considerations

In obese patients, the skin paddle may be excessively thick requiring significant flap thinning depending on the needs of the recipient site. Thinning of the VRAM can be performed safely as the epigastric perforators pass through the rectus muscle and arborize superficially within the subcutaneous tissue overlying the perforator zone. In male patients and women with an android pelvic configuration, the pelvic inlet is quite narrow which may make passage of the VRAM for pelvic reconstruction difficult, requiring thinning of the flap or selection of an alternate myocutaneous flap or the omentum to obliterate the potential pelvic space.[5]

For patients who have had many prior operations, visual identification of the perforator zone and subsequently fascial-sparing harvest may be difficult requiring a larger surface area of anterior rectus sheath to be taken with the flap. Similarly, patients with hernias or prior hernia repairs may require abdominal wall reconstruction consisting of component separation and biologic mesh repair.[4] Patients who have had prior abdominal or cardiac surgery may have had the pedicles of the VRAM sacrificed. This should be confirmed before flap elevation by angiography or by starting the dissection with exploration of the pedicle.

For patients who will require a larger skin paddle for reconstruction or have a defect farther away from the abdominal wall, an extended skin paddle can be designed to give greater reach and more flap skin surface area when utilizing a pedicled VRAM flap for reconstruction.

24.6 Positioning and Skin Markings

The patient is placed in the supine position for flap harvest. If the VRAM is being used for vaginal or perineal reconstruction, the patient's legs are placed in the lithotomy position. A vertical midline incision is planned along the linea alba with the umbilical semicircle marking placed on the side of planned flap harvest. The lateral extent of the VRAM's skin paddle should be measured before any incisions are made. With the surgeon standing at the patient's side across from the planned VRAM harvest site, place both thumbs on the linea alba and fingers on the lateral skin of the abdominal wall and roll the excess skin over the laterally advancing thumbs. Have an assistant mark where the lateral skin crosses the thumb tips. This should yield a VRAM skin paddle with a convexly curved lateral mark accompanying the vertical midline marking and containing the local perforators from the epigastric system. The cutaneous epigastric perforator zone extends on average 6 cm above to 6 cm below the umbilicus and 2 cm lateral to the linea alba to 6 cm lateral to the linea alba (▶ Fig. 24.2a).

To design an extended skin paddle VRAM, an additional superior aspect to the skin paddle is created that extends to the fifth costal interspace, parallels the costal orientation and laterally reaches to the anterior axillary line (▶ Fig. 24.2b).

For pedicled VRAM flaps intended to rotate superiorly, the same markings can be employed although careful observation of the skin below the umbilicus should be performed as the superior epigastric angiosome does not always reliably extend this far inferiorly. In some cases supercharging through microsurgical anastomosis of the inferior epigastric system to vessels within the recipient bed will be required.

24.7 Operative Technique

For the inferiorly based pedicled VRAM flap, the reconstructive team will ideally enter the abdomen before oncologic resection to protect the flap and abdominal wall during the approach. For the superiorly based pedicled VRAM flap,

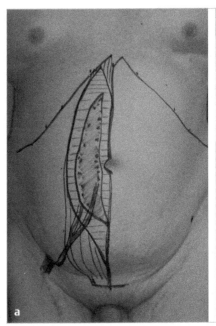
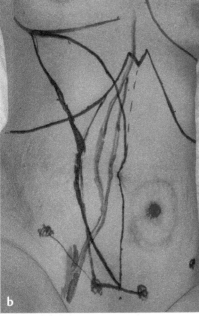

Fig. 24.2 VRAM preoperative markings. **(a)** Preoperative markings for standard VRAM skin paddle. Inferior epigastric pedicle drawn emanating from iliac system at a point half way between iliac spine and pubis. Inferior epigastric perforator zone is identified adjacent to the umbilicus. Anterior rectus fascia within the perforator zone is all that is harvested with the fascial-sparing technique. **(b)** Preoperative markings for extended VRAM skin paddle with extension parallel to costal orientation beneath the breast and extending to the anterior axillary line.

communication regarding the involvement of the internal mammary system and the eighth intercostal vessels should be performed before any extirpation or debridement of the chest begins.

A midline incision is made through skin and subcutaneous fat until the linea alba and anterior rectus fascia are identified. To perform a fascia-sparing harvest of the VRAM, dissect laterally in the subcutaneous plane until the medial row of the inferior epigastric perforators is identified. Divide the anterior fascia with scissors at the medial row perforators above the arcuate line and then angle the fascial incision toward midline as you cross the level of the arcuate line inferiorly (►Fig. 24.3a). Reflect the medial edge of the rectus muscle laterally to expose the posterior rectus fascia above the arcuate line and the transversalis fascia below the arcuate line. Divide the posterior fascia with scissors in the same orientation as the anterior fascia to create two fascial sheaths for closure above the arcuate line (►Fig. 24.3b). Divide transversalis fascia at midline and then sweep the preperitoneal fat away with finger dissection. Where abdominal oncologic resections are required, temporarily suture the anterior and posterior fascial sheaths closed with 4–0 Vicryl suture to move the rectus muscle laterally and then the abdominal extirpation can be performed (►Fig. 24.3).

The lateral VRAM skin paddle incision is made with monopolar dissection through subcutaneous fat. Subcutaneous dissection is performed medially until the lateral row perforators are identified. The anterior rectus fascial sheath is divided with scissors to isolate the anterior fascia of the epigastric perforator zone to be taken with the flap. The lateral edge of the anterior rectus sheath is elevated and the minor segmental neurovascular pedicles to the rectus muscle are divided. When the VRAM is being rotated superiorly, the inferior epigastric vessel is dissected to its iliac source in the event supercharging is required and

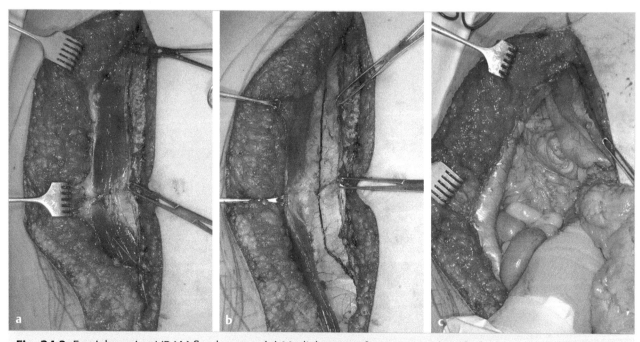

Fig. 24.3 Fascial-sparing VRAM flap harvest. **(a)** Medial row perforators are identified and anterior rectus sheath is divided and retracted medially to allow for mobilization of rectus muscle. **(b)** Once the medial edge of the rectus muscle has been moved laterally, the posterior sheath is exposed. Incising this fascia above the arcuate line (planned incision marked) creates a second fascial layer for closure. **(c)** The anterior and posterior sheath is temporarily closed to protect the flap while the intraabdominal portion of the operation proceeds. (Images courtesy of Charles E. Butler.)

the pubic insertion of the muscle is divided with electrocautery. For pelvic surgical indications when the VRAM is being rotated inferiorly, the rectus muscle is divided at the costal margin and the VRAM is elevated from costal margin to pelvic insertion until the inferior epigastric pedicle is identified entering the inferolateral aspect of the deep surface of the rectus muscle. Careful dissection of the epigastric pedicle is performed to aid in pedicle rotation.

The pelvic insertion of the rectus muscle should not need to be divided for pelvic reconstruction. When pelvic passage is required, pass the VRAM into its desired location and mark the skin paddle required for pelvic and/or vaginal resurfacing in situ. Ensure that the flap completely obliterates the dead space of the pelvic inlet while it is in position. Also verify that the inferior epigastric pedicle continues to have a strong pulse and has no tension on it while in its desired position. Transversely divide the transversalis fascia at the level of the pedicle to ensure that tension is not placed on the pedicle during fascial closure.

Withdraw the flap back to the abdomen to deepithelialize the portions of the skin paddle to be buried within the pelvis (▶Fig. 24.4a). Return the flap to its destination within the pelvis. Absorbable presacral sutures can be used to ensure that the pelvic inlet is obliterated by the deepithelialized portion of the VRAM skin paddle. Closure of the pelvic recipient site is performed by suturing the superficial fascia of the skin paddle to the muscular sling of the pelvis followed by interrupted deep dermal sutures to the muscular layer of the vagina when partial vaginal reconstruction is performed and to the perineal skin for perineal resurfacing. The distal deepithelialized extent of the skin paddle is sutured beneath the perineal skin flaps for final closure (▶Fig. 24.4b).

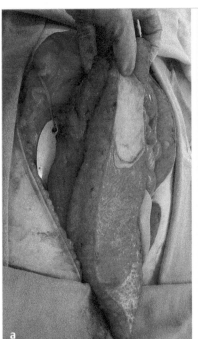
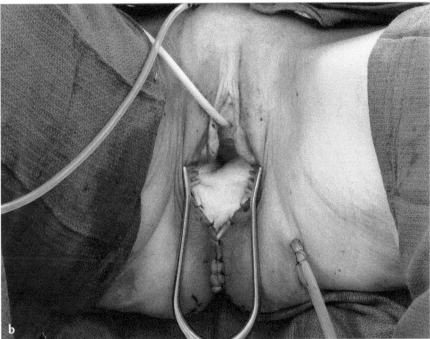

Fig. 24.4 (a) The VRAM flap has been returned to the abdomen after marking the portion to be used for posterior vaginal wall reconstruction. The portion of the flap to occupy the pelvic inlet and to be buried underneath the perineal skin flaps has been deepithelialized. (b) The VRAM flap has been delivered back into the pelvis where the posterior wall of the vagina has been reconstructed. The distal portion of the skin paddle can be seen at the introitus. The remainder has been deepithelialized and placed beneath the primarily-closed perineal skin flaps.

24.8 Donor Site Closure

The fascial sparing harvest makes abdominal donor site closure technically simpler with an improved chance at restoration of abdominal wall integrity. Permanent suture in a running or figure of eight fashion should be used for the two fascial layers above the arcuate line and in a single layer below the arcuate line. For patients who had significant scarring preventing fascial sparing closure, a unilateral component separation consisting of external oblique aponeurosis release on the side of flap harvest will allow the lateral fascial sheaths to advance medially taking tension off closure (▶Fig. 24.5a,b). Inlay mesh placement can also be used as needed to reinforce the closure in cases of prior hernia or multiple prior laparotomies. Synthetic mesh can be used above the arcuate line between the anterior and posterior sheaths. Biologic mesh is preferred when mesh reinforcement is required below the arcuate line as well to avoid synthetic mesh contributing to adhesions when contacting abdominal contents.[4] The lateral skin flap should be quilted to the abdominal wall musculature with 3–0 Vicryl suture and skin closure is performed in a standard layered technique (▶Fig. 24.5c).

24.9 Pearls and Pitfalls

- Constantly communicate with your oncologic surgeons to make sure that the epigastric pedicles are still patent and uninjured before flap harvest.
- Measure the size of the diameter of the skin paddle that can be taken before the midline incision is performed to prevent errors in measurement.

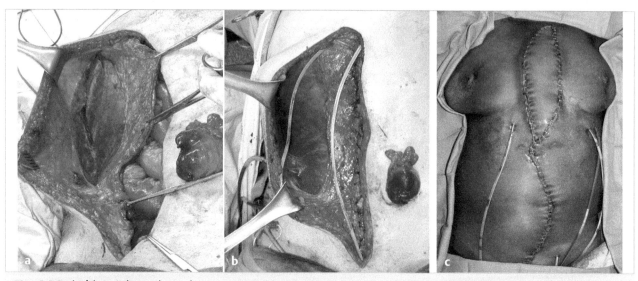

Fig. 24.5 (a,b) A right unilateral component separation is shown to aid abdominal wall closure after VRAM harvest. The external oblique aponeurosis has been divided lateral to the semilunar line and the rectus sheath fascia has been closed without tension. (Images courtesy of Charles E. Butler.) **(c)** Abdominal donor site closure. Right VRAM pedicled by the superior epigastric system with microvascular supercharging with the inferior epigastric artery and vein to the internal mammary vessels for reconstruction of a large sternal wound defect after cardiac valve replacement. A right unilateral component separation was used to assist with abdominal wound closure. Quilting sutures were used to obliterate dead space between the skin closure and the abdominal wall.

- Fascial-sparing harvest will reduce abdominal wall donor site morbidity. If fascial sparing cannot be performed due to multiple prior hernias or prior abdominal surgeries, component separation, and/or mesh reinforcement should be considered to maintain abdominal wall integrity and aid in closure.[4]
- Ensure that the epigastric pedicle feels soft without tension multiple times during the case while passing the flap and during donor site closure. Transversely divide the transversalis fascia if needed to prevent occult tension on the pedicle during abdominal wall closure.
- When rotating the VRAM flap superiorly on the superior epigastric pedicle, carefully evaluate the skin below the umbilicus to ensure that it is included in the pedicle's angiosome and is viable. Be prepared to supercharge the lower aspect of the flap by performing an anastomosis between the inferior epigastric vessels and vessels within the recipient site.

References

[1] Tobin GR, Day TG. Vaginal and pelvic reconstruction with distally based rectus abdominis myocutaneous flaps. Plast Reconstr Surg 1988;81(1):62–73

[2] Miyamoto Y, Hattori T, Niimoto M, Toge T. Reconstruction of full-thickness chest wall defects using rectus abdominis musculocutaneous flap: a report of fifteen cases. Ann Plast Surg 1986;16(2):90–97

[3] Bunkis J, Walton RL, Mathes SJ. The rectus abdominis free flap for lower extremity reconstruction. Ann Plast Surg 1983;11(5):373–380

[4] Campbell CA, Butler CE. Use of adjuvant techniques improves surgical outcomes of complex vertical rectus abdominis myocutaneous flap reconstructions of pelvic cancer defects. Plast Reconstr Surg 2011;128(2):447–458

[5] Mericli AF, Martin JP, Campbell CA. An algorithmic anatomical subunit approach to pelvic wound reconstruction. Plast Reconstr Surg 2016;137(3):1004–1017

25 Omental Flap

Donald P. Baumann

Abstract

The omental flap can be used as either a free flap or a pedicle flap for reconstruction of a posttraumatic calvarial defect. Because of the omentum flap's versatility and reliability, it has become a workhorse in reconstructive surgery. The omental flap has many applications in thoracic, abdominal, and pelvic reconstruction, as well as soft tissue resurfacing of the extremities and head and neck. In this chapter, the author covers all the bases involved in the use of the omental flap, from indications, to anatomy, to preoperative considerations, to surgical technique. Enhancing the discussion is the mention of five variations to the basic procedure.

Keywords: greater omentum, right and left gastroepiploic vessels, gastroduodenal artery, splenic artery, omental arcade, right, middle, and left omental vessels

25.1 Introduction

The omental flap can be designed as either a free flap or a pedicle flap. In 1972, Harry Buncke described the first free omental flap for reconstruction of a posttraumatic calvarial defect.[1] Because of the omentum flap's versatility and reliability it has become a workhorse in reconstructive surgery. The omental flap has many applications in thoracic, abdominal, and pelvic reconstruction as well as soft tissue resurfacing of the extremities and head and neck.

25.2 Typical Indications

- Intrathoracic defects: bronchopleural fistula, empyema, and infected vascular grafts.
- Intraabdominal defects: reconstruction of pelvic defects and reinforcement of bowel anastomoses.
- Chest wall defects: including infected sternotomy wounds.
- Soft-tissue coverage of the upper and lower extremities and head and neck region as a free tissue transfer.
- Extremity lymphedema: source of lymph node tissue transfer.

25.3 Anatomy

The **greater omentum** descends from the greater curve of the stomach and proximal duodenum passing inferiorly and anterior to the small bowel for a variable distance. It returns superiorly again to insert on the anterosuperior aspect of the transverse colon. The left border of the omentum is contiguous with the gastrosplenic ligament and the right border extends as far as the pylorus and first portion of the duodenum. The **lesser omentum** extends from the lesser curvature of the stomach and proximal duodenum to the porta hepatis of the liver. The hepatogastric and hepatoduodenal ligaments form the lesser omentum. The lesser omentum generally does not play a role in reconstructive surgery.

The size of the omental flap varies greatly with body mass index, age, sex, and prior intraabdominal infection or surgery. Omental flaps can be designed with a surface area of 25 × 50 cm² in most patients. The thickness of the flap varies significantly based on body mass index and intraabdominal fat distribution.

The main blood supply to the omental flap arises from the **right and left gastroepiploic vessels.** The right gastroepiploic artery originates from the **gastroduodenal artery** and the left gastroepiploic artery originates from the **splenic artery**. The omental flap is a type III flap by Mathes and Nahai classification. Either the right or left gastroepiploic vessels can serve as the dominant blood supply to the flap. The omentum has a rich internal vascular network within the flap consisting of an **omental arcade** and **right, middle, and left omental vessels** (▶Fig. 25.1). The omental arcade connects the right and left gastroepiploic systems. The omental arcade travels the transverse length of the omentum approximately 2 cm inferior to the greater curvature of the stomach. The right, middle and left omental vessels arise from the omental arcade and travel inferiorly with collateralization between branches.[2]

The arc of rotation of a pedicled omental flap can reach both chest and pelvis based on either the right or left gastroepiploic vessels. Decision to base the

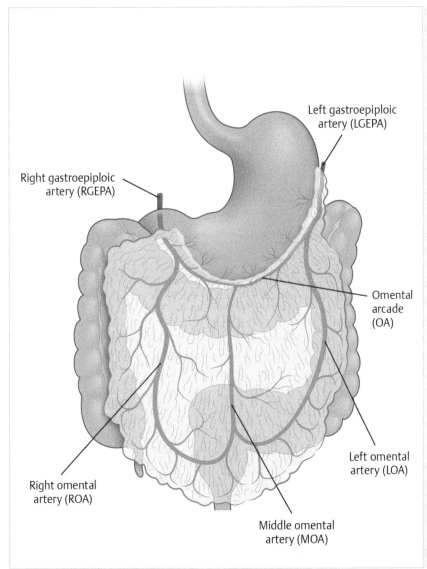

Fig. 25.1 Omental vascular anatomy. OA, omental arcade; RGEPA, right gastroepiploic artery; LGEPA, left gastroepiploic artery; ROA, MOA, LOA, right, middle, left omental arteries.

Left gastroepiploic artery (LGEPA)

Right gastroepiploic artery (RGEPA)

Omental arcade (OA)

Left omental artery (LOA)

Right omental artery (ROA)

Middle omental artery (MOA)

flap on either pedicle is determined by omental anatomy, concurrent intraabdominal surgery and laterality of defect. In designing an omental free flap the right gastroepiploic pedicle is often selected as it is slightly larger in diameter vessel than the left gastroepiploic. Care must be taken prior to pedicle division to clearly mark the artery and vein as it may be difficult to discern afterward due to the fact that the artery has a thinner wall as compared to integumentary vessels.

25.4 Variations

In general, there are three arterial branches off the gastroepiploics (the left, middle, and right) that anastomose in varying degrees at the distal aspect of the omentum. Major variations in the vascular arcade have been noted and are based on the absence or presence of the middle omental artery and the level of its bifurcation (▶ **Fig. 25.2**).[3]

- Type I—middle omental artery bifurcates near the distal omental apron.
- Type II—middle omental artery bifurcates midway between the gastroepiploic arcade and the distal omentum.
- Type III—middle omental artery bifurcates 2 to 3 cm from the gastroepiploic arcade.
- Type IV—the middle omental artery is absent with smaller accessory omental vessels in its place.
- Type V—the left omental artery is a direct branch of the splenic artery and the middle omental artery is supplied by the right gastroepiploic.

25.5 Preoperative Considerations

Preoperative planning centers around assessing the adequacy of the omental flap in terms of overall volume and ability to reach the defect. The patient's body type and prior surgery will provide insight into the availability of the omentum. Preoperative CT imaging can also be used to assess the volume of the omentum by evaluating the anterior abdominal fat compartment.

25.6 Positioning and Skin Markings

Supine positioning is preferred. The midline is marked from subxiphoid region to umbilicus. An appropriate length incision is used to gain adequate visualization in the upper abdomen. If a laparoscopic harvest is planned, four port sites are used—one infraumbilical port site, through which the flap can be delivered, two in the right flank, and one in the left.

25.7 Operative Technique

The omental flap can be harvested either by open laparotomy or minimally invasive laparoscopy based on surgeon preference and intended use of the flap. To harvest the flap a laparotomy or laparoscopy is performed to expose the upper abdominal viscera. The omentum is reflected cranially and its attachments are dissected off the transverse colon along antimesenteric border (▶ **Fig. 25.3a**). Care is taken not to injure the mesocolon and middle colic artery. Next, the omentum is reflected inferiorly and the short gastric vessels are ligated. A decision

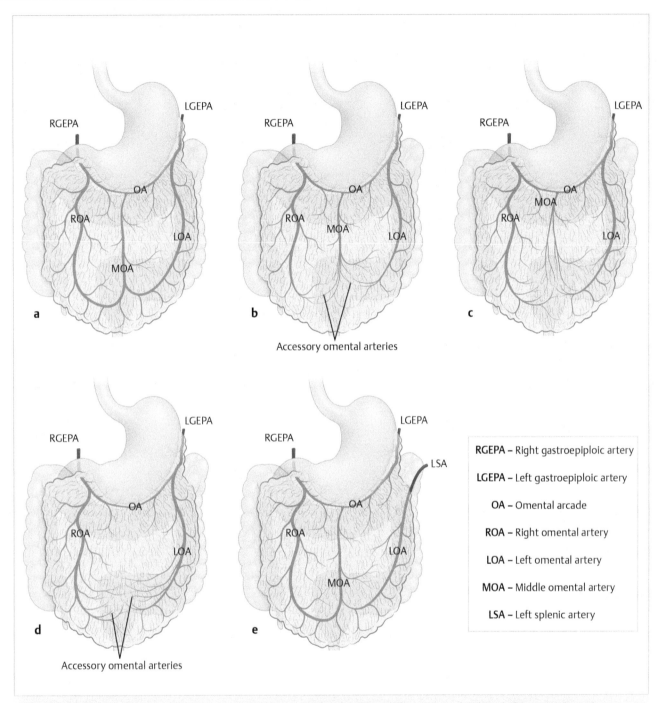

Fig. 25.2 Omental flap variations on intrinsic blood supply. **(a)** Middle omental artery bifurcates near the distal omental apron. **(b)** Middle omental artery bifurcates midway between the gastroepiploic arcade and the distal omentum. **(c)** Middle omental artery bifurcates 2 to 3 cm from the gastroepiploic arcade. **(d)** The middle omental artery is absent with smaller accessory omental vessels in its place. **(e)** The left omental artery is a direct branch of the splenic artery and the middle omental artery is supplied by the right gastroepiploic.

is made whether to design the flap on the right or left gastroepiploic vessels based on defect location. The dissection proceeds along the omental arcade toward the pedicle that will be sacrificed. ▶ **Fig. 25.3b** shows a pedicled omental flap based on the right gastroepiploic vessels (the left gastroepiploic pedicle has been ligated) in preparation for transposition into the pelvis. For an omental free flap harvest the left gastroepiploic vessels are ligated. The right gastroepiploic

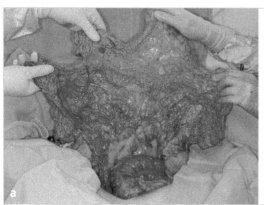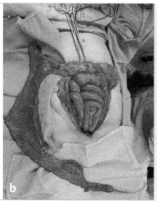

Fig. 25.3 **(a)** Intraoperative view of omental flap dissected free from transverse colon attachment. The flap is reflected cranially to illustrate the overall dimension and vascular arcades. **(b)** The omental flap has been isolated on the right gastroepiploic pedicle and divided along the omental arcade to enhance arc of rotation and flap reach to distal pelvic defect. (Image courtesy of Charles E. Butler.)

vessels are dissected proximally toward the gastroduodenal artery from the stomach to their origin to gain pedicle length for microanastomosis.[4,5]

For a pedicled flap design, the arc of rotation of a pedicled omental flap can reach both the chest and pelvis based on either the right or left gastropepiploic vessels. If additional length is needed the gastroepiploic arcade can be divided and the flap length extended. Care must be taken to ensure adequate perfusion to the distal flap before dividing the omental arcade. This is done by tracing the contributions of the right, middle, and left omental branches as they relate to the omental arcade (▶ **Fig. 25.2**). A hand-held Doppler can assist in confirming vessel location and preservation of perfusion to the distal flap after the flap is lengthened.

When transferring the omental flap into the thoracic cavity technique care must be taken in delivering the flap into the chest. A tunnel must be designed that does not compromise the flap's blood flow or allow a hernia to develop. Transferring the flap through a small cruciate incision in the diaphragm yields access into either the chest cavity or the anterior mediastinum for sternal reconstruction.

25.8 Donor Site Closure

As the omental flap can be harvested either via a midline laparotomy or minimally invasive laparoscopy donor site closure is performed with focus on adequate fascial coaptation. Consideration should be given to postoperative gastric decompression with a nasogastric tube. This prevents distention along the greater curvature of the stomach from disrupting the ligature on the short gastric vessels.

25.9 Pearls and Pitfalls

- The omental branches can be selectively divided to extend the arc of rotation and reach of the flap.
- In the omental free flap, care must be taken prior to pedicle division to clearly mark the artery and vein as it may be difficult to discern afterward due to the fact that the artery has a thinner wall as compared to integumentary vessels.
- When tunneling the flap avoid pedicle compression.

References

[1] McLean DH, Buncke HJ Jr. Autotransplant of omentum to a large scalp defect, with microsurgical revascularization. Plast Reconstr Surg 1972;49(3):268–274

[2] Liebermann-Meffert D. The greater omentum. Anatomy, embryology, and surgical applications. Surg Clin North Am 2000;80(1):275–293, xii

[3] Alday ES, Goldsmith HS. Surgical technique for omental lengthening based on arterial anatomy. Surg Gynecol Obstet 1972;135(1):103–107

[4] Maloney CT Jr, Wages D, Upton J, Lee WP. Free omental tissue transfer for extremity coverage and revascularization. Plast Reconstr Surg 2003;111(6):1899–1904

[5] Nguyen AT, Suami H, Hanasono MM, Womack VA, Wong FC, Chang EI. Long-term outcomes of the minimally invasive free vascularized omental lymphatic flap for the treatment of lymphedema. J Surg Oncol 2017;115(1):84–89

26 Free Jejunal and Supercharged Jejunal Flaps

Peirong Yu

Abstract

The small bowel has a rich blood supply, and any segment of the small bowel based on a pair of mesentery vessels can be harvested as a free flap. During the 1980s and 1990s, the free jejunal flap became the workhorse flap for pharyngoesophageal reconstruction in many centers. The small bowel can also be used for total esophageal reconstruction by transposing it to the neck. This, however, requires division of several mesentery vessels to increase its reach. Because of its segmental blood supply, division of these vessels may render the corresponding segments of small bowel ischemic. The addition of microsurgical techniques have allowed for the replacement of the entire esophagus through "supercharging." The supercharged jejunal flap has become a viable option for total esophageal reconstruction when the stomach is unavailable. This chapter guides the surgeon through the various sequential steps in the harvesting and use of the jejunal and supercharged jejunal flaps. Starting with typical indications, the discussion also covers anatomy, preoperative conditions, and the operative technique. The technique is discussed in detail for both flaps, with information about the surgical team, the work flow, harvesting, flap inset/transfer, and donor site closure.

Keywords: superior mesenteric artery, celiac artery, superior mesenteric vein, splenic vein

26.1 Introduction

The small bowel has rich blood supply. Any segment of the small bowel based on a pair of mesentery vessels can be harvested as a free flap. In fact, the first clinical free tissue transfer involved the small bowel and was reported by Seidenberg in 1959.[1] Several more successful jejunal flap reconstructions were reported in the 1960s.[2,3,4] Although these early reports demonstrated a possibility of this technique, the lack of proper magnification, microsurgical instruments, and sutures severely limited its use until the 1980s. During the 1980s and 1990s, the free jejunal flap became the workhorse flap for pharyngoesophageal reconstruction in many centers.[5,6,7,8,9,10] The small bowel can also be used for total esophageal reconstruction by transposing the small bowel up to the neck. This method, however, requires division of several mesentery vessels to increase the reach. Because of its segmental blood supply, division of these vessels may render the corresponding segments of small bowel ischemic. In 1947, Longmire[11] augmented the blood supply of the distal bowel by anastomosing a mesenteric vessel to the internal mammary artery. The addition of microsurgical techniques has allowed for the replacement of the entire esophagus through "supercharging." The supercharged jejunal flap has become a viable option for total esophageal reconstruction when the stomach is unavailable.[12,13,14,15,16]

26.2 Typical Indications

The free jejunal flap is indicated for circumferential pharyngoesophageal reconstruction following a total laryngopharyngectomy for the following:
- Primary or recurrent cancers of the hypopharynx, piriform sinus, or larynx.
- Thyroid cancer involving the esophagus.

- Benign strictures refractory to dilation, such as radiation induced strictures or ingestion of lye.
- Nonhealing pharyngocutaneous fistula following prior reconstruction and radiotherapy.

The supercharged jejunal flap is indicated for total esophageal reconstruction when gastric pull-up is not an option in the following circumstances:

1. A total or subtotal gastrectomy is required due to cancer involvement.
2. Prior gastric surgery.
3. Prior radiation to the stomach making the gastric pull-up procedure unreliable.
4. A concomitant total laryngopharyngectomy defect beyond the reach of the gastric pull-up.
5. A failed gastric pull-up procedure, which may be the most common indication.

26.3 Anatomy

The small intestine measures approximately 22 to 23 feet in length in adult. The jejunum and ileum are suspended from the posterior wall of the abdomen by the mesentery and receives blood supply from the **superior mesenteric artery** (SMA). The SMA originates from the abdominal aorta approximately 1 cm inferior to the takeoff of the **celiac artery**. It travels inferiorly passing behind the neck of the pancreas and the splenic vein, then gives rise to several jejunal and ileal arteries (▶ Fig. 26.1). These arteries divide into branches to form a series

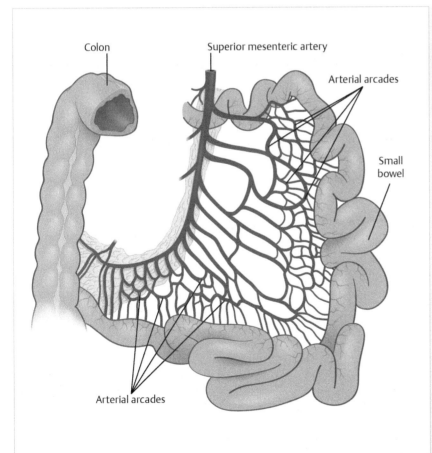

Fig. 26.1 Anatomy of the small bowel and its vascular supply. The superior mesenteric artery sends out several branches to the bowel, which form numerous vascular arcades before reaching the bowel.

of arterial arcades. The venous drainage of the small intestine accompanies the arteries through the **superior mesenteric vein**, which ultimately joins the **splenic vein** to empty into the portal system.

26.4 Variations

- The anatomy of the small intestine and its blood supply is fairly consistent.

26.5 Preoperative Considerations

Harvesting a jejunal flap involves laparotomy and bowel surgery, which by itself is a major abdominal surgery that can cause significant third spacing, fluid shift, postoperative ileus, and bowel obstruction. Therefore, careful preoperative assessment is necessary to minimize serious, even life-threatening complications. Preoperative assessment includes evaluation of the patient's cardiopulmonary, renal, and nutritional status. In addition to routine preoperative screening tests, it is often advisable to obtain pulmonary function tests, cardiac stress test, and a nutritional assessment including total serum protein, albumin, and transferrin. Each of these areas should be optimized prior to surgery. Careful planning involves a multidisciplinary team approach including head and neck surgery, general surgery or thoracic surgery, plastic surgery, critical care, nutrition, and speech pathology. Leaks and strictures may occur as well as functional swallowing difficulties. The patient and family should be well informed about these surgical risks, potential postoperative complications and functional deficits.

26.6 Positioning and Skin Markings

The flap harvesting is performed with the patient in a supine position. An upper abdominal midline incision between the xyphoid and umbilicus is used to enter the peritoneal cavity.

26.7 Operative Techniques

26.7.1 The Free Jejunal Flap

Work Flow

Pharyngoesophageal reconstruction using the free jejunal flap requires a three-team approach. The extirpative team (head and neck surgery) begins the resection and confirms the need for a circumferential pharyngoesophageal reconstruction. Approximately 1 hour before the completion of the tumor ablation, plastic surgery may start harvesting the jejunal flap. These two teams can work simultaneously without interfering with each other's progress. Two separate sets of instrument and personnel are necessary to avoid cross contamination. When the ablative surgeons are finished, the jejunal flap should be ready to be transferred. Once the flap is removed from the abdomen, the general surgical team can start reestablishing continuity of the small intestine, placing gastrointestinal tubes, and closing the abdomen. A well-organized work flow can significantly reduce operative time.

Flap Harvest

Through an upper midline laparotomy incision, a thorough intraabdominal exploration is performed to rule out any unexpected findings. The entire small bowel is examined and its vascular arcades are transilluminated using a back-lighting such as a sterile fiber optic light source (▶ Fig. 26.2a). Usually the segment of bowel corresponding to the second mesentery vessels, approximately 20 to 30 cm from the ligament of Treitz, is selected as the free jejunal flap. The length of the bowel segment is 15 to 20 cm and is marked on the mesentery close to the bowel wall with a Bovie. With backlighting, the origin of the second mesentery vessels are located. The fan-shaped mesentery between the two ends of the bowel segment and the origin of the vascular pedicle is scored with electric cautery on both sides. A window through the mesentery between the terminal vessels immediately adjacent to the bowel at each proposed line of resection is created. The mesentery and crossing vessels are clamped, divided, and ligated with 2–0 and 3–0 silk ties. Meticulous control of crossing vessels is important as even small vessels can form a significant mesenteric hematoma and threaten the safety of the flap. The vascular pedicle near its origin is cleaned of peritoneal lining, lymphatics, and fat for about 2 cm (▶ Fig. 26.2b). The vein

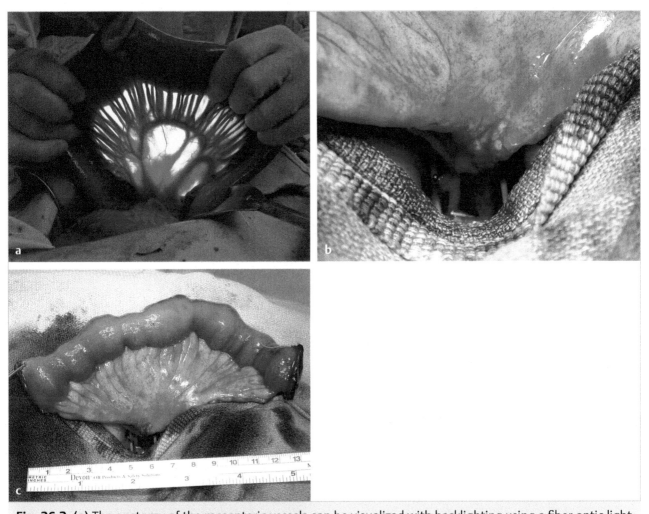

Fig. 26.2 (a) The anatomy of the mesenteric vessels can be visualized with backlighting using a fiber optic light source. (b) The mesenteric branch that serves as the pedicle of the free jejunal flap is isolated and cleaned off for approximately 2 cm from their origins. (c) Once the pedicle vessels are isolated, the jejunum is divided with a gastrointestinal stapling device.

is usually much larger than the artery. The bowel is then ready to be divided. Using a gastrointestinal stapling device, the bowel is divided perpendicular to the longitudinal axis. A marking suture is placed at the proximal resection line to ensure orientation of the loop in an isoperistaltic direction at the time of flap inset (▶Fig. 26.2). The perfusion of the jejunal flap and the adjacent bowel is inspected. A well-perfused bowel should look pink both on the mucosa and serosa without any discoloration. Pulsation of the terminal arcade vessels over the bowel wall and frequent peristalsis should be clearly visible. The bowel flap is then covered with warm and moist laparotomy pads while the recipient vessels are dissected out. Once the final preparation of the recipient site is complete, the jejunal flap is harvested. A 2–0 silk tie is placed around the base of the pedicle artery and reinforced with another tie or a hemoclip. The ischemia time of the flap is recorded. The vein is ligated in a similar fashion. Both the artery and vein are then divided. The flap is removed from the abdominal field and the area is inspected to ensure perfect vascular control. The staples lines on each end of the jejunal flap is removed and the lumen of the jejunal flap is irrigated with normal saline to remove mucus or other intestinal contents. Our experience suggests that the jejunal flap can tolerate 2 hours of warm ischemia (room temperature) without any undesirable consequences. If the recipient site is well prepared before harvesting the jejunal flap, revascularization can usually be established within an hour. Flap inset can be done after revascularization to minimize ischemia time. Alternatively, the proximal anastomosis is done first before revascularization, depending on individual surgeon's pace. If prolonged ischemia is anticipated, the bowel may be bathed in iced saline.

Flap Inset

The pharyngoesophageal defect is usually no longer than 10 cm. The straight portion of the jejunal flap is used for the reconstruction. During flap inset, the neck is returned to a neutral position without hyperextension. The proximal pharyngeal opening is significantly larger than the jejunum. Therefore, the antimesenteric border of the jejunal flap is opened longitudinally for 3 to 4 cm to create a semi end-to-side anastomosis to accommodate the size discrepancy (▶Fig. 26.3a). The author prefers using simple interrupted 3–0 Vicryl sutures for the anastomosis. The posterior wall is completed first with the anterior wall open for good visualization. A single layer anastomosis is adequate. If there is any concern for the integrity of the anastomosis, a second layer of Lampert sutures through the serosomuscular tissue can be placed. The second layer, however, can potentially narrow the lumen especially at the distal anastomosis. The proximal anastomosis is usually performed first. As the bowel is elastic, the bowel is slightly stretched without tension during the distal anastomosis. Extra bowel is divided from the main flap leaving the mesentery vessels still attached (▶Fig. 26.3a). The extra bowel is shortened to about 3 to 4 cm with two terminal mesentery vessels attached to the bowel. This segment of bowel is externalized for flap monitoring. A small window is created between the two terminal mesentery vessels and a 2–0 silk tie is placed around each vessel (▶Fig. 26.3b). The monitoring segment is sutured to the neck skin at each end of the bowel and covered with a Xeroform dressing to prevent desiccation (▶Fig. 26.3c). Flap assessment can be easily done by uncovering the Xeroform. The day before discharge, the monitoring segment is removed by tying these preplaced skin sutures.

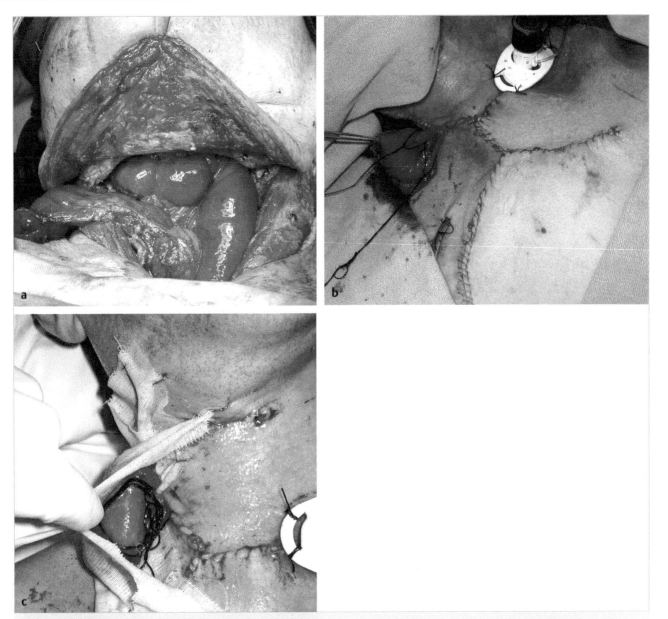

Fig. 26.3 (a) For the proximal anastomosis, the jejunum is longitudinally opened to accommodate the wide opening of the pharynx. **(b)** A small segment of bowel based on two terminal arcade vessels is externalized for monitoring purpose. A 2–0 silk tie is placed around each terminal vessel. Once the monitoring segment is ready to be removed, the mesentery vessels are tied off with these preplaced ties. **(c)** The monitoring segment of jejunum is covered with a Xeroform gauze to prevent desiccation. Flap monitoring can be easily performed by uncovering the gauze. Doppler signals can also easily be obtained from the terminal vessels.

26.8 Donor Site Closure

While the reconstructive team is working on the recipient site, the general surgery team may begin bowel anastomosis, placement of a gastrostomy tube and jejunostomy feeding tube. Small bowel continuity is commonly restored with stapling devices. A feeding jejunostomy tube is placed distal to the bowel anastomosis. The abdominal incision is then closed with layers.

26.8.1 The Supercharged Jejunal Flap

Work Flow

Establishing a fluent work flow in such a complex case is extremely important to shorten operative time and improve outcomes. The esophagectomy and gastrectomy, when necessary, are performed by the thoracic and/or general surgeons. The surgical approach is either through two incisions (abdominal and cervical) as in a transhiatal esophagectomy, or three incisions with the addition of a right thoracotomy. If a thoracotomy is required, the patient is first placed in lateral decubitus position and then switched to supine position. While the ablative surgical team is operating in the abdomen, the reconstructive surgeons can start to prepare recipient vessels in the neck. The teams then change positions. The reconstructive surgeons now prepare the jejunal flap while the ablative surgeons expose the proximal esophagus through the neck incision and remove the manubrium and clavicular head if a substernal approach is desired. The jejunal conduit is then passed through the chest and into the neck, and the teams switch positions again. The reconstructive surgeons revascularize the proximal jejunum, complete the esophagojejunal anastomosis in the neck, and fashion the monitoring segment while the other surgical team restores gastrointestinal continuity in the abdomen. When properly organized, no time is wasted for all teams involved. Clear communication between surgical teams and anesthesia regarding fluid resuscitation and avoidance of vasopressor medications is imperative as different disciplines may manage these issues differently.

Flap Harvesting

Once resection is complete, the length of the esophageal defect is measured to estimate the length of the conduit needed. The mesentery is transilluminated using a fiber optic lighting source as described earlier. The first mesenteric branch beyond the ligament of Treitz is identified and preserved to maintain blood supply to the distal duodenum and most proximal portion of jejunum, which is used to reestablish enteric continuity.

Typically, the second mesenteric branch is used for "supercharging." These vessels are dissected down to the level of the SMA and vein. Depending on the tightness of mesentery, one or two mesenteric vessels may need to be divided to increase the reach. In the simplest cases, the second mesentery vessels are divided and supercharged in the neck. The third mesentery vessels are not divided, serving as the pedicled portion of the flap (type I). The mesentery between the second and third branches is divided up to the serosal border, allowing the jejunal segment to unfurl (▶ **Fig. 26.4a**). This step helps straighten the natural sinusoidal properties of the small bowel and reduce redundancy. In most cases, however, this step alone does not yield enough length of the mesentery for the bowel to reach the neck. Therefore, the third mesenteric branch is ligated and divided (▶ **Fig. 26.4b**). The mesentery between the third and fourth mesentery vessels is divided to the level of secondary arcade vessels. These arcade vessels are preserved so that the segment of bowel normally perfused by the third mesentery vessels is now supplied by the pedicled fourth branch through intact arcade vessels (type II). This is the most common approach in our experience. If still greater length is required, such as in patients with a very long torso or a concomitant total laryngopharyngectomy, the fourth mesenteric branch can also be ligated and divided. In these cases, only the mesentery between the third and fourth branches is divided to the serosal border

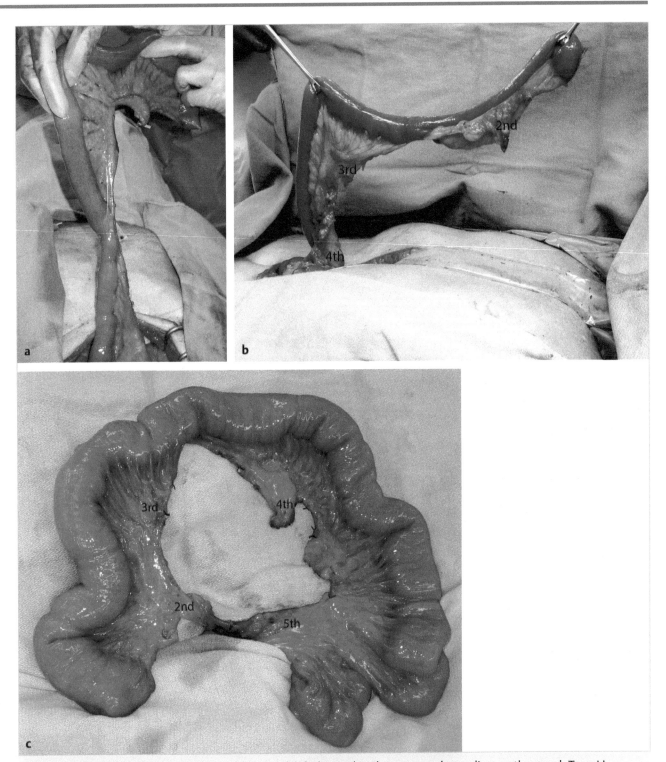

Fig. 26.4 **(a)** The supercharged jejunal flap can be fashioned in three types depending on the need. Type I is the simplest form in which the second mesentery branch is divided and supercharged in the neck while the third branch serves as the pedicled portion of the flap. The mesentery between these two branches is divided all the way to the bowel to unfurl the bowel. **(b)** The most common form is type II in which the third mesenteric branch is ligated and divided to increase the reach while the fourth branch serves as the pedicled portion of the flap. The mesentery between the second and third mesenteric vessels is divided to the serosal border of the jejunum while the arcade vessels between the third and fourth mesenteric vessels are kept intact so that the small bowel normally perfused by the third branch can be perfused by the pedicled fourth branch via these arcade connections. **(c)** If still greater length is required, both the third and fourth mesenteric branches are divided (type III). Only the mesentery between the third and fourth branches is divided to the serosal border while arcade connections are preserved between the second and third, and between the fourth and fifth branches.

while the arcade connections are preserved between the second and third, and between the fourth and fifth branches (▶ **Fig. 26.4c**). The third segment receives perfusion from the supercharged second mesentery vessels and the fourth segment receives perfusion through the pedicled fifth branch (type III).

Flap Transfer

There are two potential routes for transferring the jejunal flap to the neck: retrocardiac, which is the orthotopic route, or substernal, which is the heterotopic route that requires a portion of the manubrium, clavicular head, and first rib be removed to enlarge the thoracic inlet and avoid constriction on the jejunal conduit. The former is utilized in patients undergoing immediate reconstruction but cannot be used for delayed reconstruction as the native route is already obliterated. The latter is usually reserved for patients undergoing a delayed reconstruction after previous failed esophageal reconstruction but is also commonly used for immediate reconstruction. There are several advantages of the substernal approach:

1. Removing the manubrium, clavicular head, and part of the first rib provides excellent exposure for bowel anastomosis and recipient vessels.
2. It allows the proximal esophageal remnant to be positioned in the upper chest instead of in the neck, if oncologically feasible, easier for the jejunal flap to reach.
3. It provides excellent access to the internal mammary vessels as recipient vessels. Because of the curved nature of the mesentery, more inferior location of the recipient vessels can significantly reduce the tension of the flap and ease flap reach.

The disadvantage of the substernal route is the disruption of chest wall integrity. As increasing the mesentery length of the flap is always the "bottle neck" of this procedure, the substernal route can make the entire reconstruction easier and safer. Tension on the mesentery can cause vascular compromise or even tear the connecting arcade vessels between the perfusion zones, rendering ischemia or necrosis of the middle jejunal segment that is hidden behind the sternum. This can become a life-threatening complication if not recognized promptly.

Whether the retrocardiac or substernal route is selected, transfer is accomplished using a sterile laparoscopic camera bag to protect the conduit and prevent traction and shearing forces on the delicate arcade vessels. A chest tube is first placed in the retrocardiac or substernal route. The plastic bag is then tied to one end of the chest tube and pulled through (▶ **Fig. 26.5a**). The jejunal flap is placed inside the plastic bag with great care to avoid twisting the bowel and mesentery. The bag is the pulled to the neck while the assistant pushes the bowel flap from the abdomen to minimize traction force (▶ **Fig. 26.5b**). Once the vascular pedicle of the flap reaches the recipient vessels, the plastic bag is separated from the bowel by filling the bag with saline while pulling the bag out. This is an extremely important step as any traction on the bowel while pulling the bag out can potentially tear the connecting arcade vessels.

Once the jejunal flap is pulled up to the neck, vascular anastomoses are performed. With the substernal route, the internal mammary vessels are the ideal recipient vessels. The transverse cervical vessels are also good recipient vessels that are located low enough in the neck without the need for vein grafting. Using the carotid artery branches will most likely mandate vein grafting. Excess length of the jejunal conduit is removed and a 3 to 4 cm of proximal jejunum

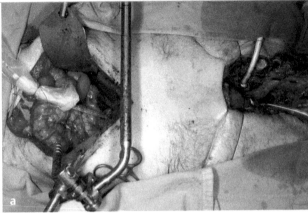

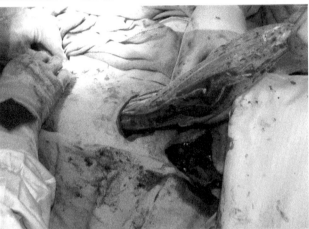

Fig. 26.5 To deliver the jejunal flap to the neck, a chest tube is first passed from the neck to the abdomen through either the retrocardiac or substernal route. **(a)** A plastic camera bag is tied to the chest tube and pulled to the neck. **(b)** The jejunal flap is then placed in the plastic bag. By pulling the bag from the neck and pushing the bowel from the abdomen, the flap is delivered to the neck without traction injury.

based on two terminal arcade vessels is exteriorized for flap monitoring as described earlier. The esophagojejunal anastomosis is then performed using a single layer of 3–0 Vicryl sutures in an end-to-end fashion. The anastomosis can also be completed with a stapling device.

Intestinal continuity is reestablished in the abdomen by the thoracic or general surgical team through a gastrojejunal anastomosis using the posterior wall of the stomach, or through a Roux-en-Y jejunojejunal anastomosis if no stomach is left. A feeding jejunostomy tube is routinely placed. Initially, we placed a nasogastric tube through the nose to the jejunal flap. After seeing perforation of the jejunum by the tube, we no longer use nasogastric tubes and have not seen any adverse effects. The midline abdominal incision is closed with heavy polypropylene sutures. Placement of neck or mediastinal drains should avoid the tip of drain touching the jejunal as bowel perforation by drains has occurred. Bilateral chest tubes are often placed as well by the thoracic surgery team.

26.9 Postoperative Care

Following free jejunal flap for pharyngoesophageal reconstruction, requirements for postoperative care are similar to that for any patient following major head and neck surgery with some special considerations. The gastrostomy tube is maintained on intermittent suction until return of active bowel sounds. Jejunostomy feeding may be initiated on the second postoperative day. A modified barium swallow study is performed to confirm healing and to assess swallowing function 7 to 14 days after surgery depending on whether previous radiotherapy was given. If satisfactory healing and function are confirmed, the patient may be started on a liquid diet, which may be advanced to a regular diet within the next several days. The feeding tube may be removed when the patient reliably demonstrates an ability to take adequate nutrition by mouth.

Total esophageal reconstruction with the supercharged jejunal flap represents a much more complex surgery, higher surgical risks, and more difficult postoperative recovery. Medical complications, particularly pleural effusion, pneumonia, and respiratory failure, are more common. Patients are monitored in a surgical intensive care unit postoperatively for careful hemodynamic and pulmonary management until they are stable enough to go to a regular floor. Tube feeding is started on return of bowel function. Barium swallow study is performed similar to free jejunal flap for pharyngoesophageal reconstruction.

26.10 Pearls and Pitfalls

- For pharyngoesophageal reconstruction with a free jejunal flap, flap insetting should be performed with the neck in a neutral position without extension and the flap slightly stretched to avoid redundancy and thus dysphagia.
- For total esophageal reconstruction with the supercharged jejunal flap, great care should be taken not to disrupt the distal arcade vessels between the mesenteric branches when pulling the flap through the chest to the neck.
- Removing the manubrium and head of clavicle to expose the internal mammary vessels while passing the jejunum via the substernal route may provide easier access to the recipient vessels and make the reconstruction simpler.

References

[1] Seidenberg B, Rosenak SS, Hurwitt ES, Som ML. Immediate reconstruction of the cervical esophagus by a revascularized isolated jejunal segment. Ann Surg 1959;149(2):162–171
[2] Roberts RE, Douglas FM. Replacement of the cervical esophagus and hypopharynx by a revascularized free jejunal autograft. Report of a case successfully treated. N Engl J Med 1961;264:342–344
[3] Nakayama K, Yamamoto K, Tamiya T, et al. Experience with free autografts of the bowel with a new venous anastomosis apparatus. Surgery 1964;55:796–802
[4] Jurkiewicz MJ. Vascularized intestinal graft for reconstruction of the cervical esophagus and pharynx. Plast Reconstr Surg 1965;36(5):509–517
[5] Hester TR, McConnel FM, Nahal F, Jurkiewicz MJ, Brown RG. Reconstruction of cervical esophagus, hypopharynx and oral cavity using free jejunal transfer. Am J Surg 1980;140(4):487–491
[6] Gluckman JL, McDonough JJ, McCafferty GJ, et al. Complications associated with free jejunal graft reconstruction of the pharyngoesophagus—a multiinstitutional experience with 52 cases. Head Neck Surg 1985;7(3):200–205
[7] Coleman JJ III, Searles JM Jr, Hester TR, et al. Ten years experience with the free jejunal autograft. Am J Surg 1987;154(4):394–398
[8] Schusterman MA, Shestak K, de Vries EJ, et al. Reconstruction of the cervical esophagus: free jejunal transfer versus gastric pull-up. Plast Reconstr Surg 1990;85(1):16–21
[9] Reece GP, Schusterman MA, Miller MJ, et al. Morbidity and functional outcome of free jejunal transfer reconstruction for circumferential defects of the pharynx and cervical esophagus. Plast Reconstr Surg 1995;96(6):1307–1316
[10] Cordeiro PG, Shah K, Santamaria E, Gollub MJ, Singh B, Shah JP. Barium swallows after free jejunal transfer: should they be performed routinely? Plast Reconstr Surg 1999;103(4):1167–1175

[11] Longmire WP Jr. A modification of the Roux technique for antethoracic esophageal reconstruction. Surgery 1947;22(1):94–100

[12] Hirabayashi S, Miyata M, Shoji M, Shibusawa H. Reconstruction of the thoracic esophagus, with extended jejunum used as a substitute, with the aid of microvascular anastomosis. Surgery 1993;113(5):515–519

[13] Heitmiller RF, Gruber PJ, Swier P, Singh N. Long-segment substernal jejunal esophageal replacement with internal mammary vascular augmentation. Dis Esophagus 2000;13(3):240–242

[14] Sekido M, Yamamoto Y, Minakawa H, et al. Use of the "supercharge" technique in esophageal and pharyngeal reconstruction to augment microvascular blood flow. Surgery 2003;134(3):420–424

[15] Sakuraba M, Kimata Y, Hishinuma S, Nishimura M, Gotohda N, Ebihara S. Importance of additional microvascular anastomosis in esophageal reconstruction after salvage esophagectomy. Plast Reconstr Surg 2004;113(7):1934–1939

[16] Poh M, Selber JC, Skoracki R, Walsh GL, Yu P. Technical challenges of total esophageal reconstruction using a supercharged jejunal flap. Ann Surg 2011;253(6):1122–1129

27 Groin/Superficial Circumflex Iliac Artery Perforator Flap

Rene D. Largo

Abstract

The groin flap is based on the superficial circumflex iliac artery and can be used as a pedicle or free flap. Currently, the flap is mainly used as a pedicle flap to cover hand and arm wounds and less frequently as a free flap owing due to its bulk, anatomical variability, and short pedicle length. The superficial circumflex iliac artery perforator flap is an evolution of the conventional groin flap and is based on a perforator of the superficial circumflex iliac artery system. This flap preserves the advantages of a groin flap with its easily concealed donor site scar but also overcomes its disadvantages of short pedicle length and bulkiness. It can be dissected in order to increase pedicle length and produce a thinner flap. This chapter discusses the procedure for using the groin flap, from indications suggesting its use, to preoperative considerations, to the surgical technique. Anatomy is covered and three variations are listed.

Keywords: superficial circumflex iliac artery perforator flap, superficial femoral artery, external iliac artery, lateral femoral cutaneous nerve

27.1 Introduction

The groin flap was first described by McGregor and Jackson in 1972 and Daniel and Taylor used it as the first successful cutaneous free flap in 1973.[1,2] The major advantage of the groin flap represents its hairless skin and inconspicuous donor site scar. The groin flap is based on the superficial circumflex iliac artery and can be used as a pedicle or free flap. Nowadays, the flap is mainly used as a pedicle flap to cover hand and arm wounds and infrequently used as a free flap mainly due to its bulk, anatomical variability, and its short pedicle length. The superficial circumflex iliac artery perforator (SCIP) flap is an evolution of the conventional groin flap and was first introduced by Koshima in 2004.[3] The SCIP flap is based on a perforator of the superficial circumflex iliac artery (SCIA) system. The SCIP flap preserves the advantages of a groin flap with its easily concealed donor site scar but also overcomes its disadvantages of short pedicle length and bulkiness. The SCIA system can be dissected further distal and the skin paddle positioned lateral to the anterior superior iliac spine (ASIS) resulting in increased pedicle length and thinner flap. The SCIP flap harvest does not require muscle or nerve dissection leading to no functional deficits and short operative time.

27.2 Typical Indications

- The groin flap is primarily a pedicled flap for coverage of dorsal hand and distal forearm wounds.
- The SCIP flap is typically used for resurfacing of up to moderate-sized skin defects that do not tolerate bulkiness and where recipient vessels are located superficially or within close proximity, such as foot, ankle, genital area, upper extremity but also the cheek, floor of mouth, tongue, or neck.

27.3 Anatomy

The **SCIA** (0.8 to 1.8 mm in diameter) and its concomitant vein arise from the femoral vessels underneath the deep fascia of the thigh about 2.5 cm inferior to the inguinal ligament dividing into superficial and deep branches about 1.5 cm from the femoral artery (▶ **Fig. 27.1**).[4] The superficial branch perforates the deep fascia immediately after its origin from the femoral artery and travels superolateral to the **ASIS**. In 15% of cases, the superficial vessel splits into two additional branches, one (superficial) supplying the skin and one (deep) supplying the fascia lata and muscle, although the superficial branch can be hypoplastic or even absent.[5] In contrast to the superficial branch, the deep branch is mostly present and long and large. The deep branch travels superolateral underneath the deep fascia, provides multiple muscle perforators and branches and finally penetrates the deep fascia at the lateral border of the sartorius muscle about 6 cm lateral to the femoral artery. The dominant perforator of SCIA is mostly located around 1.5 to 3 cm superomedial to the ASIS and measures in average 0.85 mm.[6] The SCIP flap can be based on either the superficial or deep SCIA branches or both. The SCIA may arise directly from the **superficial femoral artery**, the **external iliac artery**, or a common trunk with the deep circumflex iliac artery (DCIA). On

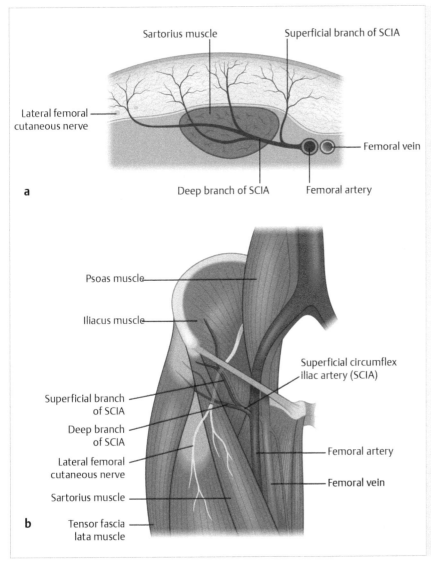

Fig. 27.1 Schematic figure of the SCIA system. (a) Cross-section. (b) Anteroposterior view.

rare occasion, the SCIA system is completely hypoplastic.[7] The **lateral femoral cutaneous nerve** crosses the arterial deep branch on top or below.

The concomitant vein of the SCIA system drains into the femoral vein. There are also cutaneous veins that run parallel to the SCIA in the superficial layer of subcutaneous tissue that ultimately drain in to the **greater saphenous vein**.

27.4 Variations

- Sartorius muscle–cutaneous groin flap.
- Chimeric flap with vascularized iliac crest bone flap (based on DCIA) and SCIP flap.
- Sensate SCIP flap based on lateral cutaneous branches of the intercostal nerves.

27.5 Preoperative Considerations

The location of the SCIA and perforators can be confirmed by hand-held Doppler ultrasonography prior to flap elevation. Alternately, the usage of preoperative color Doppler ultrasound assessment has been shown to be helpful in planning of the SCIP flap to further illustrate any hypoplasia or hyperplasia of the SCIA system.[7] Computed tomography angiography can be to illustrate the SCIA vasculature pattern.

27.6 Positioning and Skin Markings

The patient is best positioned in supine for flap harvest for most applications. The ipsilateral hip can be elevated by placing folded towels beneath the buttocks to facilitate exposure of lateral border of the flap, especially if the flap extends lateral to the ASIS.

A line is drawn between the ASIS and the pubic tubercle representing the course of the inguinal ligament. The long axis of the flap is centered on the course of the SCIA, which is located 2 to 3 cm inferior and parallel to inguinal ligament (▶ **Fig. 27.2**). The flap can be extended up to the posterior iliac spine laterally and to the femoral vessels medially. Flap dimensions measure up to 25 cm in length and up to 8 to 10 cm in width. A pinch test is performed to confirm maximal flap width for primary donor site closure. The origin of the flap pedicle is found within the triangle formed by the lateral border of the adductor longus muscle medially, inguinal ligament superiorly and the medial border of the sartorius muscle. The location of the SCIA and perforators can be confirmed by Doppler probe prior to flap elevation.

27.7 Operative Technique

27.7.1 Groin Flap

A Doppler probe can be helpful to confirm the SCIA course over the sartorius muscle to the ASIS. Flap dissection proceeds from lateral to medial. The deep fascia is incised at the lateral border of the sartorius muscle and the superficial circumflex iliac vessels are dissected to their origin.

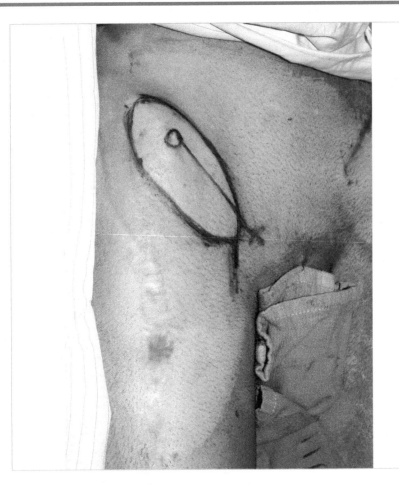

Fig. 27.2 Skin markings for a right SCIP flap, with the long axis of the flap about 2 to 3 cm below the inguinal ligament, extending from the femoral vessels medially and beyond the ASIS laterally.

27.7.2 SCIP Flap

Preoperative Doppler probe is useful for confirmation of SCIA course and its perforator location. Flap outline is based on the defect dimension and perforator location. The flap is elevated in a "freestyle" manner. The first incision is made through the inferior or superior border of the flap, allowing visualization of the superficial or deep branch and their perforators.

The SCIP flap can be harvested based on either the superficial or the deep branch of the SCIA system. The relationship between the superficial and deep system is complementary, when the superficial system is small, then the deep system is large and vice versa.[5] Once the dominant perforator is selected, the flap is elevated from lateral to medial in a suprafascial plane (▶ Fig. 27.3). The cutaneous vein in the medial part of the flap is included to overcome the sometimes too small caliber (< 0.5 mm) of the concomitant vein accompanying the flap pedicle. The superficial vein is often used alone or in combination with the concomitant vein to assure adequate venous outflow of the flap. The lateral femoral cutaneous nerve may occasionally need to be transected during flap harvest.

As a modification, the flap can also be harvested at the level of the superficial fascia preserving the deep adipose tissue of the subcutaneous fat containing lymphatics and lymph nodes.

The pedicle is somewhat short with mean length of 4.8 ± 1.3 cm (range: 3–8 cm), although microdissection of the perforator can yield to a pedicle with a mean length of 7 cm.[6]

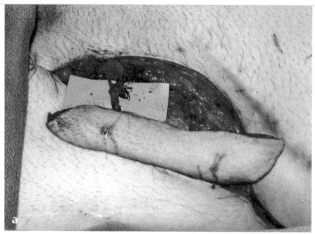

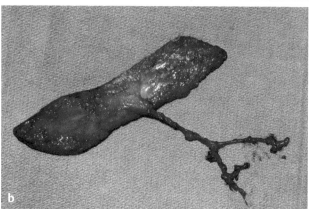

Fig. 27.3 **(a)** SCIP free flap based on a single dominant perforator arising from the superficial branch of the SCIA. **(b)** Completed dissection.

27.8 Donor Site Closure

Primary donor site closure can be achieved if the flap width is less than approximately 8 to 10 cm. A closed suction drain should be placed. Rare complications include wound dehiscence, seroma, and lymphorrhea, especially when the full thickness of subcutaneous fat is included in the SCIP flap or a groin flap is performed due to transection of lymphatics draining into the groin lymph nodes.

27.9 Pearls and Pitfalls

- The SCIP flap has lower donor site morbidity, less bulkiness, and longer pedicle length compared to the conventional groin flap.
- The SCIP flap can be elevated based on the superficial branch of the SCIA system in over 90%. If the superficial branch is absent or hypoplastic, the flap can be harvested on the deep branch of the SCIA.
- To overcome the small caliber of the concomitant vein accompanying the flap pedicle, the superficial vein is often used alone or in combination with the concomitant vein to assure adequate venous outflow of the flap.
- A major disadvantage of the SCIP flap is its limited pedicle length. If a pedicle length of more than 7 cm is needed, a vein graft mostly becomes necessary. This limitation applies often only to the artery, since the vein can be dissected out often longer than 10 cm.

References

[1] McGregor IA, Jackson IT. The groin flap. Br J Plast Surg 1972;25(1):3–16

[2] Daniel RK, Taylor GI. Distant transfer of an island flap by microvascular anastomoses. A clinical technique. Plast Reconstr Surg 1973;52(2):111–117

[3] Koshima I, Nanba Y, Tsutsui T, et al. Superficial circumflex iliac artery perforator flap for reconstruction of limb defects. Plast Reconstr Surg 2004;113(1):233–240

[4] Hsu WM, Chao WN, Yang C, et al. Evolution of the free groin flap: the superficial circumflex iliac artery perforator flap. Plast Reconstr Surg 2007;119(5):1491–1498

[5] Goh TL, Park SW, Cho JY, Choi JW, Hong JP. The search for the ideal thin skin flap: superficial circumflex iliac artery perforator flap–a review of 210 cases. Plast Reconstr Surg 2015;135(2):592–601

[6] Sinna R, Hajji H, Qassemyar Q, Perignon D, Benhaim T, Havet E. Anatomical background of the perforator flap based on the deep branch of the superficial circumflex iliac artery (SCIP Flap): a cadaveric study. Eplasty 2010;10:e11

[7] Tashiro K, Harima M, Kato M, et al. Preoperative color Doppler ultrasound assessment in planning of SCIP flaps. J Plast Reconstr Aesthet Surg 2015;68(7):979–983

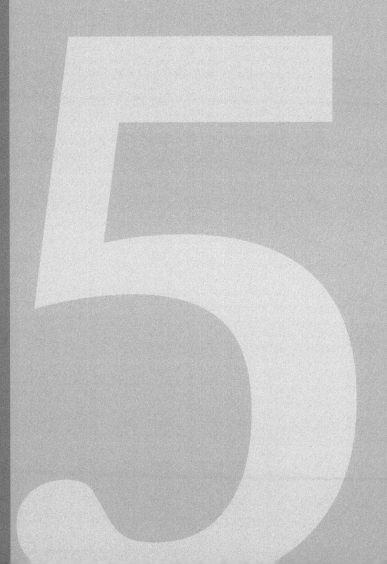

Part 5

Pelvis

28 Iliac Crest (Deep Circumflex Iliac Artery) Osseous/Osteocutaneous Free Flap

Sahil K. Kapur and Matthew M. Hanasono

Abstract

The iliac crest flap is a versatile free flap based on the deep circumflex iliac artery that is used primarily in mandibular or maxillary reconstruction and occasionally in extremity reconstruction. It has a robust blood supply with both nutrient and periosteal perforators and can be safely osteotomized to provide optimum contouring for the intended defect. It can be harvested with associated muscle (internal oblique muscle) and a skin paddle, to a height of 4 cm. The iliac crest flap can be harvested as a longitudinally split bone flap to decrease donor site morbidity. While this flap is usually harvested as a free flap, there have been reports that describe its application as a pedicled flap for the reconstruction of acetabular defects or for femoral head reconstruction in cases of ischemic necrosis. The authors guide surgeons through the constituent steps involved in the use of this flap, beginning with indications for it's use, the anatomy, preoperative considerations, and the operative technique. Three variations and three disadvantages involved in this procedure are cited.

Keywords: external iliac artery, femoral artery, anterior superior iliac spine, ascending branch, internal oblique muscle, superficial circumflex iliac artery, iliohypogasric nerve, ilioinguinal nerve, lateral femoral cutaneous nerve

28.1 Introduction

The iliac crest flap is a versatile free flap based on the deep circumflex iliac artery (DCIA) that is used primarily in mandibular or maxillary reconstruction, and occasionally in extremity reconstruction. It has a robust blood supply with both nutrient and periosteal perforators and can be safely osteotomized to provide optimum contouring for the intended defect.[1,2] It can be harvested with associated muscle (internal oblique muscle) and a skin paddle. Furthermore, it can be harvested to a height of 4 cm, considerably more than other vascularized bone flaps. The iliac crest flap can be harvested as a longitudinally split bone flap to decrease donor site morbidity. While this flap is usually harvested as a free flap, there have been few clinical reports that describe its application as a pedicled flap for the reconstruction of acetabular defects or for femoral head reconstruction in cases of ischemic necrosis.

28.2 Typical Indications

- Hemimandibular reconstruction.[3]
- Maxillary reconstruction[4]
- Long bone reconstruction (e.g., tibia).
- Acetabular or femoral head defects (as a pedicled flap).[5]

28.3 Anatomy

The iliac crest bone is perfused via nutrient and periosteal perforators originating from the **DCIA**, which forms the dominant blood supply to the flap. This vessel branches off either the **external iliac artery** or the **femoral artery**. In majority of the cases, it originates from the external iliac artery either directly beneath the inguinal ligament (41%) or cranial to it (17%). The deep inferior epigastric vessels that supply the rectus abdominis muscle originate from a similar location but travel medially. In some cases (42%), the DCIA arises caudal to the inguinal ligament, from the femoral artery.

The DCIA originates deep to the transversalis fascia and travels in a super-olateral direction toward the **anterior superior iliac spine** (ASIS). After giving rise to a large **ascending branch** that nourishes the internal oblique muscle, it pierces the transversalis fascia and enters a fibro-osseous tunnel, about 2 cm from the top of the inner lip of the crest. This tunnel is formed along the line of attachment of the iliacus and transversalis fascia. While traveling through the fibro-osseous tunnel, the DCIA gives off branches to nourish the iliac bone as well as multiple musculocutaneous perforators that pass through the transversus abdominis, internal oblique, and external oblique muscles to the overlying skin. The first of these branches originates approximately 2 cm lateral to the ASIS. Approximately 6 to 9 cm from the ASIS, the DCIA reemerges from the fibro-osseous tunnel and penetrates the transversus abdominis muscle and anastomoses with the iliolumbar artery in the plane between the internal oblique and the transversus abdominis. The artery has an approximate pedicle length of 8 to 10 cm with a diameter of 2 to 3 mm at its origin.

Skin perforators are present in 92% of the cases and are located 5 to 10.5 cm lateral to the ASIS and 0.1 to 3.5 cm (average about 0.8 cm) above the iliac crest bone.[6] Approximately 70% of the time, multiple (average of 6) small cutaneous perforators are observed. Approximately 30% of the time, the DCIA also gives off a single dominant cutaneous branch to the skin about 6.5 cm lateral to the ASIS and 1 to 2 cm superior to the iliac crest. A skin flap measuring 10 × 15 cm can be supported by this branch.[7]

A portion of the **internal oblique muscle** can be harvested with this flap based on the ascending branch that originates from the DCIA before the pedicle enters the fibro-osseous tunnel. This branch penetrates the transversalis fascia and travels in between the internal oblique and transversus abdominis muscles before anastomosing with the deep inferior epigastric artery. This branch usually lies within 1 cm from the ASIS approximately 65% of the time and within 2 to 4 cm from the ASIS approximately 15% of the time. It is replaced by multiple small branches 20% of the time. Occasionally, the ascending branch may originate from the external iliac artery and may serve as the dominant supply to the iliac bone, with only a minor contribution from the DCIA.

The **superficial circumflex iliac artery** (SCIA) serves as the minor blood supply for to the iliac crest. This vessel originates more distally from the femoral vessels. It mainly supplies the skin anterior and superior to the ASIS as well as an osseous segment near the ASIS. It usually communicates with the DCIA in the region of the iliac crest and can be used to support a larger skin paddle. The posterior aspect of the iliac crest is supplied by a deep superior branch of the superior gluteal artery.

Venous outflow for the flap follows the arterial supply. The DCIA has two venae comitantes that join together 1 to 4 cm before they empty into the external iliac or femoral vein. The vein has a pedicle length of 4 to 6 cm and is approximately 2 to 4 mm in diameter.

This flap is not sensate and does not have motor innervation. While no nerves travel with the pedicle, multiple important nerves are encountered during the dissection and should be spared. The **iliohypogastric nerve** (L1) travels between the transversus abdominis and internal oblique layers of the abdominal wall. As it transverses medially it can be encountered superior to the pedicle and medial to the ASIS. The **ilioinguinal nerve** (L1) travels between internal and external oblique muscles and can be encountered inferior to the pedicle as it travels toward the ASIS. It travels along with the spermatic cord or the round ligament. It provides innervation to the proximal medial aspect of the thigh as well as the skin on the root of the penis and scrotum in males and the skin involving the labia majora in females.

The **lateral femoral cutaneous nerve** travels caudally along the surface of the iliacus muscle. It pierces the deep fascia of the thigh 2 cm inferomedial to the ASIS. It crosses the DCIA as the vessel approaches the ASIS. If the nerve is injured during harvest it should be repaired. Injury to the nerve can result in numbness and pain along the lateral aspect of the thigh.

The iliac crest is approximately 23 cm in length. About 16 cm of this bone can harvested based on the DCIA. Approximately 4 cm of bone height can be harvested. A height of 2 cm is necessary for mandible reconstruction. The thickness of the bone varies from 1.4 cm at the ASIS to 1.7 cm at the tubercle.[8] In general, a skin paddle measuring 15 to 20 cm in length and 6 to 8 cm in width can be harvested (▶ **Fig. 28.1**).

28.4 Variations

- Duplication of the DCIA.
- Dominant ascending branch that forms the main blood supply to the bone with minor contributions from the DCIA.
- Alternate origin of the ascending branch directly from the external iliac artery.

28.5 Preoperative Considerations

Dissection of the flap can be difficult and sometimes impossible in obese patients. The skin paddle can be excessively bulky. Flap thickness and mobility can be improved by performing a perforator dissection to avoid including the external and internal oblique, and transversus abdominis muscles. In other cases, a second thinner flap such as a forearm flap may be a better solution. Alternately, the internal oblique muscle can be used as a lining flap and covered with a skin graft or allowed to mucosalize spontaneously.

28.6 Positioning and Skin Markings

The flap is harvested with the patient in supine position. A roll is placed under the contralateral hip to improve exposure while dissecting within the iliac fossa.

The skin paddle is oriented along a line drawn from the inferior tip of the scapula to the femoral artery. It is positioned such that its medial border lies at the ASIS. The superior two-thirds of the skin paddle can be positioned superior

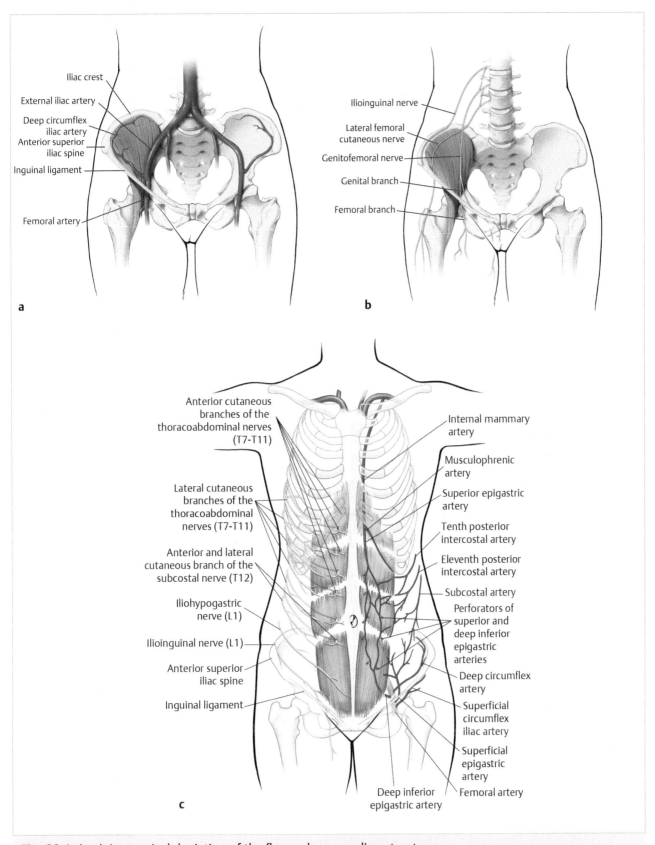

Fig. 28.1 (a-c) Anatomical depiction of the flap and surrounding structures.

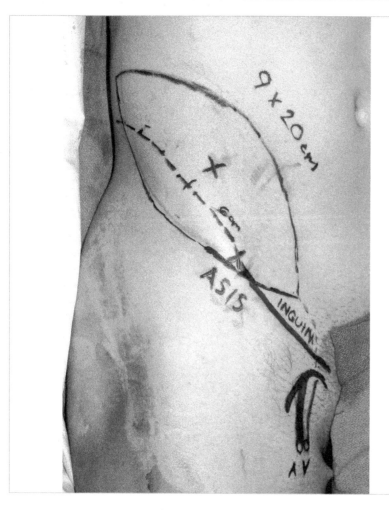

Fig. 28.2 Preoperative markings demonstrating elliptical skin paddle, inguinal ligament, ASIS, and location of the dominant perforator.

to the crest while the inferior one-third is positioned inferior to it. The paddle can measure 15 to 20 cm in length and 6 to 8 cm in width (depending on skin laxity). The most consistent skin perforator arises about 5 cm lateral to the ASIS. The skin incision is extended medially over inguinal ligament, where the pedicle dissection and harvest begin (▶ **Fig. 28.2**).

28.6.1 Operative Technique

Flap harvest technique varies based on the volume of soft tissue and thickness of bone required. The incision is first made medially approximately 1 cm superior the inguinal ligament. Soft tissue is dissected down to the transversalis fascia. The inguinal canal, round ligament, or spermatic cord are identified and retracted medially (▶ **Fig. 28.3**). The transversalis fascia, which forms the floor of the canal, is incised to expose the external iliac artery and vein. The external iliacs are dissected until the DCIA and deep circumflex iliac vein are found. As mentioned, the DCIA and deep circumflex iliac vein may occasionally arise from the femoral vessels. The pedicle is then dissected laterally toward the ASIS. Three layers of abdominal musculature, which include the external oblique, internal oblique and transversus abdominis, are incised superficial to the pedicle. Eventually, the ascending branch will be encountered, about 1 cm medial to the ASIS. The ascending branch is adherent to the deep surface of the internal oblique muscle. This branch can be used to supply a flap composed of the internal oblique muscle, if needed. Otherwise, it is ligated and divided.

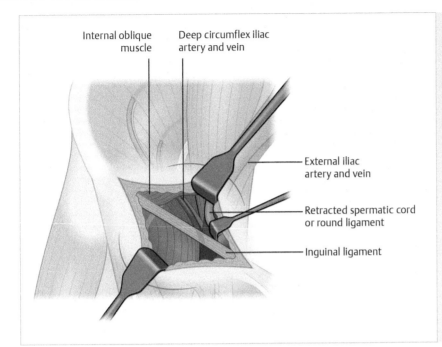

Internal oblique muscle

Deep circumflex iliac artery and vein

External iliac artery and vein

Retracted spermatic cord or round ligament

Inguinal ligament

Fig. 28.3 Illustration of skin incision and initial dissection of DCIA pedicle. Spermatic cord and round ligament is retracted as shown in the figure.

After the ascending branch is encountered, the skin incision is extended laterally and superiorly along the intended superior border of the skin paddle. Suprafascial dissection is carried out inferiorly toward the iliac crest (▶ **Fig. 28.4a**). The external oblique fascia is divided when the perforators are encountered. Perforators to the skin can come from multiple sources: intercostal vessels, lumbar vessels, or the DCIA. It is important to sufficiently trace the perforators encountered to ensure that the skin paddle includes perforators from the DCIA pedicle. Perforators originating from the intercostal or iliolumbar vessels usually have a nerve associated with them and have a posterior orientation. Perforators from the DCIA do not have an associated nerve and have a more anterior orientation. A true perforator flap is dissected if less soft-tissue bulk is needed and more skin paddle mobility is required (▶ **Fig. 28.4b**).

If a dominant perforator of 1 mm or greater in diameter is encountered, the skin paddle may be harvested as a perforator-based flap, minimizing bulk. If there are only multiple tiny perforators, then it is advisable to include several or all of them. Also, if more bulk is desirable, then a true perforator dissection is not required. In these cases, the dissection is carried down to the bone while preserving a 2 to 3 cm cuff of muscle between the skin paddle and the crest for a distance of 6 to 8 cm. This cuff of external oblique, internal oblique and transversus abdominis should contain the musculocutaneous perforators.

The properitoneal fat is then retracted medially and superiorly in order to expose the iliacus muscle and fascia. The main pedicle lies lateral to the fusion of the transversalis and iliacus fascia within a fibro-osseous tunnel adherent to the inner cortex of the iliac bone (▶ **Fig. 28.5a**). The iliacus muscle elevated off the iliac crest, inferior to the fibro-osseous tunnel containing the pedicle blood supply, in order to expose the bone sufficiently to make flap osteotomies. Care should be taken at this time not to injure the lateral femoral cutaneous nerve, which travels on the medial surface of the iliacus muscle (▶ **Fig. 28.5b**).

The inferior skin incision is made and suprafascial dissection is carried cranially toward the iliac crest. The gluteus maximus, medius, and minimus are removed from the iliac crest bone to be used in the flap to expose the inferolateral aspect

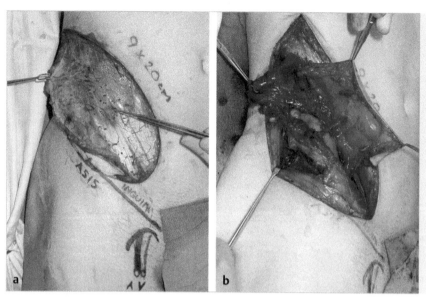

Fig. 28.4 **(a)** Suprafascial dissection over the external oblique fascia is carried until skin perforators are encountered. **(b)** True perforator flap dissection demonstrating dominant perforator perfusing the skin paddle.

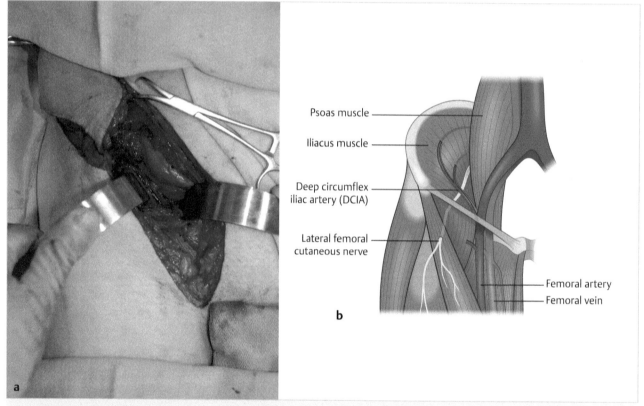

Fig. 28.5 **(a)** Retraction of the properitoneal fat to expose the DCIA pedicle. **(b)** Anatomic depiction of the lateral femoral cutaneous nerve in relation to the DCIA pedicle.

of the osteotomy if a full-thickness bone flap is planned. If only the inner cortex of bone is required the osteotomy can be designed along the crest while leaving the gluteus musculature attached to the outer lip of the crest. A segment of bone measuring up to 4 cm in height and 16 cm in length can be harvested. We prefer to outline the flap with a cutting bur then complete the osteotomies with an oscillating saw. Osteotomes may also be useful when harvesting only the inner cortex of the iliac crest. The ASIS may be left in place or harvested with the flap. If the ASIS is included in the flap, then the inguinal ligament and the origin of

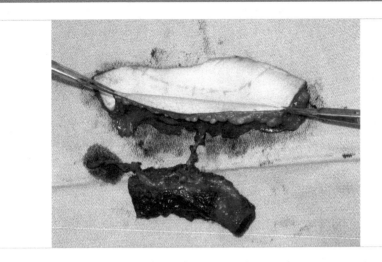

Fig. 28.6 Iliac crest free flap harvested as a true perforator flap.

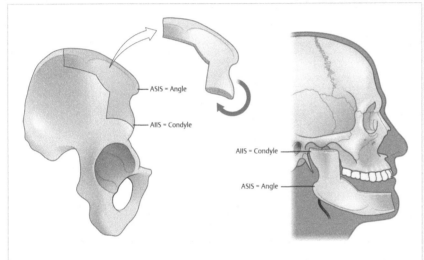

Fig. 28.7 The ipsilateral iliac crest is harvested and flipped vertically such that the ASIS forms the angle, the AIIS forms the condyle, and iliac crest rim forms the body of the neomandible.

the sartorius muscle have to be divided and should be repaired during closure. The pedicle is then dissected proximally to its origin and the flap is harvested (▶ Fig. 28.6).

An ipsilateral iliac crest flap is harvested in order to reconstruct the hemimandible. The flap is vertically flipped after harvest such that the ASIS forms the angle of the mandible and the crest forms the body of the mandible (▶ Fig. 28.7). Because the iliac crest bone is curved, it is not necessary to make any osteotomies. Closing osteotomies may be necessary to shape the iliac crest to recreate an anterior mandibular segment.

28.7 Donor Site Closure

Bone wax should be used to control bleeding, which can be significant, of the remaining bone. The iliacus fascia is sutured to the transversalis fascia. Following this, the hip is flexed and the external and internal obliques are sutured to the gluteus musculature. If a split iliac crest is harvested and the outer cortex has been left intact, holes can be drilled into this cortex to anchor the abdominal fascia. After the fascial defect has been repaired, the closure may be reinforced with an overlay prosthetic or bioprosthetic mesh to prevent hernia formation. Closed suction drains are recommended to prevent seroma formation (▶ Fig. 28.8).

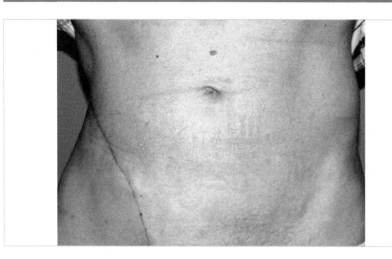

Fig. 28.8 Donor site closure.

28.8 Disadvantages

- The associated skin paddle can be very bulky, especially in the obese patient. This may necessitate the use of a second flap such as a forearm flap if a thin vascularized tissue layer is needed.
- Due to the natural curve of the bone, the iliac crest cannot provide a straight segment longer than 10 cm. This limits its use for long bone reconstruction.
- Donor site morbidity can be a significant drawback of this flap, especially if both cortices of bone are harvested. In addition to an elevated risk of donor site hernia, full-thickness harvest of iliac crest can result in aesthetic disfigurement as well as gait disturbance.

28.9 Pearls and Pitfalls

- Skin perforator anatomy is variable. Besides the variation in location, number and type of perforators, care should be taken to verify that the perforator in question arises from the DCIA. Skin perforators in this region could also originate from the lumbar artery, intercostal artery, SCIA, and the iliolumbar artery.
- The DCIA can sometimes travel in a more superficial plane between the transversus abdominis and the internal oblique muscle. In this case it can be easily mistaken for the ascending branch. Medial to lateral dissection of the pedicle helps in the identification of this variation.
- The skin paddle of the flap can be very bulky and relatively immobile over the iliac crest bone. A thinner flap with more mobility can be obtained by performing a perforator dissection, rather than including a cuff of muscle. However, in obese patients, it may be necessary to perform a second flap such as a forearm flap to provide thinner, more pliable vascularized soft tissue.
- An inner table split-cortex bone flap minimizes donor site morbidity.

References

[1] Taylor GI, Townsend P, Corlett R. Superiority of the deep circumflex iliac vessels as the supply for free groin flaps. Plast Reconstr Surg 1979;64(5):595–604

[2] Taylor GI, Townsend P, Corlett R. Superiority of the deep circumflex iliac vessels as the supply for free groin flaps. Clinical work. Plast Reconstr Surg 1979;64(6):745–759

[3] Kimata Y, Uchiyama K, Sakuraba M, et al. Deep circumflex iliac perforator flap with iliac crest for mandibular reconstruction. Br J Plast Surg 2001;54(6):487–490

[4] Brown JS, Jones DC, Summerwill A, et al. Vascularized iliac crest with internal oblique muscle for immediate reconstruction after maxillectomy. Br J Oral Maxillofac Surg 2002;40(3):183–190

[5] Karakurum G, Gülec A, Büyükbebeci O. Vascularized pedicled iliac crest graft for selected total hip acetabular reconstructions: a cadaver study. Surg Radiol Anat 2004;26(1):3–7

[6] Bergeron L, Tang M, Morris SF. The anatomical basis of the deep circumflex iliac artery perforator flap with iliac crest. Plast Reconstr Surg 2007;120(1):252–258

[7] Safak T, Klebuc MJ, Mavili E, Shenaq SM. A new design of the iliac crest microsurgical free flap without including the "obligatory" muscle cuff. Plast Reconstr Surg 1997;100(7):1703–1709

[8] Frodel JL Jr, Funk GF, Capper DT, et al. Osseointegrated implants: a comparative study of bone thickness in four vascularized bone flaps. Plast Reconstr Surg 1993;92(3):449–455, discussion 456–458

29 Singapore Flap

David M. Adelman

Abstract

The Singapore flap (also known as the pudendal thigh or vulvoperineal flap) is a pedicled fasciocutaneous flap of the proximal medial thigh. Initially, this flap was used for the correction of vesicovaginal fistulae. Thereafter, it was used for vaginal and vulval reconstruction, as well as for penile and scrotal reconstruction. Though somewhat disappointing for larger or more radical defects, flap proponents cite its thinness, ease of harvest, and partial sensation when choosing this flap. Since this flap doesn't provide bulk, it's mostly used for smaller vulvovaginal defects, rather than the more extensive defects found with exenterations. This chapter guides the surgeon through the stages of the Singapore flap procedure, beginning with typical indications, to preoperative considerations, and the surgical technique. Anatomy is discussed and four variations are listed.

Keywords: superficial perineal artery, internal pudenal vessels, deep external pudendal artery, medial circumflex femoral artery, profunda femoris, posterior labial branches of the pudendal nerve, perineal branches of the posterior cutaneous nerve of the thigh

29.1 Introduction

The Singapore flap is a pedicled fasciocutaneous flap of the proximal medial thigh. First described by Wee and Joseph, this flap was used for correction of vesicovaginal fistulae.[1] Shortly thereafter, modifications by Woods et al further demonstrated this flap's utility in vaginal reconstruction.[2] Gleeson and colleagues in 1994 published their additional experience with the Singapore flap, which was somewhat disappointing for larger or more radical defects.[3] However, by 2002, Cordeiro and colleagues had integrated this flap into their algorithm for acquired vaginal defects.[4] Flap proponents cite its thinness, ease of harvest, and partial sensation when choosing this flap. Although mostly used for vaginal and vulval reconstruction, these flaps have utility in penile and scrotal reconstruction as well. Since this flap does not provide bulk, it is mostly used for smaller vulvovaginal defects, rather than the more extensive defects found with exenterations. Although best known as the Singapore flap, the terms "pudendal thigh" and "vulvoperineal flaps" are synonymous with this reconstruction.

29.2 Typical Indications

- Posterior and/or lateral vaginal defects.
- Rectovaginal fistula repair.
- Vulvectomy.
- Perineal defects.
- Total penile reconstruction (often combined with other flaps, such as gracilis).
- Scrotal reconstruction.
- Less ideally suited for pelvic exenteration defects given its lack of bulk.

29.3 Anatomy

The Singapore flap is based on the **superficial perineal artery**, derived from the **internal pudenal vessels**, which branch from the anterior division of the internal iliac artery (▶**Fig. 29.1**). These vessels interconnect with branches of the **deep external pudenal artery** and the **medial circumflex femoral artery**, which arise from the **profunda femoris**. The **posterior labial branches of the pudendal nerve**, as well as the **perineal branches of the posterior cutaneous nerve of the thigh**, supply sensory innervation.[3] Flaps are elevated with skin, subcutaneous fat, and the deep fascia of the adductor muscles to maximize perfusion and innervation. Flaps may be 15 cm in length × 6 cm in width, or greater/lesser depending on the ability to close the donor site without tension. Although perforators to the skin are present, no special perforator dissection is required, making this flap simple to harvest.

29.4 Variations

- Unilateral or bilateral flaps may be harvested, depending on the size and scope of the defect. If bilateral, they may be sutured together in the midline prior to inset.
- The flap skin may be islanded (leaving the deep fascia intact), which follows the original description.[1] The flap is then tunneled under the vulva to reach the vaginal defect.
- Posterior flap skin may remain intact, and posterior vulva may instead be released, to avoid tunneling of flap and maximize flap perfusion.[2]
- Flaps may be based anteriorly rather than posteriorly. This modification is helpful for reconstructing anterior vaginal vulvar defects, or when the posterior perineum has been resected. Anterior flaps are perfused by the external pudendal vessels (▶**Fig. 29.1b**).

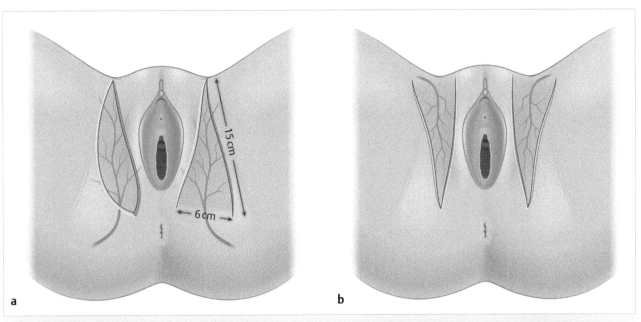

Fig. 29.1 (a) Singapore flaps based posteriorly on the superficial perineal vessels. On the patient's left, the flap skin remains attached to the donor site. The vulva may be released if needed to transpose the flap toward a vaginal defect. On the patient's right, the flap skin is islandized, which may require tunneling of the flap to reach the defect. Flap length and width are noted, but may be adjusted according to patient laxity and reconstructive needs. **(b)** Anteriorly based Singapore flaps, perfused by the external pudendal vessels. This variation may better reach anterior defects that a posteriorly based flap cannot.

29.5 Preoperative Considerations

No special preoperative studies are required. The Singapore flap tends to be relatively thin, even in obese patients. Absolute contraindications include prior flap harvest, or resection in the area of the blood supply. Relative contraindications include previous surgery or radiation to the area, or general medical comorbidities that may influence flap perfusion or healing of the donor site. Radiation tends to be given at the recipient site more often than the donor site, which makes this flap a viable option for many patients.

29.6 Positioning and Skin Markings

Lithotomy positioning is best for most applications. Skin markings are made, with the medial border lateral to the hair-bearing vulva within the thigh crease. Flap length may be up to 15 cm or more, but a longer flap may suffer from decreased perfusion distally. The width may be up to 6 cm, but should be tailored to the defect needs, and the ability to easily close the donor site without tension or significant standing cone deformity. The posterior skin margin is marked at the level of the posterior fourchette of the vulva.

29.7 Operative Technique

With the patient in lithotomy position, unilateral or bilateral flaps are marked. Flap width is adjusted to minimize the tension on primary closure of the donor site. Incisions are made with scalpel and electrocautery through skin, subcutaneous fat, and the deep fascia overlying the adductor musculature. The flap is elevated from anterior distal to proximal in the subfascial plane. The elevated flap is transposed toward the defect; if the transposition is tight, the posterior extent of the incisions can be lengthened, and/or a back-cut is made. The distal extent of the flap is secured to the defect first, to ensure sufficient length and lack of tension. The remaining flap is then approximated in layers (▶ Fig. 29.2). Bilateral flaps may be elevated simultaneously or in succession, and may be approximated to each other prior to inset into the defect.

If intraoperative concerns regarding flap perfusion arise, various clinical tests may be employed (e.g., capillary refill, indocyanine green angiography, etc.). If the distal portions appear less well perfused than the proximal ones, the distal areas may be trimmed, or the flap reinseted to the donor site and delayed.

29.8 Donor Site Closure

The donor site is closed primarily in layers. Wide undermining of the medial thigh may be necessary. The deep and superficial fascial systems should be approximated in order to reduce the tension on skin closure. Absorbable sutures may be used. Absorbable or permanent sutures may be used for skin closure, depending on surgeon preference and patient healing ability. Drains are not routinely used, but should be considered if risk for fluid collections is high. Positioning the patient with thigh adduction for 2 to 3 weeks postoperatively may reduce donor and recipient site's rates of dehiscence.

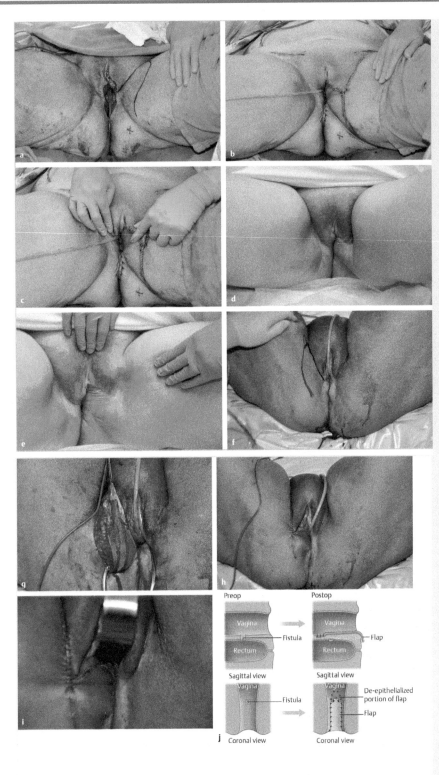

Fig. 29.2 **(a)** Patient 1 has a bilateral vulvo-vaginal defect, left side greater than right. The right side and posterior will both be closed in a complex primary fashion. A Singapore flap is designed for the left side. As the posterior vulva was resected, the flap skin may remain intact posteriorly to maximize perfusion. **(b)** Patient 1 after flap transposition and inset, with primary closure of the donor site, and complex primary repair of the right side and posterior defects. The proximal portion of the flap is used for posterior vulval reconstruction, and restores this contour well. **(c)** Patient 1, demonstrating the distal flap sutured to the remaining mucosa for full continuity of the vaginal vault. **(d,e)** Patient 1, 3 months postoperative, demonstrating excellent healing of both donor and recipient sites. Patient reports full return to activities of daily living without limitation. **(f)** Patient 2 with a postradiation rectovaginal fistula. A unilateral posteriorly based flap is designed. The skin is left intact posteriorly to maximize perfusion. **(g)** The flap is elevated, and the distal tip deepithelialized. Excellent perfusion at the dermal level is noted. Thickness of the subcutaneous tissue is also appreciable. **(h,i)** Closure of the donor site with flap inset. The right vulva was released to allow for the flap inset. The flap reconstructs the majority of the posterior vaginal wall, but is sutured to the remaining mucosa laterally and distally, with the deepithelialized tip tucked beneath. **(j)** Schematic for patient 2. A fistula exists between the posterior wall of the vagina and the anterior wall of the rectum (seen in sagittal and coronal views). The fistula is debrided and the rectal wall closed primarily. The Singapore flap is then used to reconstruct the posterior vaginal wall. The distal extent of the flap is deepithelialized and tucked under the vaginal mucosa distally, in attempts to improve healing in this previously radiated area. The flap has sufficient bulk to keep the vagina and rectum separated, but not so much that function of either is impaired.

211

29.9 Pearls and Pitfalls

- Keeping the skin intact posteriorly, rather than islandizing the flap, will maximize perfusion and promote healing in the more challenging patient.
- If intraoperative flap perfusion appears poor, flap may be delayed and transposed later.
- It is better to use bilateral flaps than try to accomplish too much with a unilateral flap. Alternatively, an inferiorly based flap, combined with a superiorly based flap, may prove effective in the properly selected patient.
- Significant tension on closure of the donor site will lead to wound healing problems. Therefore, try to maximize healing by minimizing morbidity.

References

[1] Wee JTK, Joseph VT. A new technique of vaginal reconstruction using neurovascular pudendal-thigh flaps: a preliminary report. Plast Reconstr Surg 1989;83(4):701–709
[2] Woods JE, Alter G, Meland B, Podratz K. Experience with vaginal reconstruction utilizing the modified Singapore flap. Plast Reconstr Surg 1992;90(2):270–274
[3] Gleeson NC, Baile W, Roberts WS, et al. Pudendal thigh fasciocutaneous flaps for vaginal reconstruction in gynecologic oncology. Gynecol Oncol 1994;54(3):269–274
[4] Cordeiro PG, Pusic AL, Disa JJ. A classification system and reconstructive algorithm for acquired vaginal defects. Plast Reconstr Surg 2002;110(4):1058–1065

30 Superior Gluteal Artery Perforator Flap

Ergun Kocak and Pankaj Tiwari

Abstract

Techniques for the regional advancement and rotation of myocutaneous flaps of the gluteal region have long been used for the coverage of sacral and posterior trunk defects. With the evolution of perforator flaps, the gluteal region has become a reliable donor site for autologous breast reconstruction, especially when the lower abdominal region is not an option. The author guides surgeons through the sequence of steps involved in this procedure, starting with typical indications, continuing with a discussion of anatomy, preoperative considerations, and the surgical technique. Two variations are also listed.

Keywords: internal iliac artery, anterior and posterior divisions, piriformis muscle, inferior gluteal artery, superior gluteal artery, gluteus maximus muscle

30.1 Introduction

Techniques for the regional advancement and rotation of myocutaneous flaps of the gluteal region have long been used for the coverage of sacral and posterior trunk defects. The microsurgical transfer of gluteal tissue was first reported in by Fujino et al in 1975.[1] With the evolution of perforator flaps, the gluteal region has become a reliable donor site for autologous breast reconstruction, especially when the lower abdominal region is not an option.[2]

30.2 Typical Indications

- Breast reconstruction, either immediately following or in a delayed fashion after mastectomy for breast cancer or risk-reducing mastectomy for genetic susceptibility to malignant neoplasm of the breast.
- Sacral and low trunk defects, as a pedicled flap (these techniques are not described further here).

30.3 Anatomy

The perforator vessels that supply the superior gluteal artery perforator (SGAP) flap originate from the internal iliac system (▶Fig. 30.1). The **internal iliac artery** arises from the bifurcation of the common iliac artery at the entry of the pelvis, just anterior to the sacroiliac joint. After approximately a 4 cm posteromedial course, it exits the pelvis through the greater sciatic foramen and divides into **anterior and posterior divisions**. The anterior division continues downward, anterior to the **piriformis muscle**, to give rise to several branches, including the **inferior gluteal artery**, which supplies perforators to the inferior gluteal artery perforator (IGAP) and other thigh flaps. The posterior division of the internal iliac artery pierces the sacral fascia and passes superior to the piriformis muscle. It further divides into deep and superficial branches. It is the superficial branch (**superior gluteal artery**) that courses into the **gluteus maximus muscle** belly and supplies multiple perforating branches that go on to supply the overlying fat and skin.

The superior gluteal artery enters the deep surface of the **gluteus maximus muscle** medially. Therefore, the medially located perforators are closer to the origin of the parent vessel and have a short intramuscular course. The laterally

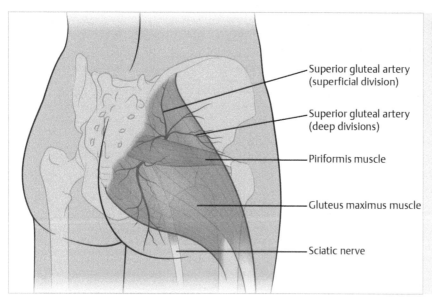

Fig. 30.1 Vascular anatomy of the superior gluteal artery, overlying skin, and pertinent anatomic landmarks.

Superior gluteal artery (superficial division)

Superior gluteal artery (deep divisions)

Piriformis muscle

Gluteus maximus muscle

Sciatic nerve

located perforators, however, travel 3 to 5 cm in the gluteus maxiumus muscle before entering the fat and skin above. As a result, the lateral perforators tend to be better choices for SGAP flap design because they provide longer pedicle length.

While the SGAP flap does not include muscle in the flap itself, several muscles with important locomotive function are encountered during flap dissection. The gluteus maximus muscle originates from the outer surface of ilium, lateral mass of sacrum, and coccyx. It inserts into the gluteal tuberosity of femur and iliotibial tract. The branches of the superior gluteal artery that give rise to the perforators of the SGAP flap run parallel to the fibers of this muscle, making it possible to dissect the pedicle by separating the muscle rather than dividing it. This minimizes injury to the gluteus maximus muscle and preserves function of this important muscle. The piriformis muscle is located deep to the gluteus maximus muscle, originating on the anterolateral surface of the sacrum and inserting on the medial aspect of the greater trochanter of the femur. This muscle serves as an important anatomic landmark in the dissection of the SGAP flap by marking the border above which the superior gluteal artery can be found exiting the pelvis and entering into the deep surface of the gluteus maximus muscle. The superior gluteal artery tends to be on the smaller side, ranging from 1.5 to 2.0 mm in diameter while the accompanying vein tends to larger, about 2.5 mm in diameter on average.

30.4 Variations

- The greatest variation is in the shape and orientation of the skin island. Most commonly, a fusiform skin island, oriented either horizontally or obliquely with the lateral-most end slightly superior, is used. Other shapes, such as a boomerang or curved shape have been described.
- Pedicled flaps of various shapes can be designed for sacral soft-tissue reconstruction.

30.5 Preoperative Considerations

The ideal patient for SGAP breast reconstruction has deflated, lax tissue in the upper gluteal region. Overweight patients with thicker, denser tissue may pose

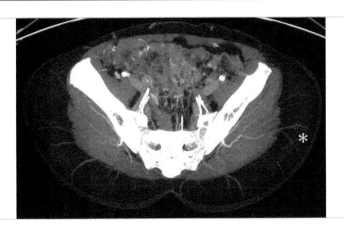

Fig. 30.2 CT angiogram of the superior gluteal artery perforators. In this axial maximum intensity projection (MIP) image, a branch of the left superior gluteal artery can be seen coursing laterally through the belly of the gluteus maximus muscle (*). It exits the muscle posterolaterally and splits into two branches shortly after entering the overlying subcutaneous tissue.

a challenge as the unyielding nature of these flaps combined with the shorter pedicle length can limit the reach of the flap vessels to the recipient mammary vessels.

Surface anatomic landmarks such as the posterior superior iliac spine (PSIS) and the greater trochanter can aid in flap design by outlining the zone where the perforator density is greatest (see Section 30.6 Positioning and Skin Markings). However, the location and number of perforators available for the design of the SGAP flap can vary significantly from patient to patient. Furthermore, the course of perforators as they travel through the muscle can be quite variable, with some taking a short, direct course to the skin and others following a more tortuous path through or around the gluteus muscle. Preoperative use of computed tomography angiography (CTA) to visualize the number and location of the dominant perforator vessels and the relative course they follow through the muscle can facilitate flap design and optimize perforator selection (▶Fig. 30.2). CTA of the gluteal region is usually done with the patient in the prone position.

Bilateral SGAP flap breast reconstruction can pose a challenge. In this setting, the time of the operation is dependent on several factors including the mastectomies, the need for multiple intraoperative position changes, and the technical difficulty of both the flap dissection and microsurgical revascularization. Using a multiteam approach flap elevation and revascularization may reduce surgical time.[3] However, if any reservations exist, staging the reconstructions to be done on different days should be considered.

30.6 Positioning and Skin Markings

Markings are applied preoperatively with the patient in the standing position (▶Fig. 30.3). The PSIS and greater trochanter are marked and a line connecting these two points is drawn. The majority of the perforators will be found near the junction of the medial two-thirds and lateral one-third of this line.[4] For breast reconstruction, the patient is positioned laterally for unilateral cases and prone for bilateral cases (see discussion regarding timing of reconstruction above). A hand-held Doppler ultrasound is used to identify perforators at the level of the skin and correlated with the preoperative CTA findings to estimate the location of the perforator(s) that will most likely be used. The proposed skin island is then marked. While designing the skin island to centralize the location of perforators is preferred, laterally located perforators are more likely to provide longer pedicle length and can be used in an off-center position in a reliable fashion. A fusiform skin island with tapered ends optimizes the closure of the defect by minimizing contour deformities at the ends of the donor site incision scar. Flap dimensions can be up to 30 cm in length and 12 cm in width,

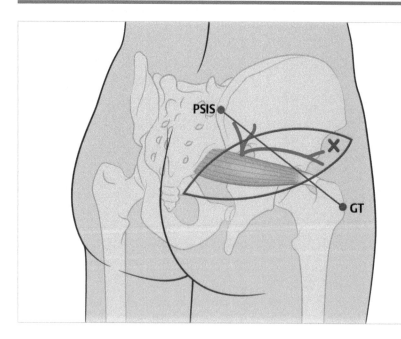

Fig. 30.3 Skin markings for the SGAP flap. The two key anatomic landmarks, the posterior superior iliac spine (PSIS) and the greater trochanter (GT), are identified and a line connecting these two points is drawn. The SGAP perforator vessels tend to be located near a point between the medial two-thirds and lateral one-third of this line. The flap can be reliably designed with the dominant perforator off center, making it possible to base the flap on more laterally located perforators to maximize pedicle length.

depending on the laxity of the gluteal region and the amount of tissue that is needed for reconstruction of the defect.

30.7 Operative Technique

The skin paddle is marked, as described earlier. The skin is first incised laterally and the flap is elevated off of the fascia from lateral to medial. The dissection starts in a suprafascial plane but is quickly transitioned into a subfascial plane when the gluteus maximus muscle is encountered. The dissection proceeds medially in this relatively avascular plane, parallel to the obliquely oriented fibers of the gluteus maximus muscle. Once the key perforators are identified, the remainder of the skin markings are adjusted if needed to optimize the perforator location and then incised. Beveling outward as the skin incisions are carried down to the fascia can increase flap volume.

The perforator is dissected from superficial to deep, following the vessels through the gluteus maximus muscle. As the dissection proceeds beyond the gluteus muscle, the deeper piriformis and gluteus minimus muscles are separated with self-retaining retractors to facilitate exposure and dissection of the vessels in this otherwise tight space. Caution should be used when retracting these muscles since excess retraction of the piriformis muscle can cause traction on the sciatic nerve, manifesting at postoperative neuropraxia.

The pedicle vessels are dissected until adequate pedicle length and vessel diameter are obtained. As mentioned, the artery can be quite small and efforts to maximize the diameter of the artery by proximal dissection should be made. After, the pedicle vessels are ligated and sharply divided, the flap donor site is closed as described later.

Like any autologous flap used for breast reconstruction, the SGAP flap is inset using a skin island that is tailored to the mastectomy defect (▶ **Fig. 30.4**). The SGAP flap, however, is typically a single perforator flap. The point where the perforator enters the deep surface of the flap is relatively inflexible and dense subcutaneous tissue of the buttock may act as a point of partial or total mechanical obstruction following flap inset for breast reconstruction requiring careful technique during flap inset.

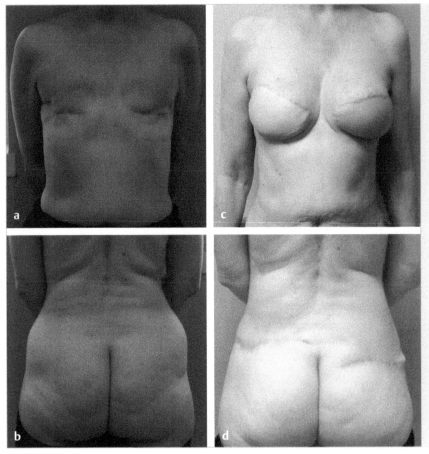

Fig. 30.4 (a,b) Preoperative and (c,d) postoperative appearance of a delayed, staged SGAP flap breast reconstruction.

30.8 Donor Site Closure

The donor site is approximated using several layers of absorbable sutures. The muscle and fascia are closed with interrupted figure-of-eight sutures. A closed suction drain is placed superficial to the muscle and deep to the subcutaneous tissue. The superficial fascial system is approximated, followed by closure of the skin with deep dermal and skin sutures.

Postoperative donor site contour deformities are not common. In bilateral cases, the buttocks may appear "lifted," especially for patients who have laxity and excess skin preoperatively. For unilateral cases, minor asymmetry between the flap donor side and the normal side may result, but rarely require corrective interventions. Cases of asymmetry or deformity can be addressed with autologous fat grafting of the donor side or suction lipectomy of the contralateral side at a later time if they do occur.

30.9 Pearls and Pitfalls

- Unilateral SGAP can be done consistently and efficiently for either delayed or immediate breast reconstruction cases. On the other hand, bilateral cases present a more challenging situation. Staging the reconstruction of the two sides should be considered if there is any concern.
- Generally, the flap is designed around a single perforator vessel. More than one perforator can be incorporated in the flap design, but the integrity of the gluteus maximus muscle should be considered and only minimal muscle damage should be tolerated.

- The relatively short pedicle length of the SGAP flap increases the risk of traction injury. This is mainly a concern when the flap is used for breast reconstruction immediately following mastectomy. In this setting, it is not uncommon for the mastectomy pocket to be aggressively dissected, especially laterally. This lateral space can be tailored to the flap dimensions and obliterated using several rows of quilting-style sutures placed between the lateral chest wall fascia and the deep surface of the overlying skin. Further flap stability can be obtained by suturing the flap to the deep surface of the medial mastectomy skin or to the chest wall laterally.

References

[1] Fujino T, Harasina T, Aoyagi F. Reconstruction for aplasia of the breast and pectoral region by microvascular transfer of a free flap from the buttock. Plast Reconstr Surg 1975;56(2):178–181

[2] Allen RJ, Tucker C Jr. Superior gluteal artery perforator free flap for breast reconstruction. Plast Reconstr Surg 1995;95(7):1207–1212

[3] DellaCroce FJ, Sullivan SK. Application and refinement of the superior gluteal artery perforator free flap for bilateral simultaneous breast reconstruction. Plast Reconstr Surg 2005;116(1):97–103, discussion 104–105

[4] Gagnon AR, Blondeel PN. Superior gluteal artery perforator flap. Semin Plast Surg 2006;20(2):79–88

31 Inferior Gluteal Artery Perforator Flap

Mark Schaverien

Abstract

The gluteal artery perforator flaps are usually reserved as secondary options for women that desire free autologous flap breast reconstruction, who do not have sufficient abdominal tissues or an abdomen suitable for free abdominal flaps. They may also be the preferred option in women with significant soft tissue of the buttock or those with significant functional demands of the abdomen who wish to avoid abdominal donor site morbidity. The major advantages of the perforator flaps include reduced donor site morbidity and longer pedicle, thus avoiding the need for vein grafts. The in-the-crease variation of the inferior gluteal artery perforator flap has the distinct advantage of coming from an excellent donor site, with a scar that is hidden in the gluteal fold and is well concealed by clothing. It is particularly advantageous for women with smaller breast size, as well as the younger patient with genetic risk factors for breast cancer who elects prophylactic mastectomy but may lack sufficient abdominal tissue for bilateral reconstruction. This chapter covers everything involved in this reconstructive procedure from start to finish, beginning with typical indications, to anatomy, to preoperative considerations, to the operative technique. Two variations are also mentioned.

Keywords: superior gluteal artery, inferior gluteal artery, internal iliac artery, piriformis muscle, posterior superior iliac spine, ischial tuberosity

31.1 Introduction

The gluteal artery perforator flaps are usually reserved as secondary options for women that desire free autologous flap breast reconstruction, yet have insufficient abdominal tissues or an abdomen unsuitable for free abdominal flaps. They may also be the preferred option in women with significant excess soft tissue of the buttock when compared with the abdomen, or in those with significant functional demands of the abdomen that wish to avoid abdominal donor site morbidity.

Fujino was the first to introduce gluteal tissue as a myocutaneous free flap for breast reconstruction in 1975.[1] Le-Quang performed the first breast reconstruction with an inferior gluteal myocutaneous flap in 1978; however, the use of this flap was limited by the short pedicle with frequent requirement for vein grafting and donor site morbidity.[2] The use of inferior and superior gluteal artery perforator (IGAP and SGAP, respectively) flaps for breast reconstruction, based on the inferior and superior gluteal artery perforators, respectively, with preservation of the gluteus maximus muscle, was first described by Allen and colleagues in 1993.[3,4] The major advantages of the perforator flaps include reduced donor site morbidity and longer pedicle avoiding the need for vein grafts. The same group introduced the in-the-crease IGAP flap. This flap has the distinct advantage of an excellent donor site with a scar that is hidden in the gluteal fold and is well concealed by clothing with minimal contour change to the buttock.[4] It is particularly advantageous for women with smaller breast size, as well as the younger patient with genetic risk factors for breast cancer who elects prophylactic mastectomy but may lack sufficient abdominal tissue for bilateral reconstruction. The weight of tissue harvested from the buttock is usually slightly in excess of the mastectomy weight, with mean flap weight approximately 400 g (range: ~ 200–600 g). Compared with the SGAP flap, the in-the-crease IGAP flap has a longer pedicle and typically results in less distortion of the gluteal region.

31.2 Typical Indications

- Breast reconstruction (free flap).
- Perineal reconstruction (pedicled flap).
- Posterior thigh reconstruction (pedicled flap).

31.3 Anatomy

The **superior and inferior gluteal arteries** are terminal branches of the **internal iliac artery** and exit the pelvis above and below the **piriformis muscle** to supply the upper and lower halves of the gluteus maximus muscle, respectively. The inferior gluteal artery accompanies the greater sciatic nerve, the internal pudendal vessels, and the posterior femoral cutaneous nerve, and gives off perforating vessels that penetrate the muscle to supply the overlying fat and skin of the lower buttock. Between two and four perforating vessels originating from the inferior gluteal artery will be located in the lower half of the gluteus maximus.[5]

The junction of the lower and middle thirds of a line drawn between the **posterior superior iliac spine** (PSIS) and outer part of the **ischial tuberosity** (I) marks the point of emergence of the inferior gluteal artery from the lower part of the greater sciatic foramen. The piriformis muscle is located along the midpoint of a line drawn between the PSIS and the coccyx and the superior edge of the greater trochanter. Perforators will be located in the area below piriformis muscle and above inferior gluteal crease, lateral to the vertical line PSIS–I (▶ **Fig. 31.1**).

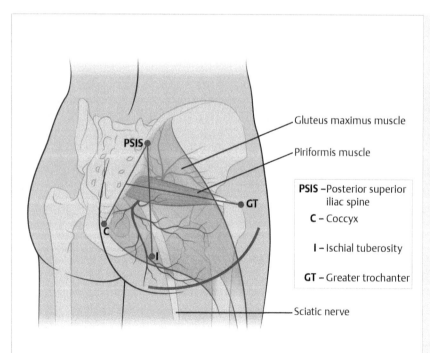

Gluteus maximus muscle

Piriformis muscle

PSIS – Posterior superior iliac spine

C – Coccyx

I – Ischial tuberosity

GT – Greater trochanter

Sciatic nerve

Fig. 31.1 Anatomical landmarks for design of the inferior gluteal artery perforator flap. Perforators will be located in the area below piriformis muscle and above inferior gluteal crease, lateral to the vertical line from the posterior superior iliac spine to the ischial tuberosity. C, coccyx; I, ischial tuberosity; PSIS, posterior superior iliac spine.

Perforators closer to the medial aspect of the buttock have short intramuscular lengths, whereas those located laterally travel obliquely through the gluteus maximus muscle and tend to give longer pedicle lengths. After giving off perforators in the buttocks, the inferior gluteal artery descends into the thigh accompanied by the posterior femoral cutaneous nerve. The **posterior femoral cutaneous nerve** innervates the skin of the perineum and posterior surface of the thigh and leg. At the origin from the internal iliac vessels the caliber of the inferior gluteal artery is around 2 mm and the vein around 3.5 mm. The IGAP flap pedicle length is typically 7 to 10 cm.

31.4 Variations

- Pedicled transverse flap design for reconstruction of defects of the posterior thigh.
- V–Y pedicled advancement flap for reconstruction of abdominoperineal resection (APR) defects.

31.5 Preoperative Considerations

Preoperative imaging with computed tomographic angiography or magnetic resonance angiography allows selection of the best perforators and reduces time taken to harvest the flap.[6] A hand-held Doppler probe is then used to confirm the location of the inferior gluteal artery perforators preoperatively with the patient placed in the same position as for surgery.

31.6 Positioning and Skin Markings

The gluteal fold is marked with the patient in the standing position, and the inferior limit of the flap is marked 1 cm inferior and parallel to the gluteal fold. The superior limit is drawn approximately 7 cm cephalad to this. The length of the flap parallels the gluteal fold and is typically approximately 18 cm in length (▶ Fig. 31.2). The adipose tissue to be beveled at the cephalad and caudal aspects to recruit additional soft tissue with the flap is also marked.

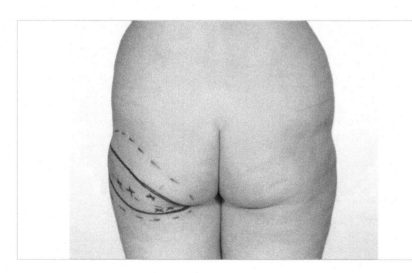

Fig. 31.2 Preoperative markings. The gluteal fold is marked with the patient in a standing position, and the inferior limit of the flap is marked 1 cm inferior and parallel to the gluteal fold. The superior limit is drawn approximately 7 cm cephalad to this. The length of the flap parallels the gluteal fold and is approximately 18 cm in length. The adipose tissue that is to beveled at the cephalad and caudal aspects to recruit additional soft tissue with the flap is also marked.

31.7 Operative Technique

For unilateral breast reconstruction, the patient is placed in the lateral position to harvest the flap. This will require supine positioning at the start of the case for mastectomy and recipient vessel preparation, and at the end for microvascular anastomosis and flap inset. Some authors advocate lateral decubitus positioning for unilateral reconstruction, allowing vessel exposure, flap harvest, and flap inset without position change. Simultaneous bilateral IGAP flap harvest in the prone position is performed for bilateral breast reconstruction, then following donor site closure the patient is returned to the supine position for microvascular anastomosis and flap inset.

Once the patient is positioned, the skin incisions are carried out into the subcutaneous fat, then beveled outward at the cephalad and caudal aspects to recruit additional soft-tissue width and volume down through the fascia to the gluteus maximus muscle circumferentially. Care is taken at the caudal aspect to protect the posterior femoral cutaneous nerve since injury will result in paresthesia of the posterior thigh and leg. Care is also taken not to transgress into the ischial fat pad overlying the ischial tuberosity medial to the gluteus maximus muscle as this can lead to discomfort when sitting. The sciatic nerve should never be visualized.

The flap is elevated from lateral to medial in the subfascial plane (▶ Fig. 31.3b). The flap is elevated in a perpendicular direction to the fascial septa arising from the muscle fibers, with care taken not to damage the perforators that arise within these septa. Although a single large perforator will adequately perfuse the flap, it is preferable to harvest two perforators for improved flap perfusion, particularly venous drainage. Once suitable perforators are identified, the muscle is spread in the direction of its fibers and dissection continues until both the artery and vein are of sufficient size to be anastomosed to the recipient vessels and the pedicle of sufficient length (▶ Fig. 31.3c,d). Usually, the artery is smaller than the internal mammary artery and is the limiting factor. Typically, an artery of 2.0 to 2.5 mm and a vein of 3.0 to 4.0 mm in diameter are sufficient for anastomosis. The last few centimeters of the dissection are the most time consuming and complex due to the presence of multiple side branches, and care must be taken not to inadvertently ligate the main pedicle prematurely.

31.8 Donor Site Closure

The skin and fat overlying the gluteus maximus muscle and posterior thigh are undermined superiorly and inferiorly suprafascially to allow layered approximation of the donor site to prevent a contour deformity. The donor site is closed in layers over a suction drain. The scar should be hidden in the gluteal crease (▶ Fig. 31.4).

31.9 Pearls and Pitfalls

- The optimal patient has a pear-shaped body habitus, with relatively large buttocks and small breast size.
- Harvest of at least two separate perforators is advised to allow for additional venous drainage in case of venous congestion.
- A significant drawback of using the IGAP for free flap breast reconstruction is the long operative time due to position changes and tedious pedicle dissection.

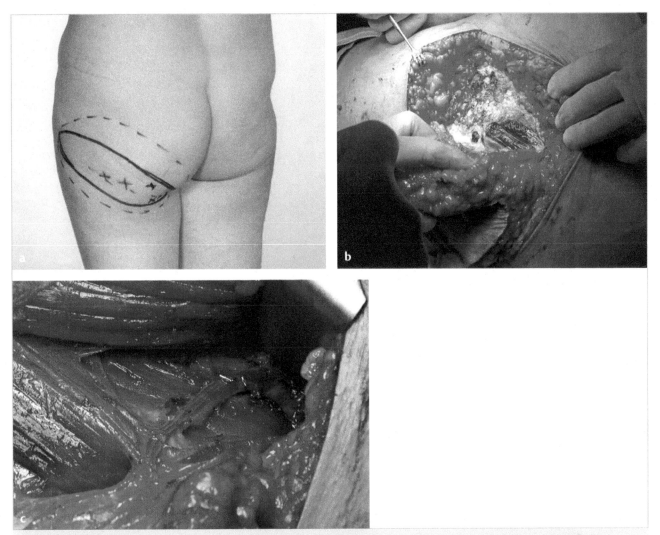

Fig. 31.3 (a) Flap harvest. Incisions are carried out into the subcutaneous fat, then beveled outward at the cephalad and caudal aspects to recruit additional soft tissue down through the fascia to the gluteus maximus muscle circumferentially. The flap is elevated from lateral to medial in the subfascial plane in a perpendicular direction to the fascial septa arising from the muscle fibers allowing perforators to be identified. **(b)** Once suitable perforators are identified, the muscle is spread in the direction of its fibers without division of the muscle and dissection continues until both the artery and vein are of sufficient size to be anastomosed to the recipient vessels in the chest and the pedicle of sufficient length. **(c)** The last few centimeters of the dissection are the most time consuming and complex due to the presence of multiple side branches, and care must be taken not to inadvertently ligate the main pedicle prematurely. **(d)** Although a single large perforator will adequately perfuse the flap, it is preferable to harvest two perforators in case there is a requirement for additional venous drainage due to flap venous congestion.

- Unlike the soft and pliable tissues of the lower abdominal region, the gluteal subcutaneous fat is firmer and denser. This makes the flap more difficult to shape into a breast mound and improvement of contour deformities using fat grafting may be required secondarily.
- Asymmetry between the buttocks following unilateral flap harvest may necessitate secondary liposuction to the contralateral buttock.
- Care must be taken to avoid injury to the posterior femoral cutaneous nerve at the inferior margin of the flap. This can lead to permanent paresthesia of the posterior thigh and leg.

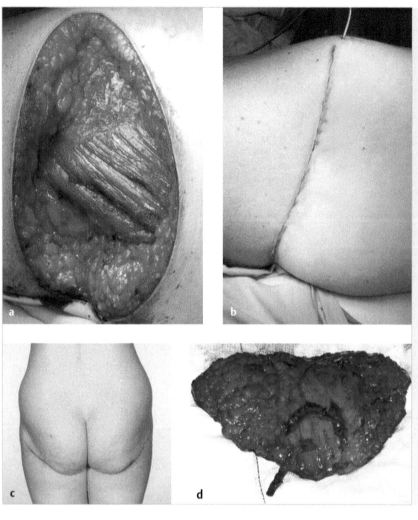

Fig. 31.4 **(a)** The skin and fat overlying the gluteus maximus muscle and posterior thigh are undermined superiorly and inferiorly to allow layered approximation of the donor site to prevent a contour deformity. The donor site is closed in layers over a suction drain. The scar is hidden in the gluteal crease. **(b,c)** Donor site appearance following bilateral skin-sparing mastectomies and immediate reconstruction with IGAP flap. Note good symmetry of the buttocks with minimal contour deformity and with scars hidden in the gluteal crease.

References

[1] Fujino T, Harasina T, Aoyagi F. Reconstruction for aplasia of the breast and pectoral region by microvascular transfer of a free flap from the buttock. Plast Reconstr Surg 1975;56(2):178–181

[2] Le-Quang C. Two new free flaps developed from aesthetic surgery II. The inferior gluteal flap. Aesthetic Plast Surg 1980;4(1):159–168

[3] Guerra AB, Metzinger SE, Bidros RS, Gill PS, Dupin CL, Allen RJ. Breast reconstruction with gluteal artery perforator (GAP) flaps: a critical analysis of 142 cases. Ann Plast Surg 2004;52(2):118–125

[4] Allen RJ, Levine JL, Granzow JW. The in-the-crease inferior gluteal artery perforator flap for breast reconstruction. Plast Reconstr Surg 2006;118(2):333–339

[5] Ahmadzadeh R, Bergeron L, Tang M, Morris SF. The superior and inferior gluteal artery perforator flaps. Plast Reconstr Surg 2007;120(6):1551–1556

[6] Vasile JV, Newman T, Rusch DG, et al. Anatomic imaging of gluteal perforator flaps without ionizing radiation: seeing is believing with magnetic resonance angiography. J Reconstr Microsurg 2010;26(1):45–57

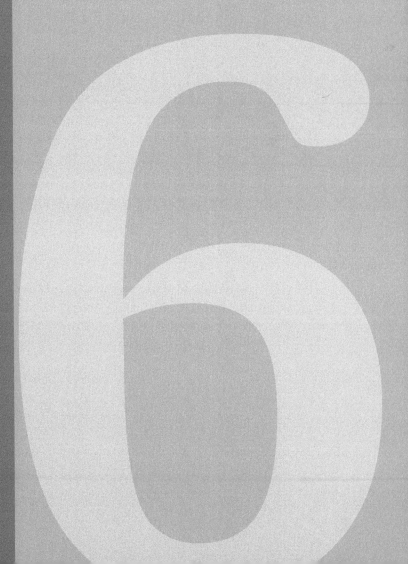

Part 6

Upper Extremity

32 Lateral Arm Flap

Edward I. Chang

Abstract

The lateral arm flap is most commonly used for reconstruction of the head and neck and extremity defects, and can be transferred as a free or pedicled flap for reconstruction of upper arm and shoulder defects. The flap can be harvested as a perforator flap or as a fasciocutaneous flap. The lateral arm flap has not emerged as a workhorse flap due to concerns regarding pedicle length and caliber, but it can be a useful option when a relatively thin and pliable flap is needed. This chapter discusses the indications for the use of the lateral arm flap, the anatomy involved, the preoperative considerations, and the operative technique. Two variations and donor site closure are described.

Keywords: radial collateral artery, profunda brachii, lateral antebrachial cutaneous nerve, radial nerve

32.1 Introduction

The lateral arm flap is most commonly used for reconstruction of head and neck as well as extremity defects, and can be transferred as a free flap or as a pedicled flap for reconstruction of upper arm and shoulder defects.[1,2] The flap can be harvested as a perforator flap or as a fasciocutaneous flap. The lateral arm flap has not emerged as a workhorse flap due to concerns regarding pedicle length and caliber but can be a useful option when a relatively thin and pliable flap is needed.[3]

32.2 Typical Indications

- Soft-tissue defects of the upper arm and shoulder can be reconstructed with a pedicled lateral arm flap.
- Soft-tissue defects of the upper or lower extremity needing soft pliable tissue for coverage of exposed structures such as bone, tendon, nerve, or vessels.
- Head and neck defects including reconstruction of partial pharyngeal, floor of mouth, tongue, or other soft tissue defects.

32.3 Anatomy

The lateral arm flap is a fasciocutaneous flap that can be harvested as a true perforator flap or as a fasciocutaneous flap based on the **radial collateral artery** which is a branch of the **profunda brachii** artery that ultimately anastomoses with the radial recurrent artery near the elbow. The radial collateral artery pedicle becomes superficial toward the lateral epicondyle allowing the flap to be harvested as a fasciocutaneous flap; however, reliable perforators arise more proximally to supply the skin overlying the lateral arm region. The main pedicle travels in the septum between the biceps brachii muscle and the triceps muscle (▶Fig. 32.1). The **lateral antebrachial cutaneous nerve** is a branch of the radial nerve that travels in close proximity to the main pedicle and often needs to be divided in order to free the pedicle and flap from the arm.[3] The

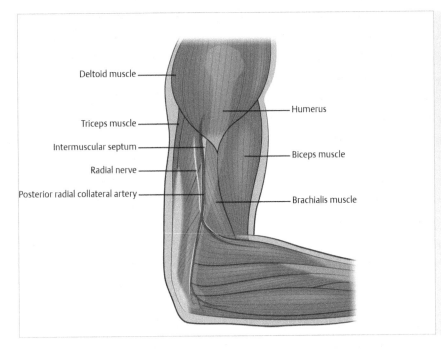

Fig. 32.1 The pedicle to the lateral arm flap lies in the septum between the triceps and biceps brachii muscle. The pedicle may travel on the surface of the humerus lying very close to the radial nerve, which should be preserved and protected during the dissection.

lateral antebrachial cutaneous nerve can also be used to create a sensate flap both for a pedicle flap to the upper arm or in the setting of a free tissue transfer. Patients commonly report an area of numbness in the distribution of the nerve following flap harvest, but this is well tolerated and has minimal functional deficits.

The **radial nerve**, however, is also in close proximity to the main pedicle and travels along the spiral groove of the humerus running posterior to anterior. The radial nerve must be identified prior to ligating the lateral antebrachial cutaneous nerve. In certain circumstances, the pedicle and the radial nerve are densely adherent to the periosteum of the humerus. A periosteal elevator is useful in performing the dissection to minimize any trauma to the pedicle or the radial nerve.

As the pedicle proceeds proximally, the pedicle will proceed in a deep and posterior vector, which defines the limit of the dissection. The deltoid insertion can be released in order to achieve more pedicle length and diameter if necessary. Anatomical studies have demonstrated a reliable pedicle length of approximately 7 cm with an average arterial diameter of 1.7 mm and an average venous diameter of 2.5 mm.[3] There are usually between one and three septocutaneous perforators, which we term the A, B, and C perforators. The perforators may not always join the main pedicle and anatomical variants have been found where one of the perforators may arise from a separate pedicle. This is reminiscent of perforators arising from the transverse oblique branch that has been described during harvest of the anterolateral thigh (ALT) flap.

32.4 Variations

- An osteocutaneous flap can be harvested to include a portion of the humerus with the overlying skin paddle of the lateral arm flap.
- A chimeric flap can also be harvested to include not only the overlying skin paddle, as well as the humerus, but also a cuff of the triceps muscle to add additional soft tissue bulk to the flap.

32.5 Preoperative Considerations

Flap selection will often be determined by patient's body habitus, and the lateral arm tissue often provides bulk that is slightly thicker than a forearm-based flap but thinner than a thigh-based flap. For many head and neck defects, a thigh-based flap, such as the ALT flap, is more amenable to a two-team approach than the lateral arm flap and is one reason why the ALT flap is often preferred.[4, 5] However, for lower extremity reconstruction, the lateral arm would be well suited for simultaneous flap harvest and recipient site preparation. The flap is harvested from the nondominant arm when possible.

32.6 Positioning and Skin Markings

The patient is placed in the supine position, and the patient's arm is shaved and should be prepped circumferentially allowing full range of motion of the arm. The arm from which the flap is to be raised is typically placed across the patient's torso during the flap harvest. The landmarks for the flap harvest are the deltoid insertion and the lateral epicondyle. A line connecting these two points establishes the flap meridian and closely approximates the septum between the biceps and triceps muscle. The flap is usually centered longitudinally over this line and a pinch test is performed to determine the maximum width of the flap that permits primary closure. Alternatively, up to about half the circumference of the upper arm can be used for the flap and a skin graft can be used to close the donor site. Three consistent perforators, termed A, B, and C, are located approximately 7, 10, and 12 cm from the deltoid insertion, respectively.[3] The flap is centered over one or more of these perforators (▶Fig. 32.2). The dissection starts posteriorly and proceeds anteriorly until perforators are

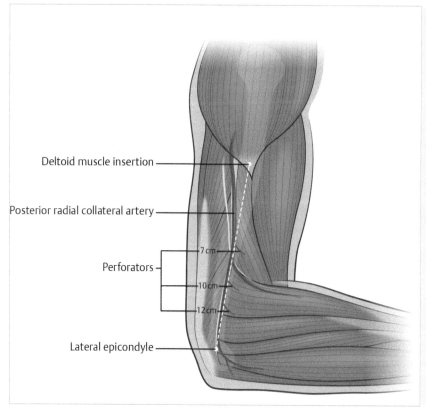

Deltoid muscle insertion

Posterior radial collateral artery

Perforators

7 cm

10 cm

12 cm

Lateral epicondyle

Fig. 32.2 A line connecting the deltoid insertion and the lateral epicondyle closely approximates the septum between the triceps and biceps, and cutaneous perforators arising from the posterior radial collateral artery can be reliably located at 7, 10, and 12 cm from the deltoid insertion.

visualized, so performing the initial dissection while sitting down is usually more comfortable for the surgeon.

32.7 Operative Technique

Refer to Video 32.1 for an example of the operative technique for the lateral arm perforator flap. Once the flap dimensions are marked, the posterior skin incision is made and dissection is carried down to the deep fascia that invests the biceps and triceps muscles. The fascia is incised and the dissection proceeds in the subfascial plane over the triceps muscle. As the dissection proceeds toward the septum, the perforators should be easily visualized. The perforators are carefully traced to the main pedicle that lies in between the biceps and the triceps. Once the main pedicle has been visualized, the distal pedicle can be ligated, and the pedicle can be dissected more proximally for length and caliber.

During this portion of the dissection, the lateral antebrachial cutaneous nerve is often seen traveling superficial to the main pedicle. This nerve should be preserved until the pedicle is clearly freed from the underlying tissue, which will then expose the radial nerve. At this time, the anterior incision can be made and dissection again proceeds through the skin, down to fascia, and then through the fascia into the subfascial plane. The planes of the anterior and posterior dissection should join allowing the flap to be freed from the arm. During the flap elevation, it is critical to pay careful attention so that the radial nerve is not injured (▶ Fig. 32.3). A no-touch technique is recommended and small vessels should be clipped and cut, rather than divided with either monopolar or bipolar electrocautery.

At this point, the lateral antebrachial nerve often needs to be divided to free the pedicle from the surrounding tissue. The nerve can be dissected proximally to its takeoff from the main radial nerve if a sensate flap is desired. The flap is then elevated from distal to proximal freeing the pedicle from the surrounding tissue. The deltoid insertion can be partially released in order to gain additional exposure to obtain more pedicle length and caliber.

32.8 Donor Site Closure

The donor site should be inspected for hemostasis and to make certain that the radial nerve has not been injured during the dissection. The divided septal fascia between the biceps and triceps muscle should not be reapproximated as this can lead to compression of the radial nerve. A closed suction drain is placed into the donor site. The incision is then closed primarily in layers. In the setting that a larger skin paddle is harvested that can allow primary closure, a skin graft can be utilized to resurface the defect.

32.9 Pearls and Pitfalls

- A subfascial dissection is performed in order to identify the perforators supplying the overlying skin paddle both from the posterior and anterior approach. Perforators are reliably located using landmarks of

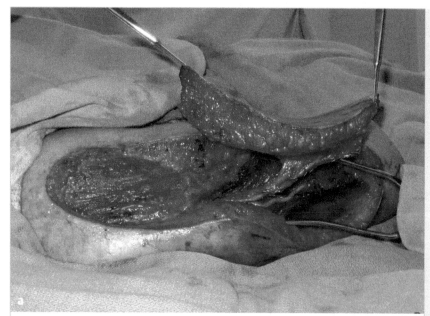

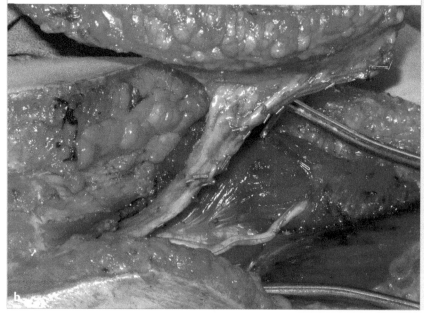

Fig. 32.3 (a) Lateral arm flap after the dissection is complete. (b) Close-up view. The radial nerve often runs very close to the pedicle of the lateral arm flap; however, the lateral antebrachial cutaneous nerve will need to be divided in order to harvest the flap.

the deltoid insertion and the lateral epicondyle. The A, B, and C perforators are typically located at 7, 10, and 12 cm from the deltoid insertion between the biceps and triceps muscles.

- A no-touch technique is recommended during the flap harvest to minimize any trauma or injury to the radial nerve. Avoid the use of cautery during the flap harvest as this can cause inadvertent injury to the nerve resulting in significant donor site morbidity.
- Release of the deltoid insertion will allow greater exposure for more proximal dissection of the pedicle to increase both the length and caliber of the pedicle.

References

[1] Hwang K, Lee WJ, Jung CY, Chung IH. Cutaneous perforators of the upper arm and clinical applications. J Reconstr Microsurg 2005;21(7):463–469

[2] Jordan SW, Wayne JD, Dumanian GA. The pedicled lateral arm flap for oncologic reconstruction near the shoulder. Ann Plast Surg 2015;74(1):30–33

[3] Chang EI, Ibrahim A, Papazian N, et al. Perforator mapping and optimizing design of the lateral arm flap: anatomy revisited and clinical experience. Plast Reconstr Surg 2016;138(2):300e–306e

[4] Busnardo FF, Coltro PS, Olivan MV, et al. Anatomical comparison among the anterolateral thigh, the parascapular, and the lateral arm flaps. Microsurgery 2015;35(5):387–392

[5] Klinkenberg M, Fischer S, Kremer T, Hernekamp F, Lehnhardt M, Daigeler A. Comparison of anterolateral thigh, lateral arm, and parascapular free flaps with regard to donor-site morbidity and aesthetic and functional outcomes. Plast Reconstr Surg 2013;131(2):293–302

33 Radial Forearm Fasciocutaneous/Osteocutaneous Free Flap

Mark W. Clemens

Abstract

Small- and moderate-sized postoncologic defects of the head and neck can result in swallowing difficulty and impaired functional outcomes, if reconstructed with large bulky flaps that occlude the oropharynx. Because of its thin size, pliability, and reliable anatomy, the radial forearm free flap remains an essential workhorse for pharyngeal, tongue, floor of mouth, and orbital reconstruction, as well as for resurfacing modest-sized cutaneous defects throughout the body. The radial forearm fasciocutaneous/osteocutaneous free flap procedure is one of the most performed free flaps worldwide for head and neck reconstruction. This chapter focuses on the pertinent indications, anatomy, preoperative considerations, operative technique, and expected outcomes of the radial forearm fasciocutaneous/osteocutaneous free flap procedure.

Keywords: radial artery, ulnar artery, superficial palmar artery, deep palmar artery, cephalic cubital vein, basilic cubital vein, median cubital vein, medial antebrachial cutaneous nerve, lateral antebrachial cutaneous nerve, musculocutaneous nerve

33.1 Introduction

Small- and moderate-sized postoncologic defects of the head and neck can result in swallowing difficulty and impaired functional outcomes if reconstructed with large bulky flaps that occlude the oropharynx. Because of its thin size, pliability, and reliable anatomy, the radial forearm free flap (RFFF) remains an essential workhorse for pharyngeal, tongue, floor of mouth, and orbital reconstruction as well as for resurfacing modest-sized cutaneous defects throughout the body. The RFFF was first described by Drs. Guofan Yang and Yuzhi Gao of the Shenyang Military Hospital in 1981,[1] and has become one of the most performed free flaps worldwide for head and neck reconstruction.[2,3] The RFFF may be raised as a fasciocutaneous or osteocutaneous free flap depending on the reconstructive needs of the ablative site. This chapter will focus on the pertinent anatomy, indications, technique, and outcomes of the RFFF flap.

33.2 Typical Indications

- Cutaneous defects of the neck, face, scalp, groin, and upper extremity.
- Pharyngeal wall either as a cutaneous patch for partial pharyngeal defect or tube fabrication for pharyngoesophageal reconstruction.[2]
- Small- to moderate-sized oral and oropharyngeal defects.
- Upper extremity and hand wounds, either by pedicled or reverse pedicled.
- Scalp, forehead, and facial defects.
- Orbital wall lining.
- Double tube fabrication for total penile reconstruction.

33.3 Anatomy

The RFFF is a fasciocutaneous flap of variable size harvested from the fore-arm skin overlying the radial vessels. The dominant blood supply of the RFFF is the **radial artery** (▶ **Fig. 33.1a**). The radial artery anatomy is constant and reliable. The radial artery is supplied by the brachial artery, which bifurcates into the ulnar and radial artery. The forearm is composed of three muscle groups: the "mobile wad" in the posterior compartment of the forearm (bra-chioradialis, extensor carpi radialis longus, and extensor carpi radialis brevis muscles), the flexor–pronators in the anterior compartment of the forearm

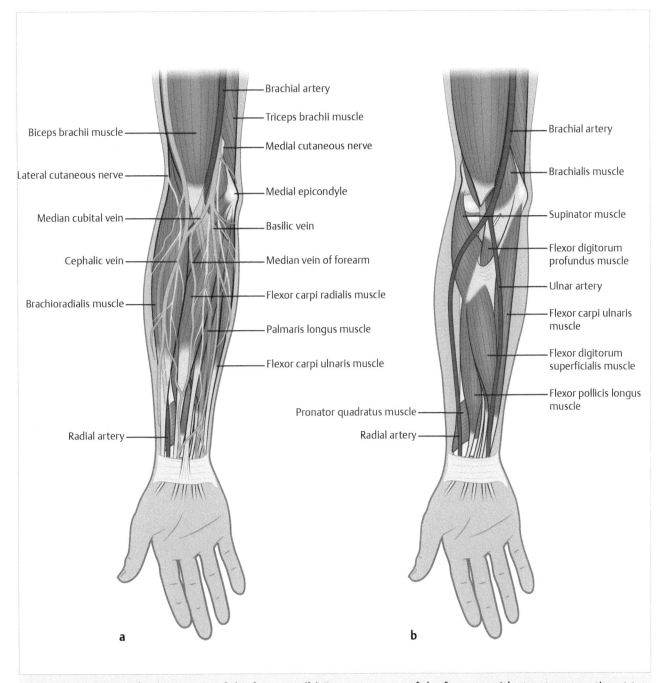

Fig. 33.1 **(a)** Superficial anatomy of the forearm. **(b)** Deep anatomy of the forearm with structures pertinent to the radial forearm free flap.

(pronator teres, pronator quadratus, flexor carpi radialis, flexor digitorum superficialis and profundus, palmaris longus, and flexor carpi ulnaris muscles), and the posterior extensor compartment containing the extensor muscles. The radial artery follows a course in the fascial plane between the brachioradialis, radial extensors, and the pronator teres (▶ **Fig. 33.1b**). The forearm skin extends from 2 cm distal to the elbow crease to the wrist crease and is supplied by perforators from the radial and **ulnar artery**. Either arterial system by itself is sufficient to carry the entire overlying volar forearm skin and up to one-third of the radial posterior surface as a flap. The ulnar and radial artery anastomose through the **superficial and deep palmar arteries**. In the proximal third of the forearm, the radial artery lies between the brachioradialis and the pronator teres, in the middle third it lies between the brachioradialis and flexor carpi radialis muscles, and in the distal third it is subcutaneous and, therefore, palpable. Distally at the level of the wrist, the radial artery runs beneath the abductor pollicis longus and extensor pollicis brevis, which traverses the "anatomical snuff box." In the proximal forearm, the radial artery branches, giving off the radial recurrent artery and the inferior cubital artery. The radial artery gives rise to perforating vessels every 1 to 2 cm in the distal forearm.

The venous drainage is via paired venae comitantes that accompany the radial artery. Despite having valves, numerous interconnections between the two veins allow for retrograde elevation of the flap. The deep venae comitantes are the main venous drainage of the RFFF and should be anastomosed when a free flap is required.[4] Additional superficial venous drainage of the forearm is provided by the **cephalic, basilic, and median cubital veins**. The superficial venous system can be elevated with the flap and can usually be used as an alternate drainage system. Alternately, both venous systems can be anastomosed separately or together if dissected proximally to where the superficial systems join with the deep system at the cubital fossa. In practice, anastomosis of the deep system is sufficient in the overwhelming majority of cases.

The **medial and lateral antebrachial cutaneous nerves** are the sensory nerve supply to the RFFF and may be elevated with the flap to provide a sensate skin paddle. However, the flap is usually not harvested as a sensate flap. The medial cutaneous nerve courses with the basilic vein and the lateral antebrachial cutaneous nerve is a continuation of the **musculocutaneous nerve** and accompanies the cephalic vein. The **radial nerve** is the dominant motor nerve to the forearm extensors and is supplied by small branches off of the radial artery.

33.4 Variations

- Elevation as an adipofascial flap.
- Composite bone and skin reconstruction (e.g., for mandibular reconstruction) by modification with elevation as an osteocutaneous flap.[5]
- Foot reconstruction by modification with elevation of vascularized tendons.

33.5 Preoperative Considerations

Physical examination should be performed to assess the patient's general condition, the forearm skin integrity, noting any previous scars or surgeries which may have damaged the radial artery, and an Allen's test to confirm sufficient ulnar artery perfusion of the hand in the absence of radial perfusion. A small number of patients may be radial artery dominant and in that situation, the contralateral limb, an ulnar artery flap, or an alternative flap should alternatively be chosen. If both limbs have identical radial perfusion, preference is commonly given to the patient's nondominant writing hand.

33.6 Positioning and Skin Markings

The patient is placed into a supine position with the preferred arm placed on an arm board extension from the main bed. The course of the radial artery is determined by palpating the artery or can be confirmed by a Doppler examination. The tumor ablation site defect (▶Fig. 33.2a) is measured and these dimensions are transposed onto the forearm starting from the second wrist crease and centered over the radial artery (▶Fig. 33.2b,c). The radial artery courses within the lateral intermuscular septum up to the center of the antecubital fossa.

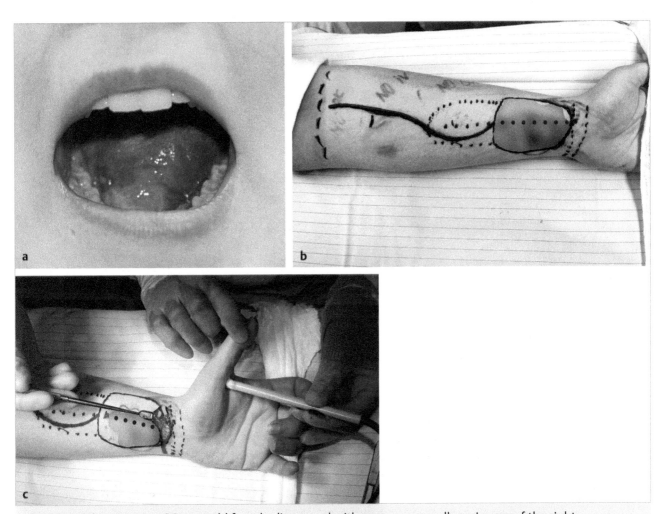

Fig. 33.2 **(a)** Patient is a 36-year-old female diagnosed with a squamous cell carcinoma of the right hemitongue and floor of mouth. She requires surgical resection and free flap reconstruction. She has recurrent disease status post prior resection and local radiation therapy. Preoperative tumor is demonstrated. **(b)** Patient's left forearm demonstrates preoperative flap markings for resurfacing of the tongue and floor of mouth. **(c)** The radial artery is visualized and occluded, and arterial flow from the ulnar artery to the thumb is confirmed by Doppler examination.

For larger defects, the entire skin of the forearm from the wrist to the elbow flexion crease can be raised as part of the flap. This type of large flap elevation is more applicable for situations such as forequarter amputations requiring a fillet of forearm flap coverage. The significant morbidity that would be associated with a fillet of forearm makes this impractical outside of this extreme situation. Most commonly, a strip of forearm skin is raised from approximately 3 × 5 cm to 6 × 12 cm. Small flaps less than 2 cm in width may be closed primarily obviating the need for a skin graft. The cephalic vein lies radial to the pedicle and can be incorporated in larger flaps. Note even when the cephalic vein is large, the venous output is secondary to the radial venae comitantes and should not be utilized in place of the main pedicle unless a clear anastomosis between the superficial and deep venous system can be demonstrated.

Skin paddles should be designed over the distal aspect of the forearm where the skin is thinnest. A proximal adipofascial flap of the midforearm can be incorporated into the flap design, which can be used to provide additional soft-tissue bulk to obliterate communications between the neck and oral cavity.

Osteocutaneous flaps are raised by incorporating a thin segment of the distal radius bone.[5] Segments up to 12 cm in length have been described; however, increasing bone harvest increases the patient's risk of a postoperative fracture. The radial artery supplies vascularity to the radial bone from the pronator teres to the radial styloid.

Hand defects can be reconstructed with the radial forearm flap raised as a retrograde pedicle flap. The venae comitantes are a valved system; however, numerous branching communications allow for retrograde flow. The retrograde pedicled flap for hand defects is amendable to elevation under an axillary or subclavian nerve block.

33.7 Operative Technique

Refer to Video 33.1 for an example of the operative technique for the radial forearm free flap. Dissection of the RFFF begins with incision of the distal end of the flap along the proximal wrist crease exposing the radial artery and venae comitantes. Once the pedicle has been visualized, it is occluded and perfusion to the hand from the ulnar artery is verified with a Doppler to the base of the thumb (►**Fig. 33.2c**). Flap elevation under a tourniquet allows for a relatively bloodless dissection. The tourniquet is elevated to approximately 50 mm Hg above systolic blood pressure after limb exsanguination. Dissection continues on the ulnar border of the flap in a subfascial plane down the tendons of the forearm with care taken to leave the paratenon intact (►**Fig. 33.3a**). The plane of dissection is superficial to the palmaris longus but may incorporate this tendon if desired. The radial artery and venae comitantes are identified and approached cautiously to ensure incorporation into the flap. Next, the radial skin incision is performed in a similar fashion with ligation of superficial veins. The cephalic vein may be incorporated and elevated with the flap for additional venous outflow; however, this vein represents a secondary venous drainage system and is not necessary to incorporate nor a replacement for the venae comitantes. The cutaneous branch of the radial nerve should be identified and preserved, since ligation is prone to neuroma formation and results in loss of sensation over the radial aspect of the dorsum of the hand.

Once the skin paddle of the flap has been raised, a "lazy S" incision is made from the flap over the course of the radial artery to 1 cm below the antecubital fossa. An adipofascial proximal extension of the flap can be raised at this point which gives additional soft-tissue bulk and can help with obliterating any communication between the oral cavity and neck. For sensate flaps, either the lateral cutaneous nerve of the forearm running along with the cephalic vein or the medial cutaneous nerve centrally located in the forearm should be identified and elevated with the flap. The radial artery and venae comitantes are identified by reflecting the brachioradialis radially. The pedicle dissection proceeds up to the antecubital fossa from its origin at the brachial artery (▶Fig. 33.3b). At this point, the flap recipient site is prepared with preparation of vessels, followed by pedicle ligation and vessel anastomosis (▶Fig. 33.3c; ▶Fig. 33.4a).

33.8 Variations

The vascular pedicle of the RFFF lies within the lateral intermuscular septum which courses from the styloid process to deep to the brachioradialis. Division of this septum should be performed in a distal-to-proximal manner deep to

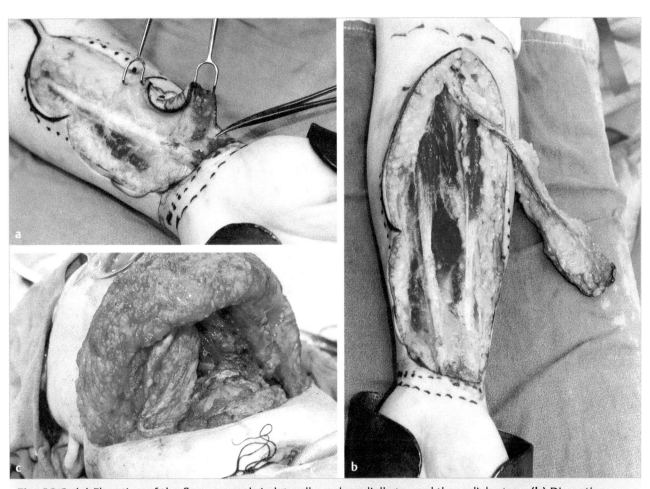

Fig. 33.3 **(a)** Elevation of the flap proceeds in laterally and medially toward the radial artery. **(b)** Dissection proceeds in a subcutaneous plan until radial artery is encountered and the dissection runs deep to the artery and venae comitantes. The flap is elevated along with the radial vessels up to the antecubital fossa. **(c)** Note a small amount of subcutaneous fat is elevated with the pedicle which will be placed to obliterate the tunnel communicating between the oral and neck cavity.

the vascular pedicle to facilitate fasciocutaneous flap elevation. However, small branches from the pedicle pass down to the periosteum of the radial bone and these are preserved when harvesting an osteocutaneous flap. Radial bone may be harvested proximally from the insertion of the pronator teres to distally at the radial styloid. The septum between the periosteum and the radial artery must be preserved and addition of a small cuff of flexor muscle helps preserve this communication. Once the desired length of radial bone is exposed, osteotomies are performed creating a keel-shaped vascularized bone graft. For mandibular defects requiring bony angulation, wedge osteotomies may be performed so long as the larger flat periosteal surface is kept in continuity. Large osseous defects may require bone grafting with cancellous bone chips to the donor site and/or prophylactic radial bone plating.

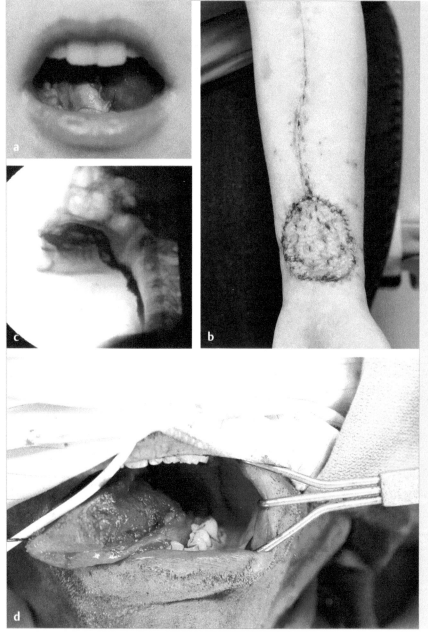

Fig. 33.4 (a) Patient is shown approximately 6 weeks following tumor ablation and reconstruction. (b) Her forearm defect was reconstructed with a full-thickness skin graft harvested from her groin crease. (c) Swallow study performed at 6 weeks demonstrates excellent swallowing without evidence of regurgitation or contrast leakage. (d) Patient is a 64-year-old man diagnosed with squamous cell carcinoma of his left tongue. Following resection of tumor, patient has a defect of one-third of the anterior tongue extending back to the lateral pharyngeal wall.

(Continued)

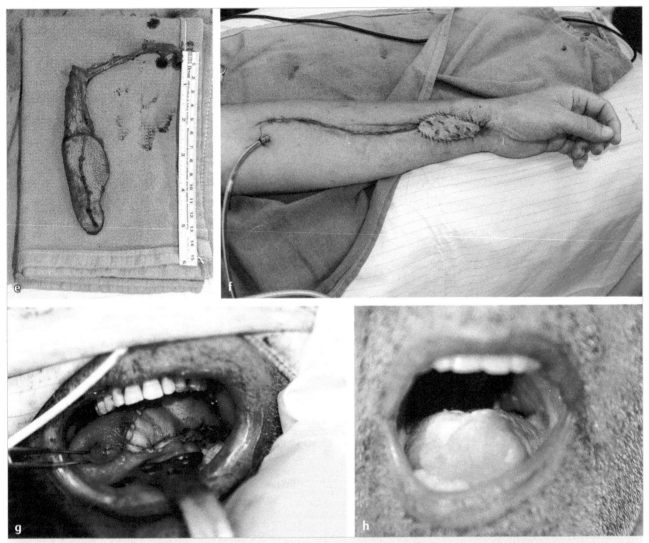

Fig. 33.4 (*Continued*) **(e)** A left-sided radial forearm free flap was elevated with a small fat pad and radial vessels. **(f)** Patient's donor forearm defect was reconstructed with a full-thickness skin graft from his groin crease. **(g)** Immediate inset of the flap into the tongue and pharyngeal defect is shown. **(h)** Patient is shown at 1 year postoperative with complete healing and has intelligible speech following speech therapy.

33.9 Donor Site Closure

Grafting of the radial artery with a vein graft may be considered in radially dominant patients, but is not necessary the majority of the time. RFFF flaps less than 2 cm in width may be closed primarily with undermining of the skin medially and laterally. The majority of RFFF donor defects require reconstruction with either a split- or full-thickness skin graft. Full-thickness skin grafts heal with a more aesthetic appearance, and should be harvested in a non–hair-bearing portion of the groin crease and pie-crusted prior to placement (▶ Fig. 33.4a–c). Skin grafts may be fixed in place with a tie over bolster, foam bolster, or a negative-pressure wound dressing. A postoperative splint is utilized to immobilize the wrist joint for 4 to 6 days until the bolster is removed. Following elevation of osteocutaneous flaps, protective splinting is employed for 6 weeks (▶ Fig. 33.4d–h).

33.10 Pearls and Pitfalls

- Preoperative evaluation with an Allen test to ensure adequate ulnar perfusion of the hand is essential prior to ligation of the radial artery. Check and recheck.
- The dominant blood supply of the RFFF is the deep system of the venae comitantes and cannot be substituted by the cephalic vein alone.
- During elevation of the RFFF flap, tendon paratenon must be preserved to prevent scar tethering of the tendons and allow for a vascular bed for skin grafting.
- Osteocutaneous flaps should incorporate no more than 25% of the radial bone to prevent pathological fractures postoperatively.

References

[1] Yang G, Chen B, Gao Y, et al. Forearm free skin flap transplantation:56 cases [in Chinese]. Zhonghua Yi Xue Za Zhi 1981;61:139–141

[2] Song R, Gao Y, Song Y, Yu Y, Song Y. The forearm flap. Clin Plast Surg 1982;9(1):21–26

[3] Harii K, Ebihara S, Ono I, Saito H, Terui S, Takato T. Pharyngoesophageal reconstruction using a fabricated forearm free flap. Plast Reconstr Surg 1985;75(4):463–476

[4] Demirkan F, Wei FC, Lutz BS, Cher TS, Chen IH. Reliability of the venae comitantes in venous drainage of the free radial forearm flaps. Plast Reconstr Surg 1998;102(5):1544–1548

[5] Soutar DS, Widdowson WP. Immediate reconstruction of the mandible using a vascularized segment of radius. Head Neck Surg 1986;8(4):232–246

34 Ulnar Artery Perforator Flap

Albert H. Chao and Matthew M. Hanasono

Abstract

Fasciocutaneous flaps based on the ulnar artery, were initially described as the ulnar forearm flap, and they eventually resulted in a true perforator flap known as the ulnar artery perforator flap. The thinness, pliability, and relative hairlessness of the ulnar artery perforator flap make it a good option for certain types of reconstruction, such as oral and oropharyngeal defects involving the floor of the mouth, buccal mucosa, and tongue, as well as resurfacing of the hand and fingers. In addition, the flap has minimal donor site morbidity, owing to a location away from flexor tendons, and inconspicuous resulting scar, making it a useful alternative to the radial forearm flap. The ulnar artery perforator flap is most commonly performed as a microvascular free flap, but it has also been used as a pedicled flap for upper extremity defects. This chapter guides the surgeon through each step of the procedure in the use of the ulnar artery perforator flap, from typical indications, to anatomy, to preoperative considerations, to the surgical technique. Two variations and donar site closure are all discussed.

Keywords: ulnar artery, flexor digitorum superficialis muscle, flexor digitorum profundus muscle, common interosseous artery, flexor carpi ulnaris muscle

34.1 Introduction

Fasciocutaneous flaps based on the ulnar artery were first described in 1982 by Song et al.[1] as the ulnar forearm flap. Improved understanding of the vascular anatomy of this region later led to the ability to perform a true perforator flap known as the ulnar artery perforator (UAP) flap. The thinness, pliability, and relative hairlessness of the UAP flap make it a good option for certain types of reconstruction, such as oral and oropharyngeal defects including floor of mouth, buccal mucosa, and tongue, as well as resurfacing of the hand and fingers. In addition, the flap has minimal donor site morbidity, owing to a location away from flexor tendons and inconspicuous resulting scar, making it a useful alternative to the radial forearm flap.[2] The UAP flap is most commonly performed as a microvascular free flap, but has also been described for use as a pedicled flap for upper extremity defects.[3]

34.2 Typical Indications

- Oral and oropharyngeal defects, including floor of mouth, buccal mucosa, and following partial and hemiglossectomy.
- Upper extremity defects, including of the hand and fingers as a free flap, and of the forearm, elbow, and upper arm as a pedicled flap.
- Subtotal and total nasal reconstruction as a lining flap but as a second choice to the radial forearm flap due to a shorter pedicle length.

34.3 Anatomy

The **ulnar artery** is the primary arterial blood supply to the medial aspect of the forearm. It arises from the brachial artery and terminates in the superficial palmar arch, which joins with the superficial branch of the radial artery. It is palpable on the anterior and medial aspect of the wrist and is accompanied by paired venae comitantes. In the proximal forearm, it travels between the **flexor digitorum superficialis (FDS) and flexor digitorum profundus (FDP) muscles**, and gives rise to the **common interosseous artery** approximately 2 to 3 cm after its origin, which should be preserved during flap harvest. The ulnar artery then courses between the FDS and **flexor carpi ulnaris (FCU) muscle** in the distal forearm. Two to three skin perforators consistently originate from the ulnar artery (▶ **Fig. 34.1**).[4] These perforators have been named perforators A, B, and C, based on their location. The A perforator is located approximately 7 cm proximal to the pisiform, or one-fourth of the forearm length from the pisiform. The B perforator is located approximately 4 cm proximal to the A perforator, and the C perforator located roughly 5 cm proximal to the B perforator. The long axis of the flap should initially be centered on the B perforator, which is the most consistent of all three types of perforators and present in 95% of individuals. The A and B perforators are generally all septocutaneous, while C perforators are most often septocutaneous (91%) but occasionally take a musculocutaneous course through the FCU.

The UAP flap has both a deep and superficial venous system. The deep system consists of the venae comitantes, which travel alongside the ulnar artery and are considered the primary venous drainage of the UAP flap. The venae comitantes are generally of good caliber (2–4 mm) and are satisfactory for microvascular tissue transfer. The superficial venous drainage is provided by the **basilic vein**, which is usually larger in caliber than the venae comitantes, but is often out of the territory of the skin paddle design due to its relatively posterior location.

The ulnar artery travels with the **ulnar nerve** in the distal two-thirds of the forearm where it lies radial to the nerve, and great care should be exercised during pedicle dissection in this region to prevent nerve injury. The **medial antebrachial cutaneous nerve** (MABC) travels with the basilic vein in the proximal forearm, and then divides into anterior and ulnar branches more distally, which provide sensory innervation to the anteromedial and posteromedial aspects of the forearm, respectively. The MABC can be harvested with the UAP flap when a sensate flap is needed.

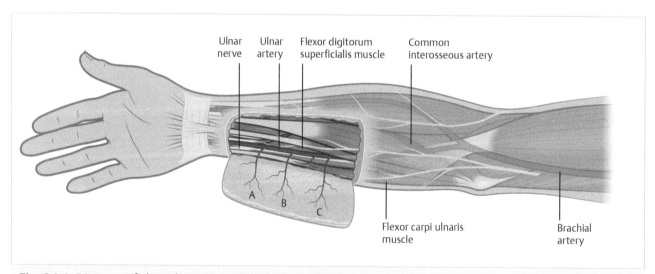

Fig. 34.1 Diagram of clinical anatomy. FDS, flexor digitorum superficialis.

34.4 Variations

- Myocutaneous flap with inclusion of a portion of the FCU by preserving muscular perforating branches from the ulnar artery.
- Osteomyocutaneous flap with ulnar bone. Inclusion of the FCU is necessary in this case, as it provides the myoperiosteal blood supply to the ulna. An approximately 12-cm-long and 0.75-cm-thick segment of bone can be harvested with the UAP flap.

34.5 Preoperative Considerations

The nondominant arm is selected as the flap donor site when possible. An Allen test should be performed preoperatively in order to determine whether the patient demonstrates ulnar dominance, in which case the contralateral side or an alternative flap should be considered.

34.6 Positioning and Skin Markings

The patients are positioned supine with their upper extremity placed on an arm table. A line connecting the pisiform at the wrist crease and the volar aspect of the medial epicondyle of the humerus is drawn (▶ Fig. 34.2). The flap skin paddle is tentatively centered on this line along the radial–ulnar axis, as most perforators are located on this line or slightly ulnar to it, and on the B perforator

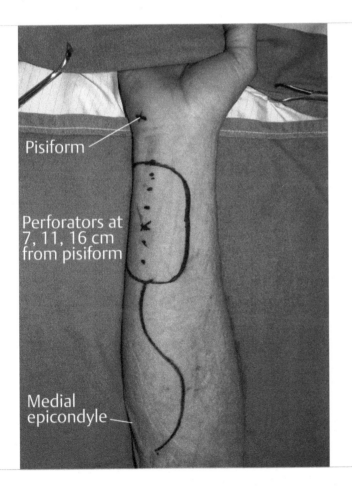

Fig. 34.2 Photograph of preoperative markings.

Pisiform

Perforators at 7, 11, 16 cm from pisiform

Medial epicondyle

along the proximal–distal axis. Skin paddle dimensions of up to approximately 10 × 15 cm can be harvested reliably. To minimize tendon exposure, a point 5 cm proximal to the wrist crease is marked to indicate the distal-most extent that the flap should be harvested. The procedure is performed under tourniquet control without exsanguination in order to facilitate perforator identification and dissection.

34.7 Operative Technique

Refer to Video 34.1 for an example of the operative technique for the ulnar artery perforator flap. An incision is first made on the radial aspect of the skin paddle, and then suprafascial dissection is performed ulnarly until the perforators within the septum between the FCU and FDS are visualized (▶ Fig. 34.3). It is helpful to mark the precise locations of the perforators entering the flap on the skin paddle surface with permanent suture and adjust the flap design, if necessary, to ensure adequate blood flow to the flap based on the actual locations of the perforators. Slightly radial to the perforators, the fascia is incised and the septum is isolated, exposing the ulnar vessels and nerve. The perforators arising from the ulnar vessels are preserved, while the rest of the septum can be left intact or incised if necessary. The remaining skin paddle incisions are then made and the flap is dissected suprafascially on the ulnar side up to the septum, then the fascia is again divided millimeters away so that the deep compartment is entered and the septum and blood vessels can be isolated.

Distally, it is advisable to perform an intraoperative Allen test to confirm adequate perfusion to the hand by the radial artery. The ulnar artery and venae comitantes at the distal aspect of the flap are then ligated and divided. If there are musculocutaneous perforators, intramuscular dissection through the FCU is performed, or a small cuff of muscle included. The ulnar vessels are then gently separated from the ulnar nerve in a distal-to-proximal direction. Avoidance of electrocautery and monopolar diathermy is preferred during this portion of the procedure to prevent injury to the ulnar nerve, with use of clips when possible to control muscular branches. A linear incision is then made from the proximal aspect of the skin paddle toward the antecubital fossa to provide exposure

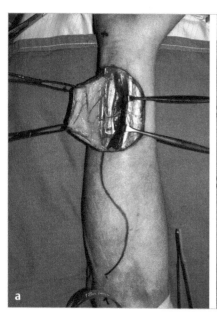
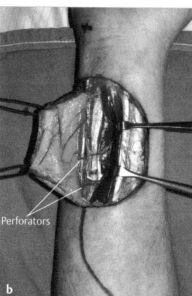

Fig. 34.3 **(a)** Dissection is performed from radial to ulnar until the ulnar blood vessels and their septocutaneous perforators are identified. **(b)** Close-up showing septocutaneous perforators arising from the ulnar artery.

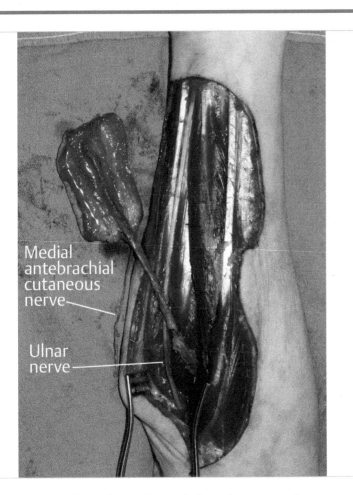

Fig. 34.4 Completed ulnar artery perforator flap, including harvest of the medial antebrachial cutaneous nerve.

for further dissection of the ulnar vessels up to the level of bifurcation with the common interosseous artery, as well as for dissection of the MABC to be included with the flap, if desired (▶ Fig. 34.4).

34.8 Donor Site Closure

Closure of the donor site typically requires skin grafting, although primary closure is possible for narrow flaps in patients with sufficient skin laxity. Note that graft take of the UAP flap donor site is usually superior that that of the radial forearm flap donor site because skin grafting is performed over flexor muscle bellies rather than tendons (▶ Fig. 34.5).

34.9 Pearls and Pitfalls

- The perforator anatomy of the UAP flap is consistent, and the distal perforators almost always have a septocutaneous course that facilitates flap elevation.
- An Allen test should be performed in order to identify potential ischemic consequences to the hand associated with flap harvest. Ulnar artery–dominant circulation to the hand is a contraindication to use of this flap, and, conversely, the UAP flap is preferred over the radial forearm flap when there is evidence of radial artery dominance.
- Use of a tourniquet without exsanguination can facilitate perforator identification and dissection.

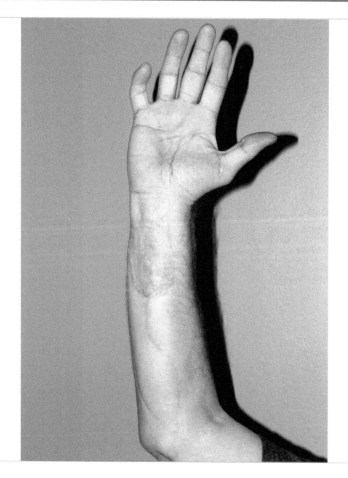

Fig. 34.5 Donor site appearance after reconstruction with a split-thickness skin graft.

- In the distal two-thirds of the forearm, avoidance of electrocautery and monopolar diathermy during pedicle dissection can help prevent injury to the ulnar nerve.
- The vascular pedicle of the UAP flap is typically shorter than that of the radial forearm flap.

References

[1] Song R, Gao Y, Song Y, Yu Y, Song Y. The forearm flap. Clin Plast Surg 1982;9(1):21–26
[2] Sieg P, Bierwolf S. Ulnar versus radial forearm flap in head and neck reconstruction: an experimental and clinical study. Head Neck 2001;23(11):967–971
[3] Wei Y, Shi X, Yu Y, Zhong G, Tang M, Mei J. Vascular anatomy and clinical application of the free proximal ulnar artery perforator flaps. Plast Reconstr Surg Glob Open 2014;2(7):e179
[4] Yu P, Chang EI, Selber JC, Hanasono MM. Perforator patterns of the ulnar artery perforator flap. Plast Reconstr Surg 2012;129(1):213–220

Part 7

Lower Extremity

35 Anterolateral Thigh Flap

Aladdin H. Hassanein and Justin M. Sacks

Abstract

The anterolateral thigh has become a workhorse flap because of its versatility, large skin paddle, the ability for a two-team approach, reliable anatomy, the potential to be sensate, and a favorable donor site morbidity. It is typically harvested as a fasciocutaneous perforator flap. It is most frequently transferred as free tissue for soft-tissue defects ranging from scalp to lower extremity, but it can be used as a pedicled flap for abdominal, lower extremity, and perineal reconstruction. In this chapter, the authors provide surgeons with the sequence of steps involved in the anterolateral thigh flap procedure. Typical indications are first given, followed by anatomy, preoperative considerations, and the surgical technique. Six variations and donor site closure are also discussed.

Keywords: anterior superior iliac spine, descending branch of the lateral femoral circumflex artery, profunda femoris artery, lateral femoral cutaneous nerve

35.1 Introduction

The anterolateral thigh (ALT) flap was first described by Song et al in 1984.[1] The ALT has become a workhorse flap because of its versatility, large skin paddle, the ability for a two-team approach, reliable anatomy, the potential to be sensate, and favorable donor site morbidity. It is typically harvested as a fasciocutaneous perforator flap. The ALT is most frequently transferred as free tissue for soft-tissue defects ranging from scalp to lower extremity, but it can be used as a pedicled flap for abdominal, lower extremity, and perineal reconstruction.[2,3,4,5]

35.2 Typical Indications

- Scalp defects.
- Oropharynx and hypopharyngeal defects.
- Abdominal wall soft-tissue defect (pedicle or free).
- Perineal reconstruction (pedicle).
- Phalloplasty (pedicle or free).
- Distal third leg wounds.
- Cutaneous defect anywhere on the body requiring skin resurfing with thin fasciocutaneous flap (e.g., axilla, upper/lower extremity, back, chest, etc.).

35.3 Anatomy

The ALT flap includes the fasciocutaneous area overlying the axis from the **anterior superior iliac spine** (ASIS) to the lateral patella (▶Fig. 35.1). Perforating branches of the **descending branch of the lateral femoral circumflex artery** (LFCA) supply the flap. The LFCA arises from the proximal **profunda femoris artery** and divides into the ascending, transverse, and descending branches. The descending branch of the LFCA travels deep to the rectus femoris muscle in the intermuscular septum between the rectus femoris and vastus lateralis muscle. The vastus lateralis muscle is lateral to the rectus femoris and medial to the tensor fascia lata (TFL). The perforators of the LFCA that perfuse the flap commonly are mostly musculocutaneous (80%) with a course through the vastus

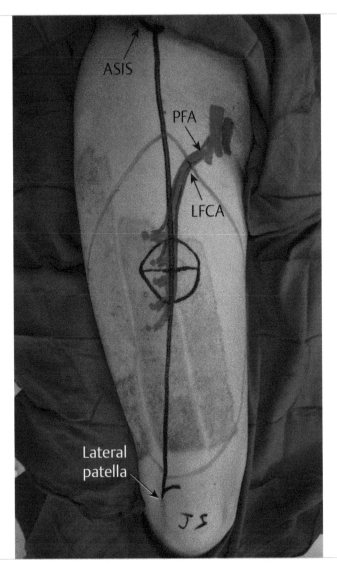

Fig. 35.1 Anatomy of anterolateral thigh flap. ASIS, anterior superior iliac spine; PFA, profunda femoral artery; LFCA, lateral femoral circumflex artery. The pedicle to the flap is the descending branch of the LFCA.

lateralis muscle.[2,3] If present, septocutaneous perforators are most frequently found proximally. The primary perforator ("B" perforator) is usually found at the midpoint between the axis from the ASIS to the lateral patella.[3] An "A" perforator frequently is located 5 cm proximal to the "B" perforator, and a "C" perforator 5 cm distal.[3] Venous drainage of the flap is through venae comitantes that accompany the LFCA. The caliber of the LFCA is approximately 2 to 3 mm and the vein is slightly larger. Distally the LFCA communicates with the superior genicular artery above the patella. The **lateral femoral cutaneous nerve** (L2–L3), which emerges from the deep fascia 10 cm below the ASIS, can be included to provide sensory innervation.[2] Typical skin paddle width to allow for primary closure is 8 cm, although larger flaps have been described. The pedicle length is approximately 8 cm but can vary depending on which perforator is chosen. The more distal the perforator, the longer the pedicle. If there is concern for perfusion, then two or more perforators can be harvested. Additionally, two or more independent skin islands can be designed around separate perforators.

35.4 Variations

- Myocutaneous flap (includes the vastus lateralis muscle).
- Chimeric flap including rectus femoris and/or tensor fascia lata.
- Sensate flap (with lateral femoral cutaneous nerve).

- Superthin flap (suprafascial dissection, thinned postharvest except 2 cm radius around perforator).
- Reversed pedicle flap for knee defects.
- Adipofascial flap.

35.5 Preoperative Considerations

An ALT flap used for cutaneous defects/skin resurfacing may be excessively thick in obese patients.[4] An adipofascial flap with a skin graft or other thinner fasciocutaneous flaps (e.g., radial forearm, or medial sural artery flap) should be considered in these patients. The skin paddle can be eccentrically designed around the perforator to increase and enhance the pedicle reach at the recipient site. A flap width greater than 8 to 10 cm typically cannot be closed primarily and requires skin grafting. Preoperative tissue expansion may be considered in an electively planned case that will require a wide flap if skin grafting is not desired.

35.6 Positioning and Skin Markings

The supine position is ideal for most indications. The ASIS and lateral patella are marked and serve as the reference axis of the flap (▶ Fig. 35.2). The patient's

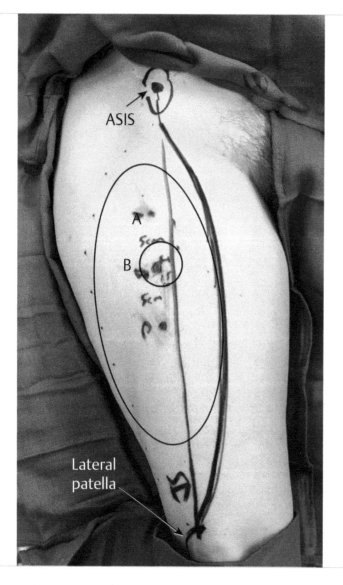

Fig. 35.2 Markings for anterolateral thigh flap. A line connecting the anterior superior iliac spine (ASIS) and lateral patella is drawn. Perforator "B" is typically found 1.5 cm posterior to the midpoint of the line. Perforator "A" and "C" are 5 cm proximal and distal to perforator "B," respectively. One-third of the flap is marked anterior to the ASIS–lateral patella axis.

legs should be positioned so that the toes point anteriorly for the markings, which can be facilitated by a clamped towel to secure the feet together, will facilitate identification of the septum and will be a key anatomical landmark for designing the skin paddle for the flap. The midpoint between the line connecting the ASIS and lateral patella is marked. The main perforator "B" usually is found within a 3-cm radius of the midpoint of the ASIS–lateral patella axis, most often 1.5 cm posterior to midpoint of the line. Perforator "A" typically is located 5 cm proximal to perforator "B," and perforator "C" is 5 cm distal. A hand-held Doppler probe is used to locate the perforator signal on the skin. The skin island classically is drawn in a lenticular shape and skewed around the axis so that one-third of the flap is anterior to the ASIS–lateral patella line (A–P line) and two-thirds of the flap is posterior to this line.

35.7 Operative Technique

Refer to Video 35.1 for an example of the operative technique for the anterolateral thigh free flap. The anterior marking of the flap is incised initially and the dissection proceeds laterally subfascially over the rectus femoris muscle to intermuscular septum between the rectus femoris muscle and the vastus lateralis muscle. The septum is opened, which is facilitated by retracting the rectus femoris medially (▶ **Fig. 35.3a**). The descending branch of the LFCA lies in the septum posterior to the rectus femoris. Care must be taken while opening of the septum to avoid injury to the pedicle and perforators. The descending branch of the LFCA is exposed and its perforating vessels are identified. The perforator(s) are chosen to supply the flap. If an adequate septocutaneous perforator is present, it is preferred to simplify the dissection. If the perforators are musculocutaneous, a large perforator with a simple intramuscular course is favored. The posterior marking is adjusted if necessary based on the location of the perforator and the posterior portion of the flap is incised and elevated medially toward the perforator. A perforator dissection is performed through the vastus lateralis muscle (if a musculocutaneous perforator is chosen) to the LFCA takeoff from the profunda femoral artery.

The descending branch of the LFCA is ligated at the portion distal to the flap. One or more nerve branches to the vastus lateralis are found adjacent to the pedicle and may need to be sacrificed to mobilize the pedicle. However, they can be repaired primarily during the donor site closure with neurorrhaphy. The LFCA branch to the rectus femoris and nerve should be preserved. If there are no suitable ALT flap perforators or if they are diminutive, then the anteromedial thigh (AMT) flap should be considered. In this instance, the perforators to this medial thigh-based flap typically arise off the rectus femoris branch of the descending branch of the lateral circumflex femoral vessels. In the majority of situations, the ALT flap perforators will be sufficient. However, understanding the potential variability of the thigh vascular anatomy is critical once a thigh is decided upon for flap harvest. An inverse relationship between size and number of ALT and AMT perforators exists and when ALT perforators are inadequate, the AMT perforators are typically useable.[6] Once the vascularity of the flap is deemed appropriate, the vascular pedicle is clipped and the flap is transferred (▶ **Fig. 35.3b–f**).

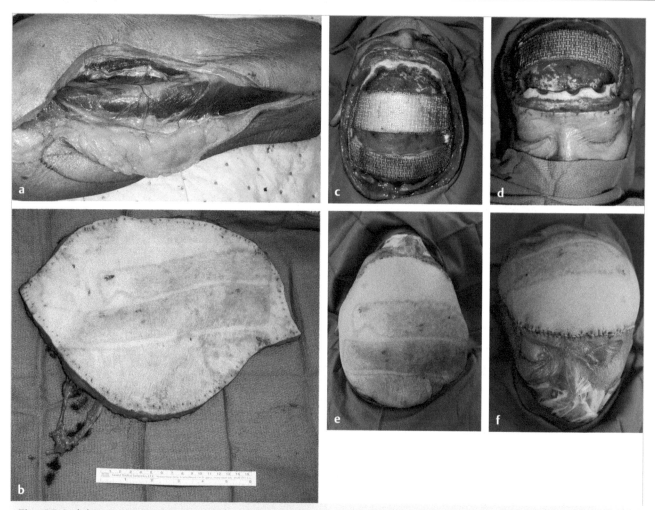

Fig. 35.3 **(a)** Harvesting the anterolateral thigh flap. The medial incision is made and subfascial dissection proceeds laterally. The septum between the rectus femoris and vastus lateralis is opened to find the descending branch of the lateral femoral circumflex artery. The perforator is chosen. A musculocutaneous perforator must be dissected through the vastus lateralis. **(b)** A harvested anterolateral thigh flap. **(c,d)** A 66-year-old male with a scalp defect following resection of a recurrent angiosarcoma. **(e,f)** A large anterolateral thigh flap inset over a scalp defect.

35.8 Donor Site Closure

The donor site can usually be closed primarily if the width is less than 8 cm. A skin graft may be required for wider flaps. "Purse-stringing" closure of the donor site can reduce the skin defect required for skin grafting. This is done with an absorbable running dermal 2–0 or 3–0 suture. A closed suction drain is placed in the donor site. A vacuum-assisted closure device placed over an interface dressing is used in the cases that require split-thickness skin grafting. Full-thickness skin grafting can be used in the cases where the thigh cannot be closed primarily and there is excess skin from the skin flap harvest that would otherwise be discarded.

35.9 Pearls and Pitfalls

- If no significant LFCA perforating vessels are found, (1) the medial thigh can be explored for perforators or the (2) ALT flap can be taken with the vastus lateralis muscle thereby increasing the chances of harvesting the skin paddle with extremely small vascular perforators.
- There are good functional outcomes and acceptable morbidity if the vastus lateralis is sacrificed and the other three quadriceps muscles are preserved.

References

[1] Song YG, Chen GZ, Song YL. The free thigh flap: a new free flap concept based on the septo-cutaneous artery. Br J Plast Surg 1984;37(2):149–159

[2] Xu DC, Zhong SZ, Kong JM, et al. Applied anatomy of the anterolateral femoral flap. Plast Reconstr Surg 1988;82(2):305–310

[3] Yu P. Characteristics of the anterolateral thigh flap in a Western population and its application in head and neck reconstruction. Head Neck 2004;26(9):759–769

[4] Seth R, Manz RM, Dahan IJ, et al. Comprehensive analysis of the anterolateral thigh flap vascular anatomy. Arch Facial Plast Surg 2011;13(5):347–354

[5] Pang J, Broyles JM, Berli J, et al. Abdominal- versus thigh-based reconstruction of perineal defects in patients with cancer. Dis Colon Rectum 2014;57(6):725–732

[6] Yu P, Selber J, Liu J. Reciprocal dominance of the anterolateral and anteromedial thigh flap perforator anatomy. Ann Plast Surg 2013;70(6):714–716

36 Anteromedial Thigh Flap

Alexander F. Mericli and Jesse C. Selber

Abstract

The anteromedial thigh flap is used infrequently, mainly owing to its variable and inconsistent anatomy. There are no obvious advantages of the anteromedial thigh flap over the anterolateral thigh flap. The anatomical location, donor site morbidity, and cutaneous thickness are identical. The usefulness of the anteromedial thigh flap stems from the fact that the vascular anatomy of the thigh is reciprocally dominant between the anterolateral and anteromedial perforators. Therefore, the anteromedial thigh flap is important to be familiar with for situations when the anterolateral thigh demonstrates absent or inadequate perforators. In this chapter, the authors guide surgeons through the entirety of the anteromedial thigh flap procedure, beginning with typical indications, to a discussion of anatomy, to preoperative considerations, and the operative technique itself. A listing of four variations and notes on donor site closure round out the discussion.

Keywords: pedicle flap, free flap, descending branch lateral circumflex femoral descending artery, skin paddle

36.1 Introduction

In 1984, Song and colleagues first described the anteromedial thigh (AMT) flap in conjunction with the anterolateral thigh (ALT) flap.[1] Despite this fact, the flap is used infrequently, mainly owing to its variable and inconsistent anatomy. There are no obvious advantages of the AMT flap over the ALT flap. The anatomical location, donor site morbidity, and cutaneous thickness are identical. The usefulness of the AMT flap stems from the fact that the vascular anatomy of the thigh is reciprocally dominant between the anterolateral and anteromedial perforators.[2,3] Therefore, the AMT flap is important to be familiar with for situations when the ALT demonstrates absent or inadequate perforators.

36.2 Typical Indications

- Regional use as pedicle flap:
  - Groin.
  - Mons.
  - Thigh.
  - Knee.
- Distant use as free flap:
  - Head and neck.
  - Upper extremity.
  - Lower extremity.

36.3 Anatomy

In the Western population, 4.3% of thighs will have no ALT perforators and 26% will only have one perforator. However, in patients where there are no ALT perforators, there is nearly a 100% chance that adequate AMT perforators are present.

Furthermore, in situations where there is only one ALT perforator, in 75% of these thighs, there is a useable AMT perforator.[4] Therefore, if a multipaddle flap is required and only one perforator is present for the ALT flap, then a second skin paddle can be designed using the AMT tissues (▶Fig. 36.1). The AMT perforator extends from the rectus femoris muscle branch of the **descending branch of the lateral femoral circumflex vessels**. After sending a branch to the rectus femoris muscle, the pedicle emerges medial to the rectus femoris, in the proximal thigh, between the rectus femoris and sartorius muscles. The pedicle continues to travel distally between the rectus femoris and vastus medialis muscles. The distal end of the pedicle then penetrates the deep fascia to become a cutaneous perforator, supplying the skin and subcutaneous tissues of the AMT.

AMT perforators can alternately arise directly from the **superficial femoral artery**. The perforators from the superficial femoral artery are short (3–5 cm) and are more distal compared to those from the rectus femoris branch. Therefore, in order for the AMT flap to be clinically useful, its perforators must arise from the rectus femoris branch; this allows for a vascular pedicle similar in length and diameter to that of the ALT flap. Yu and Selber found AMT perforators associated with the rectus femoris branch in 51% of thighs.[5] Most thighs with adequate AMT perforators had only a single perforator.

In the flap's original description by Song, the surface location of the AMT perforators was described as being in the triangular intermuscular space formed by the rectus femoris, sartorius, and vastus medialis.[1] Yu and Selber provide a more quantitative description, based on the "ABC" system of perforator anatomy.[5] They found that when a line is drawn connecting the **anterior superior iliac spine** (ASIS) and the superomedial border of the **patella** (AP line), the B perforator exists on the midpoint of this line. If additional perforators are present

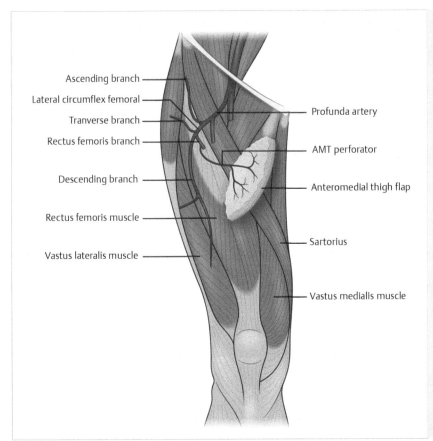

Fig. 36.1 Relevant anatomy of the anterolateral and anteromedial thigh flaps. The lateral femoral circumflex artery branches into a descending branch and the branch to the rectus femoris muscle. The descending branch continues inferiorly between the rectus femoris and vastus lateralis muscles to supply the tissues of the anterolateral thigh. The rectus femoris branch enters the deep surface of the rectus femoris muscle before splitting into perforators, which emerge between the rectus femoris and sartorius or vastus medialis muscles to supply the tissues of the anteromedial thigh flap.

Ascending branch
Lateral circumflex femoral
Tranverse branch
Rectus femoris branch
Descending branch
Rectus femoris muscle
Vastus lateralis muscle

Profunda artery
AMT perforator
Anteromedial thigh flap
Sartorius
Vastus medialis muscle

(A and/or C perforators), then they can be found 5 cm proximal or distal to the location of the B perforator. On the x-axis, the AMT perforators are located, on average, 3.2 cm medial to the AP line, corresponding to the intermuscular space between the rectus femoris and sartorius/vastus medialis muscles.

The associated skin paddle is more anterior compared to the ALT; similar to the ALT, the donor site usually will require skin grafting for closure if the cutaneous component of the flap is wider than 8 to 9 cm.

36.4 Variations

- Pedicled flap.
- Free flap.
- Combined with ALT territory and rectus femoris muscle ("subtotal thigh flap").
- Combined with ALT as chimeric flap.

36.5 Preoperative Considerations

During the initial history and physical examination, the patient's bilateral thighs should be examined. Scars from previous injuries or surgeries as well as the subcutaneous thickness of the lateral and anterior thigh tissues should be noted; a lower extremity vascular examination should be performed. If the thigh subcutaneous fat is more than 2 cm thick, then a different flap may be a better option. The location of the ALT and/or AMT perforators can be estimated with hand-held Doppler ultrasonography; the ALT perforators will be most easily found running in the palpable septum between the rectus femoris and vastus lateralis muscles.[2] If no ALT perforators can be found, then the region of the AMT flap should be examined. As described previously, the AMT perforators exist at the midpoint of the AP line, on average 3.2 cm medial to it. If the patient has a history of peripheral vascular disease and/or if a multiple skin paddle flap is anticipated, then a preoperative computed tomography angiography (CTA) should be considered. CTA of the thigh has been shown to accurately predict the location of thigh perforators in relation to other anatomical structures and may assist in preoperative planning (▶ Fig. 36.2).[6]

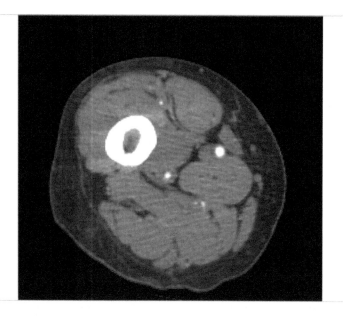

Fig. 36.2 Computed tomographic image demonstrating an anterolateral thigh (ALT) and anteromedial thigh (AMT) perforator in the same slice. The ALT perforator is located between the rectus femoris and vastus lateralis muscles, whereas the AMT perforator is between the rectus femoris and sartorius muscles.

36.6 Positioning and Skin Markings

The patient should be placed in the supine position with the thighs adducted and bilateral hips internally rotated. In order to maintain this position intra-operatively, the bilateral feet are padded in order to prevent pressure injury, and secured to each other. The ASIS and superolateral border of the patella are marked and a line connecting these two points is made (the AP line). If the AP line is considered the y-axis, then the B perforator for the ALT flap as well as the B perforator for the AMT flap exist at the midpoint of this line; the A and C perforators exist 5 cm proximal and distal to the midpoint, respectively. On the x-axis, the ALT perforators are located on average 1.5 cm lateral to the AP line and the AMT perforators are located on average 3.2 cm medial to the AP line. Provisional marks are placed in these locations. Typically, the initial incision for a thigh flap is designed in parallel with the AP line, 1.5 to 2 cm medial. From this incision, the anterolateral thigh can be explored for adequate and appropriate perforators; if none are present, then through this same incision the anteromedial thigh can be explored for a possible AMT flap.

36.7 Operative Technique

A line is drawn connecting the ASIS and the superolateral border of the patella. Perforator B is marked at the midpoint of the AP line, 1.5 cm lateral to it; perforators A and C are marked 5 cm proximal and 5 cm distal to perforator B, respectively. The medial border of the ALT flap design is typically 1.5 to 2 cm medial to the AP line; this corresponds with the lateral border of the AMT flap design (▶Fig. 36.3a). A straight anterior incision is made and dissection proceeds suprafascially to explore the cutaneous perforators in the ALT flap territory. If no viable perforators are found, or if a chimeric ALT/AMT flap is to be designed, then through the same incision the AMT territory perforators are explored. Similarly, a subfascial dissection is performed extending medially over the rectus femoris muscle and sartorius–vastus medialis muscles. The intermuscular space between the rectus femoris and vastus medialis/sartorius muscles can be easily entered to explore the origin of the perforators. In order to be clinically useful as an AMT flap, the perforators must join the rectus femoris branch of the lateral femoral circumflex descending artery and vein. If the AMT perforators emerge from the superficial femoral artery, then an AMT flap is generally not possible. If a chimeric ALT/AMT is required, then the pedicle is dissected as proximally as possible, to where the lateral femoral circumflex descending artery and vein emerge from the profunda femoral vessels; a common trunk will be found here, immediately before branching into the rectus femoris/AMT pedicle and lateral femoral circumflex descending/ALT pedicle (▶Fig. 36.3b). Depending on the requirements of the defect, the AMT flap can be raised as fasciocutaneous flap, as myocutaneous flap with a section of rectus femoris muscle, or as a subtotal thigh flap including all the rectus femoris and vastus lateralis muscles as well as the fasciocutaneous tissues of the ALT.

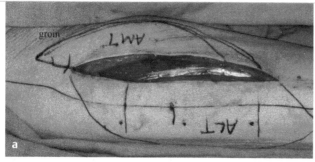

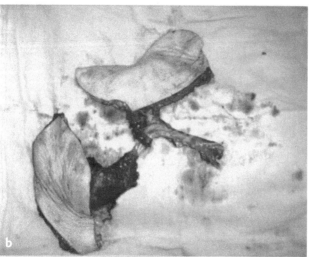

Fig. 36.3 **(a)** The location of the anteromedial thigh is directly medial to the tissues used for the anterolateral thigh flap. The AMT perforators exist 3.2 cm medial to the AP line. **(b)** Chimeric ALT/AMT flap.

36.8 Donor Site Closure

The donor site generally should close primarily if it is 8 to 9 cm in width or less. Anything wider usually requires a skin graft. Occasionally, conservative subcutaneous undermining is required for a tension-free closure. Overzealous closure of the donor site to avoid a skin graft can result in muscle ischemia, soft-tissue necrosis, and even compartment syndrome. The incision is closed in layers, reapproximating the Scarpa's fascia, deep dermis, and superficial dermis. One or two drains are imperative to reduce the possibility of a seroma.

36.9 Pearls and Pitfalls

- The AMT flap offers no advantage over the ALT flap.
- The AMT flap is useful when there are no ALT perforators, when the ALT perforators are too small and therefore inadequate, and/or when there is only one ALT perforator and a multiple skin paddle flap is required.
- There is a reciprocal dominance between the ALT and AMT perforators.
- In order to be clinically useful, the AMT perforators must arise from the rectus femoris muscle branch of the lateral femoral circumflex artery; a flap cannot be designed using vessels coming from the superficial femoral artery.
- Similar to the ALT flap, if the AMT donor site is wider than 8 to 9 cm, then a skin graft will likely be required for donor site closure.

References

[1] Song YG, Chen GZ, Song YL. The free thigh flap: a new free flap concept based on the septocutaneous artery. Br J Plast Surg 1984;37(2):149–159

[2] Hong JP, Kim EK, Kim H, Shin HW, Hwang CH, Lee MY. Alternative regional flaps when anterolateral thigh flap perforator is not feasible. J Hand Microsurg 2010;2(2):51–57

[3] Yu P, Selber J, Liu J. Reciprocal dominance of the anterolateral and anteromedial thigh flap perforator anatomy. Ann Plast Surg 2013;70(6):714–716

[4] Yu P. Characteristics of the anterolateral thigh flap in a Western population and its application in head and neck reconstruction. Head Neck 2004;26(9):759–769

[5] Yu P, Selber J. Perforator patterns of the anteromedial thigh flap. Plast Reconstr Surg 2011;128(3):151e–157e

[6] Garvey PB, Selber JC, Madewell JE, Bidaut L, Feng L, Yu P. A prospective study of preoperative computed tomographic angiography for head and neck reconstruction with anterolateral thigh flaps. Plast Reconstr Surg 2011;127(4):1505–1514

37 Rectus Femoris Muscle Flap

Alexander F. Mericli and Charles E. Butler

Abstract

The rectus femoris muscle can be used as a pedicled or free flap for reconstructing a variety of defects. As a pedicled flap, it will easily reach the lower abdomen, mons pubis, lateral hip, perineum, and groin. The flap can be harvested as a myocutaneous or muscle-only flap, depending on the requirements of the defect. Depending on the size of the defect, the rectus muscle can be designed as an isolated flap or can be combined with other components of the lateral femoral circumflex vascular axis (vastus lateralis, anterolateral thigh skin and subcutaneous tissue, iliotibial band, and/or tensor fascia lata muscle) for the creation of a subtotal thigh flap. Although the rectus femoris is recognized as a useful flap, debate continues regarding its associated donor site morbidity. Several authors have reported no loss of knee extension capacity or strength following harvest of this flap, but other studies have reported a qualitative loss in either range, motion or strength. The only quantitative study found knee range of motion to be unaffected after use of the rectus femoris flap. This chapter covers all the salient elements of the surgical procedure, beginning with indications for use of the flap, anatomy, preoperative considerations, the operative technique, and concluding with donor site closure. Four variations to the procedure are also mentioned.

Keywords: Lateral femoral circumflex artery, superficial femoral artery, pedicled muscle flap, pedicled myocutaneous flap, free subtotal thigh flap, innervated rectus femoris flap

37.1 Introduction

The rectus femoris muscle can be used as pedicled or free flap for reconstruction of variety of defects. As a pedicled flap, it will easily reach the lower abdomen, mons pubis, lateral hip, perineum, and groin.[1,2,3,4,5] The flap can be harvested as a myocutaneous or muscle-only flap, depending on the requirements of the defect. Depending on the size of the defect, the rectus muscle can be designed as an isolated flap, or can be combined with other components of the lateral femoral circumflex vascular axis (vastus lateralis, anterolateral thigh skin and subcutaneous tissue, iliotibial band, and/or tensor fascia lata muscle) for the creation of a subtotal thigh flap. Although the rectus femoris is recognized as a useful flap, debate continues regarding its associated donor site morbidity. Several authors have reported no loss of knee extension capacity or strength following harvest of this flap.[2,5] Other studies have reported a qualitative loss in either range, motion, or strength. The only quantitative study found knee range of motion to be unaffected after use of the rectus femoris flap.[2]

37.2 Typical Indications

- Pedicled: reconstruction of the groin, perineum, ischium, and inferior abdomen.
- Free: reconstruction of the abdominal wall, chest, and head and neck.

37.3 Anatomy

The rectus femoris is part of the quadriceps muscle complex. The muscle is bordered by the vastus medialis medially, the vastus lateralis laterally, and the vastus intermedius on its deep surface. The sartorius muscle crosses obliquely over the rectus femoris muscle proximally. It is a bipennate muscle with two distinct muscle bellies (▶ **Fig. 37.1a**). The muscle originates from both the anterior inferior iliac spine and the anterior rim of the acetabulum and therefore functions to both flex the hip and extend the knee, via its insertion onto the patella. The vascular supply of the rectus femoris is consistent with that of a type II muscle flap, as defined by Mathes and Nahai. The major pedicle is a proximal branch of the **lateral femoral circumflex artery**. The branch to the rectus femoris muscle emerges 1 to 2.5 cm distal to where the lateral femoral circumflex artery branches from the profunda femoris artery. The pedicle enters the muscle on its deep and lateral surface. After sending a branch to the rectus femoris muscle,

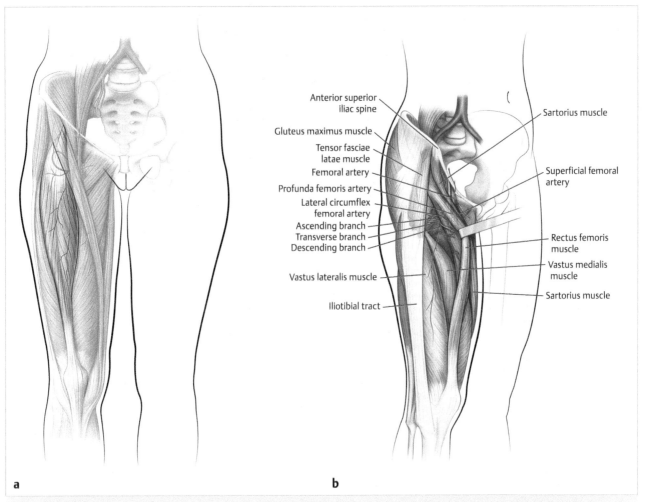

a   b

Fig. 37.1 **(a)** Muscular anatomy of the anterior thigh. **(b)** Anatomy of the lateral femoral circumflex vascular tree. Note the major and minor pedicles to the rectus femoris muscle. The flap can only be based on the more proximal major pedicle; the minor pedicles are generally not sufficient to sustain the flap. (From Zenn MR, Jones GE. Reconstructive Surgery: Anatomy, Technique, and Clinical Applications. New York: Thieme Medical Publishers; 2012.)

the lateral femoral circumflex neurovascular bundle continues inferiorly, traveling in the septum between the vastus lateralis and rectus femoris muscle, to supply the vastus lateralis and is the vascular basis of the anterolateral thigh flap. The minor pedicle(s) are one to three small branches from the **superficial femoral artery**, distally. Generally, the minor pedicles are not independently sufficient to support complete flap viability (▶ **Fig. 37.1b**). The major and minor pedicle arteries are accompanied by paired venae comitantes that drain into the lateral circumflex femoral vein and superficial femoral vein, respectively.

37.4 Variations

- Pedicled muscle flap.
- Pedicled myocutaneous flap.
- Pedicled or free subtotal thigh flap (rectus femoris myocutaneous flap + anterolateral thigh flap).[1]
- Innervated rectus femoris flap for dynamic abdominal wall reconstruction.[3]

37.5 Preoperative Considerations

Special attention should be paid to a past history of any abdominal, groin, or thigh surgeries or injuries. If peripheral vascular disease is suspected, a computed tomographic angiogram should be considered to verify perfusion of the rectus femoris muscle. The tentative reconstructive plan should be discussed with all involved surgical services (i.e., vascular surgery for groin wounds, general surgery for abdominal wall reconstruction cases, etc.).

37.6 Positioning and Skin Markings

The patient is placed in the supine position with the bilateral legs internally rotated at the hip. The legs are secured in this position at the forefoot with a combination of tape and foam to relieve pressure. Markings are placed on the anterior superior iliac spine and the midpoint of the upper border of the patella; a line connecting these two points represents the central axis of the rectus femoris muscle (▶ **Fig. 37.2**). For a muscle-only rectus flap, either one or two incisions are designed along the central axis of the muscle. For a more minimally invasive approach, the two-incision technique is used: a short distal incision is planned for the distal thigh to allow disinsertion of the muscle from the patella. This incision is directly overlying the rectus femoris muscle and 6 to 8 cm in length. A separate incision is designed more proximally, over the region of the major pedicle. This incision will allow for more proximal dissection and will facilitate tunneling of the muscle into the abdominal defect, if a pedicled flap is planned. If a minimally invasive approach is not necessary, an incision is made over the central anterior axis of the thigh, directly overlying the rectus femoris muscle, from groin to distal thigh. If a cutaneous component is to be included with the flap, then the skin paddle is designed as an ellipse directly overlying the muscle; a skin paddle up to 8 cm in width can generally be designed and the thigh still closed primarily in most patients.

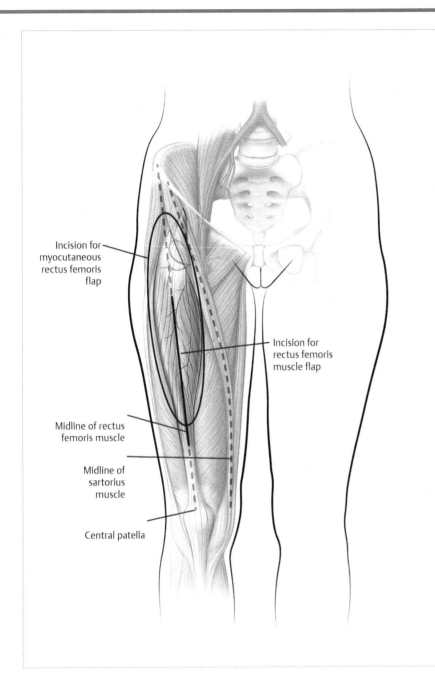

Fig. 37.2 Illustration depicting the surgical markings necessary for a muscle-only rectus femoris flap (*yellow line*) and myocutaneous flap (*solid black line*). (From Zenn MR, Jones GE. Reconstructive Surgery: Anatomy, Technique, and Clinical Applications. New York: Thieme Medical Publishers; 2012.)

Incision for myocutaneous rectus femoris flap

Incision for rectus femoris muscle flap

Midline of rectus femoris muscle

Midline of sartorius muscle

Central patella

37.7 Operative Technique

For a muscle-only flap, an incision is made centered over the long axis of the muscle. If a skin paddle is desired, then an incision is made around the circumference of the ellipse. With a large skin paddle, it is useful to suture the edges of the skin to the muscle fascia once the flap is elevated to prevent any shearing of the skin during dissection. For a muscle-only flap, the first incision should be made 4 to 6 cm proximal to the patella. Dissection is carried down through the subcutaneous adipose tissue and through the deep fascia overlying the muscle belly. Blunt dissection is used to free the muscle along its medial and deep surfaces. Laterally and distally, the plane between the rectus femoris muscle and vastus lateralis muscle is often ill-defined. The distal muscle belly is disinserted from the patella, leaving 2 to 3 cm of tendon with the muscle flap to assist with inset suturing. The muscle is dissected proximally, freeing it from its medial, lateral, and deep attachments. Several groups of vessels from the superficial femoral artery and vein (the minor pedicles) will be encountered entering the muscle's deep surface which should be divided and ligated. Either the incision is extended proximally up to the groin, or for a more minimally invasive approach, a separate incision is made overlying the groin and the disinserted muscle is passed from the distal incision and into the proximal incision (▶Fig. 37.3a). A lighted retractor can be helpful with this step of the dissection. The sartorius muscle will be found obliquely crossing over the muscle, from superior lateral to inferior medial. The main pedicle enters the rectus femoris muscle on its deep and lateral surface at the level of the sartorius (▶Fig. 37.3b). The pedicle (about 2–5 cm in length) is dissected up to the junction of the profunda femoris artery in order to gain additional pedicle length in the case of a free flap and rotational freedom in the case of a pedicled flap. The nerve to the muscle is divided to avoid undesirable contraction during knee extension. Passing the flap deep to the sartorius (subsartorial transposition) will allow for approximately 5 cm of additional advancement (▶Fig. 37.3b). For a groin wound, the flap can be inset into the defect with its deep surface facing anteriorly and native groin skin closed over the muscle flap (▶Fig. 37.3c). Alternatively, the proximal muscle origin can be released to islandize the flap for a rotational inset. For a myocutaneous flap, the skin paddle can be inset as dictated by the requirements of the defect (▶Fig. 37.3d).

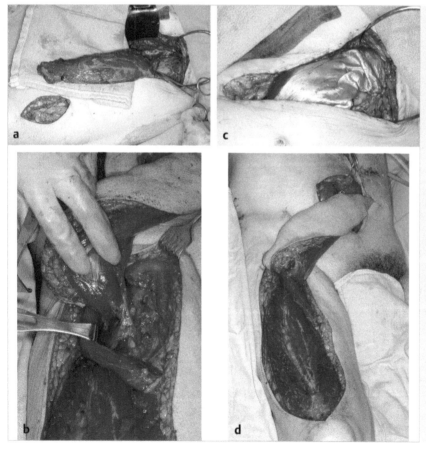

Fig. 37.3 (a) Minimally invasive rectus femoris muscle flap harvest with limited distal incision. (b) The rectus muscle is passed deep to the sartorius muscle for an additional 5 cm of advancement. Note the location of the major pedicle, entering the deep surface of the muscle. (c) When the flap is designed as a pedicled muscle flap for groin reconstruction, the flap can be positioned so that the deep surface of the muscle faces anteriorly. If sufficient native groin skin is present, then the skin can be directly closed over the muscle flap. (d) For a myocutaneous variant, the flap can be rotated and inset as far superior as the lower abdomen or mons pubis.

37.8 Donor Site Closure

Reconstructing the quadriceps tendon complex is an extremely important step of this operation and cannot be underestimated. Doing so will help to minimize the noted donor site morbidity and loss of terminal knee extension. Buried interrupted permanent sutures are typically used to approximate the vastus lateralis tendon to the tendon of the vastus medialis, thus centralizing the moment arm of the remaining quadriceps tendon. It is not uncommon to extend this tenorrhaphy for 15 cm proximally. The soft tissues of the thigh should be closed in layers, over one or two drains. The patient should be placed in a knee immobilizer splint after donor site closure, with the knee in extension. This splint should be worn during ambulation for 3 to 6 weeks. Ambulation is encouraged as early as the first postoperative day with weight bearing as tolerated.

37.9 Pearls and Pitfalls

- The patient's legs should be internally rotated at the hip during both preoperative marking and surgery.
- The flap is most commonly used as a pedicled flap, but also can be designed as free flap. Because of the short pedicle length, if a free flap is required, vein grafting may be necessary.
- As a pedicled flap, the muscle should be passed deep to the sartorius muscle for an additional 5 cm of advancement.
- Donor site morbidity is limited to decreased eccentric quadriceps strength. Range of motion is unaffected.
- The majority of donor site morbidity can be obviated by performing a vastus medialis lateralis tenorrhaphy, using a knee immobilizer during the postoperative period, and engaging a physical therapy regimen.

References

[1] Lin SJ, Butler CE. Subtotal thigh flap and bioprosthetic mesh reconstruction for large, composite abdominal wall defects. Plast Reconstr Surg 2010;125(4):1146–1156

[2] Caulfield WH, Curtsinger L, Powell G, Pederson WC. Donor leg morbidity after pedicled rectus femoris muscle flap transfer for abdominal wall and pelvic reconstruction. Ann Plast Surg 1994;32(4):377–382

[3] Koshima I, Nanba Y, Tutsui T, Takahashi Y, Itoh S, Kobayashi R. Dynamic reconstruction of large abdominal defects using a free rectus femoris musculocutaneous flap with normal motor function. Ann Plast Surg 2003;50(4):420–424

[4] Alkon JD, Smith A, Losee JE, Illig KA, Green RM, Serletti JM. Management of complex groin wounds: preferred use of the rectus femoris muscle flap. Plast Reconstr Surg 2005;115(3):776–783, discussion 784–785

[5] Sbitany H, Koltz PF, Girotto JA, Vega SJ, Langstein HN. Assessment of donor-site morbidity following rectus femoris harvest for infrainguinal reconstruction. Plast Reconstr Surg 2010;126(3):933–940

38 Gracilis Muscle/Myocutaneous Flap

Sameer A. Patel

Abstract

The gracilis flap has many applications as either a pure muscle flap, a myocutaneous flap, or either a pedicled or free flap. It was first used for reconstruction of the rectal sphincter, and subsequently used as a myocutaneous flap for vaginal reconstruction, which established its utility for pelvic and perineal reconstruction. With advances in microsurgical techniques, the gracilis saw use as a free flap for reconstruction of head and neck defects and for other indications as well. This chapter covers the sequential steps in the procedure involving this flap, from typical indications, to anatomy, to peroperative considerations, to the surgical technique, and, finally, to donor site closure.

Keywords: ischiopubic ramus, pes anserinus, medial tibial condyle, adductor longus muscle, semimembranosus muscle medial circumflex femoral artery, profunda femoris artery, superficial femoral artery

38.1 Introduction

The gracilis flap has many applications as either a pure muscle flap or a myocutaneous flap, and as either a pedicled or a free flap. It was first described for reconstruction of the rectal sphincter in the early 1950s by Pickrell et al.[1] Subsequent application as a myocutaneous flap for vaginal reconstruction established its utility for pelvic and perineal reconstruction.[2] With the advances in microsurgical techniques in the 1970s, Harii et al reported its use as a free flap for reconstruction of head and neck defects.[3] Since that time, many other indications for the gracilis flap have been described.

38.2 Typical Indications

- Dynamic facial reanimation in cases of facial paralysis as a free muscle flap with cross-facial nerve grafting.
- Soft-tissue defects of the upper and lower extremity as a free muscle or myocutaneous flap including coverage of exposed hardware.
- Breast reconstruction as a free transverse upper gracilis (TUG) flap.
- Pelvic and perineal reconstruction including vaginectomy defects, abdominoperineal resection (APR) defects, pelvic exenteration defects, and vulvar defects.

38.3 Anatomy

The gracilis muscle is a long thin muscle which begins broader proximally and tapers distally. Its primary function is to adduct the hip and thigh, but it also contributes to medial rotation and flexion of the hip as well as flexion of the knee. The muscle originates at the **ischiopubic ramus** (symphysis pubis and inferior pubic ramus) and inserts as a structure termed the **pes anserinus** onto the medial tibia just below the **medial tibial condyle**. The pes anserinus represents the confluence of the tendons of the sartorius, gracilis, and

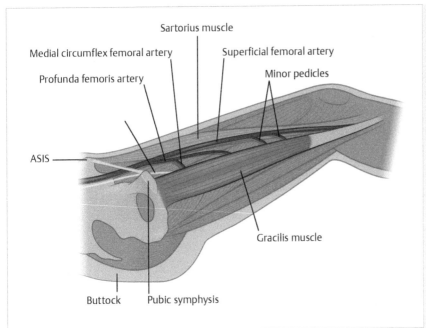

Fig. 38.1 Anatomy of the gracilis muscle.

semitendinosus muscles. The muscle is bordered anteriorly by the **adductor longus muscle** and posteriorly by the **semimembranosus muscle**. It is important not to confuse the sartorius muscle for the gracilis muscle, especially when evaluating the muscles distally in the leg. One will note that the sartorius muscle inserts medially on the knee but as one follows it proximally, it inserts laterally on the anterior superior iliac spine (▶Fig. 38.1).

The gracilis is a Mathes and Nahai type II muscle with a dominant pedicle and additional minor pedicles distally. The dominant pedicle branches from the **medial circumflex femoral artery** (a branch of the **profunda femoris artery**) and travels deep to the adductor longus to enter the proximal third of the muscle approximately 10 cm below the pubic tubercle. Approximately 7 cm of pedicle length can be harvested for free tissue transfer. The artery is accompanied by paired venae comitantes. Generally, there are two to three additional minor pedicles (branches of the profunda femoris artery proximally and **superficial femoral artery** distally) distally which are divided during flap harvest. The venae comitantes travel with the artery.

When harvested as a myocutaneous flap, it is important to note that the majority of the perforators to the skin overlying the gracilis muscle enter in the proximal third of the skin paddle in the region where the pedicle enters the muscle.[3,4,5,6] This may explain why the distal-most portion of a vertically oriented skin paddle is oftentimes unreliable and is why a transverse upper skin paddle is favored if possible. If a vertically oriented skin paddle is necessary, incorporating all available perigracilis fascia and fat may maximize the number of perforators captured and result in improved skin paddle viability.[7]

The muscle is innervated by the anterior branch of the obturator nerve. Prior to entering the muscle belly, the nerve may divide into two separate segments. This is particularly important when used for facial reanimation.

38.4 Variations

There are no additional variations.

38.5 Preoperative Considerations

Careful evaluation of the donor site is critical to ensure that there is no potential compromise of the pedicle or the muscle. If a myocutaneous flap is planned, distribution of the fat on the medial thigh should be evaluated to assess volume, particularly for breast reconstruction. In cases of vaginal or vulvar reconstruction, thickness of the overlying skin should be evaluated. If the skin paddle is deemed to be too bulky, consideration can be given to harvest of muscle only with overlying skin grafting.

38.6 Positioning and Skin Markings

Depending on the indication it is being used for, the gracilis flap may be harvested in either lithotomy or in the "frog-leg" position with the hip externally rotated and the knee flexed. The lithotomy position works well for cases in which the flap is to be used for pelvic or perineal reconstruction. For indications other than perineal or pelvic reconstruction, positioning the patient in the frog-leg position is most ideal. This provides adequate exposure and ease of harvest. This positioning can be used when a myocutaneous flap with a vertical skin paddle or a transverse upper skin paddle is being harvested. Draping and surgical preparation should extend from the pubic symphysis superiorly to the upper portion of the tibia inferiorly.

Preoperative markings should be made with the patient in standing position prior to entering the operating room. Markings are different for muscle-only flaps versus myocutaneous flaps. In thin patients, the gracilis muscle belly may be palpated and marked. However, in patients who are obese, this may not be possible. In this case, the long axis of the muscle can be located by placing a line from the ischium to the medial condyle of the knee. In some cases, the adductor longus muscle, which is a much bulkier muscle, can be palpated by having the patient actively adduct the thigh against resistance. The posterior border of the adductor longus may be marked, and a second line approximately two to three fingerbreadths posterior to this approximates the long axis of the gracilis muscle (▶ Fig. 38.2). The vascular pedicle is usually located about 10 cm inferior to the pubic tubercle.

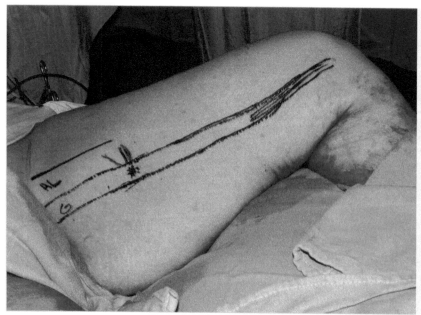

Fig. 38.2 Skin markings for the gracilis muscle flap with the left knee flexed and hip externally rotated. The gracilis muscle is posterior to the adductor longus muscle, which is usually palpable. The vascular pedicle enters the muscle belly about 10 cm inferior to the pubic tubercle.

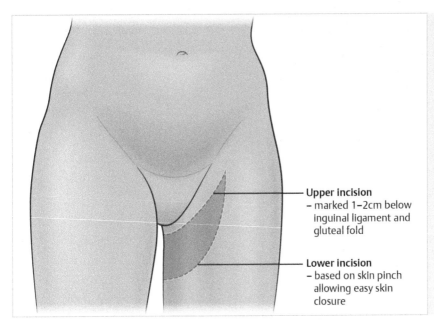

Fig. 38.3 Skin markings for the TUG free flap.

Upper incision
– marked 1–2cm below inguinal ligament and gluteal fold

Lower incision
– based on skin pinch allowing easy skin closure

For myocutaneous flaps, preoperative markings vary depending on the orientation of the skin paddle. For the TUG flap, a transverse skin paddle is marked overlying the upper third of the muscle. The anterior border of the flap is medial to the femoral neurovascular bundle. The posterior border of the flap is the posterior midline of the inferior buttock fold. The superior border is 1 to 2 cm below the inguinal crease and the inferior gluteal fold. The width of the skin paddle should be determined using a pinch test, with the widest part of the skin ellipse just posterior to the posterior edge of the gracilis muscle. A skin paddle up to 11 cm wide and 25 cm long can be harvested (▶ **Fig. 38.3**). If a longitudinal skin paddle is desired, the skin paddle should be designed to overlie the belly of the gracilis muscle. Again, in this case, it is important to incorporate the proximal third of the skin as well as the perimuscle fascia and fat.

38.7 Operative Technique

Flap harvest begins with the appropriate positioning as described. When used as a muscle flap without a skin paddle, either as a pedicled flap or a free flap, an incision is made directly overlying the muscle. Dissection is carried down to the level of the muscle fascia and the fascia is incised. The fascia is elevated off the underlying muscle anteriorly to identify the border between the gracilis and the adductor longus muscle. The fascia is then elevated posteriorly to identify the posterior border of the muscle. At this point, a plane is created between the adductor longus muscle and the gracilis muscle (▶ **Fig. 38.4a**). Distally, small segmental branches will be identified traveling to the muscle. The dominant pedicle will be seen entering the proximal third of the muscle traveling in the loose areolar plane between the adductor and the gracilis. The muscle tendon may then be divided distally and the muscle elevated off the deep surface. In cases where the muscle is to be pedicled for perineal reconstruction, the proximal muscle may be kept intact to minimize the possibility of twisting the muscle. If it is to be used as a free flap, the proximal muscle can be divided from its origin once the recipient site is prepared (▶ **Fig. 38.4b**).

If a myocutaneous flap is required, flap harvest begins by careful attention to the skin markings. For the TUG flap, a transverse skin paddle is marked overlying the upper third of the muscle. The superior incision should be 1 to 2 cm

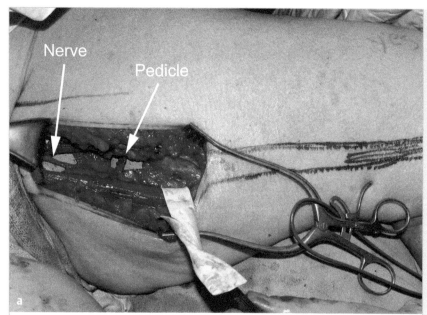

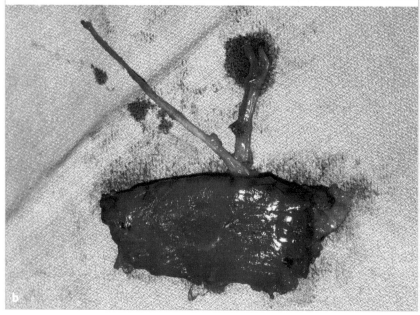

Fig. 38.4 (a) Dissection of the gracilis muscle. The pedicle is found 10 cm below the pubic tubercle and the nerve enters the muscle belly about 1 cm superior to the pedicle. (b) Dissected gracilis muscle free flap with vascular pedicle and nerve to be used for facial reanimation. Note that entire width of the muscle was not harvested.

below the inguinal ligament and extend posteriorly. The skin paddle should be centered over the muscle. A "pinch test" is performed to determine where the lower border of the skin paddle should be, assuring that closure will be feasible without undue tension. Elevation of the flap begins anteriorly. The plane of dissection is just deep to Scarpa's fascia initially. The great saphenous vein will be encountered and is preserved if possible during the anterior dissection. Medial to the saphenous vein, the plane of dissection deepens to include the deep fascia covering the adductor longus. Once the posterior border of the adductor longus is identified, the fascia is incised and the pedicle is identified in the same loose areolar plane as described above. The muscle can then be divided distal to the pedicle, and posterior dissection can then be performed. Again the skin and subcutaneous tissue is elevated until the posterior border of the gracilis is identified. The majority of the fat included with this flap is obtained from the portion of the skin paddle posterior to the gracilis muscle. The TUG flap can then be transferred as a free flap for reconstruction, most often for breast reconstruction.

If a longitudinal skin paddle is desired, the skin paddle should be designed to overlie the belly of the gracilis muscle. Again, in this case, it is important to incorporate the proximal third of the skin as well as the perimuscle fascia and fat (▶Fig. 38.5). This will allow for increased reliability of the middle and distal portions of the skin paddle. The anterior incision is made and carried down to the fascia. The fascia overlying the adductor longus is then incised and incorporated with the flap harvest. The anterior border of the gracilis is then identified as described for a muscle-only flap. Posteriorly, fascia is again included overlying the semimembranosus muscle until the posterior border of the gracilis is identified. The gracilis can then be divided distally and elevated off of the deep surface. It will be necessary to divide the minor pedicles coming from the superficial femoral and profunda femoris arteries.

38.8 Donor Site Closure

The donor site should be closed over a closed suction drain. In those cases where a skin paddle is harvested, a layered closure should be performed to minimize

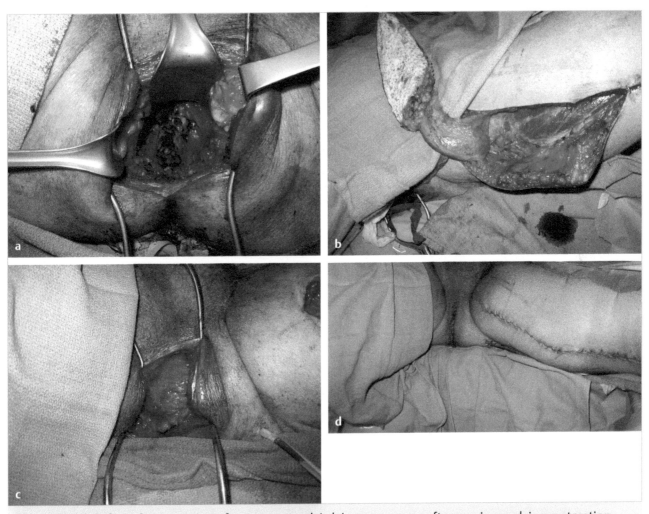

Fig. 38.5 (a) Defect after resection of a recurrent pelvic leiomyosarcoma after previous pelvic exenteration and radiation therapy. Note the large cavity in the perineum. **(b)** Gracilis flap elevated with overlying skin paddle. The skin paddle was deepithelialized. **(c)** The deepithelialized skin paddle and muscle is tunneled into the defect to obliterate the large dead space. **(d)** Final closure and donor site.

(Continued)

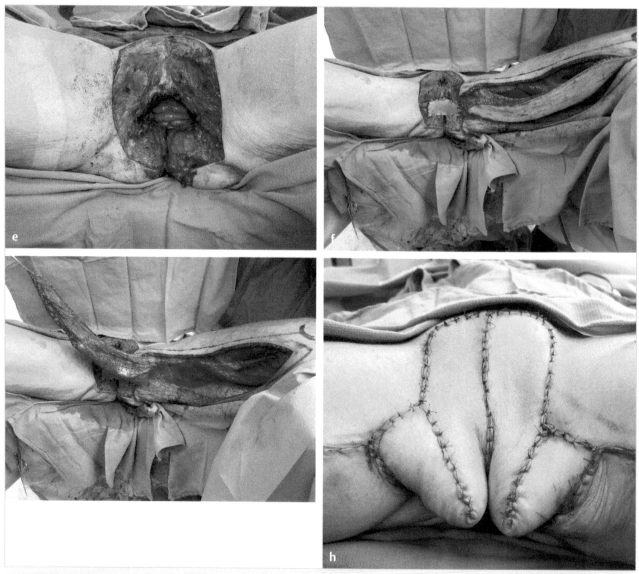

Fig. 38.5 (*Continued*) (**e**) Large perineal and pelvic defect extending into the peritoneal cavity after pelvic exenteration. (**f**) Acellular dermal matrix used to seal off abdominal contents. Note harvest of the gracilis myocutaneous flap with longitudinal skin paddle. (**g**) Flap elevated with pedicle isolate. Note the sartorius and adductor longus muscles. (**h**) Flaps rotated into the defect to provide coverage. (**e-h** courtesy of Eric I-Yun Chang.)

the likelihood of dehiscence, including the superficial fascial layer, deep dermal layer, and subcuticular layer.

38.9 Pearls and Pitfalls

- Preoperative marking is critical with the patient in standing position, particularly in obese patients in whom a skin paddle is planned.
- For the TUG flap, the saphenous vein is preserved and only a modest amount of fat is included with the skin paddle anterior to the gracilis muscle belly, with the larger amount of fat being obtained from posterior to the gracilis muscle belly.

- For a longitudinally oriented skin paddle, harvest skin over the proximal third of the muscle and include the perigracilis fat and fascia. If the proximal skin is not necessary, it may be deepithelialized and buried under the native skin bridge.

References

[1] Pickrell K, Georgiade N, Maguire C, Crawford H. Correction of rectal incontinence; transplantation of the gracilis muscle to construct a rectal sphincter. Am J Surg 1955;90(5):721–726

[2] McCraw JB, Massey FM, Shanklin KD, Horton CE. Vaginal reconstruction with gracilis myocutaneous flaps. Plast Reconstr Surg 1976;58(2):176–183

[3] Harii K, Ohmori K, Sekiguchi J. The free musculocutaneous flap. Plast Reconstr Surg 1976;57(3):294–303

[4] Yousif NJ, Matloub HS, Kolachalam R, Grunert BK, Sanger JR. The transverse gracilis musculocutaneous flap. Ann Plast Surg 1992;29(6):482–490

[5] Juricic M, Vaysse P, Guitard J, Moscovici J, Becue J, Juskiewenski S. Anatomic basis for use of a gracilis muscle flap. Surg Radiol Anat 1993;15(3):163–168

[6] Giordano PA, Abbes M, Pequignot JP. Gracilis blood supply: anatomical and clinical re-evaluation. Br J Plast Surg 1990;43(3):266–272

[7] Whetzel TP, Lechtman AN. The gracilis myofasciocutaneous flap: vascular anatomy and clinical application. Plast Reconstr Surg 1997;99(6):1642–1652, discussion 1653–1655

39 Transverse Upper Gracilis Flap

Anson Nguyen, Stacy Wong, and Michel Saint-Cyr

Abstract

The gracilis myocutaneous flap has been utilized to reconstruct a variety of defects. It has also been used for breast reconstruction, reconstruction of the pelvic/genitoperineal region as a pedicled flap, and for reconstruction of the head and neck, breast, and upper and lower extremities as a free flap. It has been adapted by many surgeons into a transverse design to avoid necrosis of the distal skin paddle. The transversely oriented flap, named the transverse upper gracilis flap, is mainly used as a free flap for autologous reconstruction of small-to-medium volume breasts. It is best suited in cases where the abdomen is contraindicated as a donor site, or for those who wish to avoid abdominal, buttock, or back scars. The transverse upper gracilis flap is limited by the small volume of harvest and donor site complications, including contracture of the thigh scar and subsequent labial spreading. Modifications to improve this flap involve posteriorly extended harvest of the flap and various design alterations based on improved knowledge of vascular anatomy. This chapter directs the reader to the major concerns in the use of the transverse upper gracilis flap, from typical indications, to anatomy, to preoperative considerations, to surgical technique. Four variations come in for special mention, and the discussion concludes with information on donor site closure.

Keywords: flap, myocutaneous, gracilis, transverse, breast reconstruction

39.1 Introduction

Since its introduction in 1975, the gracilis myocutaneous flap has been utilized for the reconstruction of a variety of defects. It was later applied to breast reconstruction in 1992 using a vertical skin paddle.[1] The gracilis myocutaneous flap has been used for reconstruction of the pelvic/genitoperineal region as a pedicled flap and for reconstruction of the head and neck, breast, and upper and lower extremities as a free flap. It has been adapted by many surgeons into a transverse design to avoid necrosis of the distal skin paddle. The transversely oriented flap, named the transverse upper gracilis (TUG) flap, is mainly used as a free flap for autologous reconstruction of small-to-medium volume breasts. It is best suited in cases where the abdomen is contraindicated as a donor site, or for those who wish to avoid abdominal, buttock, or back scars. Limitations of the TUG flap are related to small volume of harvest and donor site complications, including contracture of the thigh scar and subsequent labial spreading. Modifications to improve this flap involve posteriorly extended harvest of the flap and various design alterations based on improved knowledge of vascular anatomy.

39.2 Typical Indications

- Primary use:
  - Autologous breast reconstruction of small-to-medium volume breasts.

- Other uses:
  - Head and neck reconstruction.
  - Upper and lower extremity reconstruction.
  - Pelvic/genitoperineal reconstruction.

39.3 Anatomy

The TUG flap consists of the gracilis muscle and an overlying skin paddle from the upper medial thigh. The gracilis is a thin, strap-like adductor of the leg, which originates from the ischiopubic ramus and inserts onto the medial tibia at the pes anserinus. It is the most superficial of the medial thigh muscles and is located posteromedial to the adductor longus (▶ **Fig. 39.1**).

The proximal, dominant pedicle of the TUG flap arises from the **medial circumflex femoral artery** or directly off the **profunda femoris** and is accompanied by two venae comitantes of similar size (▶ **Fig. 39.2**). It enters the gracilis muscle approximately 10 ± 2 cm below the pubic tubercle, measures 1 to 2 mm

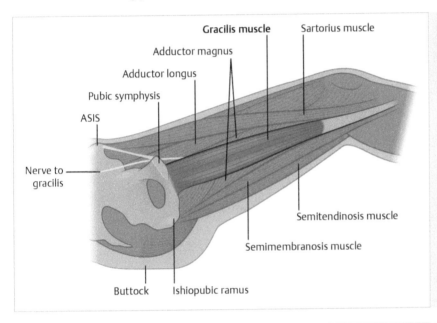

Fig. 39.1 Medial thigh muscular anatomy showing the location of the gracilis muscle. ASIS, anterior superior iliac spine.

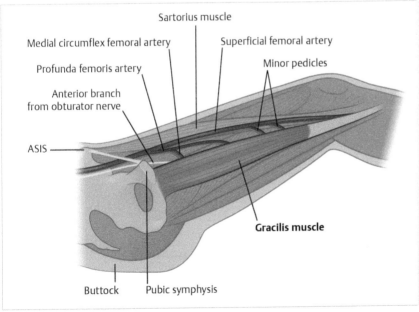

Fig. 39.2 Vascular anatomy of the gracilis muscle.

in diameter, and is typically found under the **adductor longus muscle**. A length of 6 to 8 cm can typically be obtained. A variation is a double main pedicle. The distal vascular pedicle(s) of the gracilis muscle arise from the **superficial femoral vessels**. Choke vessels, which are connections between vascular territories without an intervening capillary bed, exist between the main pedicle and surrounding cutaneous vasculature, particularly the superficial femoral artery. The vascularity extends more posteriorly than anteriorly, as well as vertically in the region overlying the gracilis muscle.[1]

Prior to entering the muscle, the main pedicle is divided into three to six branches, which continue to the cutaneous tissues through the muscle as musculocutaneous branches or through the intermuscular septum between the adductor longus and gracilis as septocutaneous branches. The musculocutaneous perforators are more numerous, distributed more proximally, and of smaller caliber than the septocutaneous perforators.[2] These perforators have a tendency to orient in a transverse fashion, which led to the transverse design of the TUG flap. Linking vessels connect adjacent perforasomes, and cognizance of these vessels in modified flap designs can enhance distal tip survival.[3]

Innervation of the TUG flap consists of the **anterior branch from the obturator nerve** to gracilis carrying motor cutaneous sensory fibers. This nerve is deep to the vessels and typically divided unless the gracilis is used as a functional muscle transplant. During dissection, the posterior branch of the **greater saphenous vein** is also ligated and divided, whereas the anterior branch of the saphenous vein should be spared. A skin paddle of 12 × 25 cm may be obtained, especially with extension of the paddle posteriorly, and various modifications have been described to reliably increase the volume of the harvest.[3]

39.4 Variations

- Bilateral stacked TUG flaps for unilateral breast reconstruction.[4]
- Combined TUG and profunda artery perforator flap.
- Perforator flap, with sparing of a functional gracilis muscle.[2]
- Modifications in design:
  - Horizontal extension TUG: extension of the skin paddle posteriorly to a point midway between the medial midaxial line and the posterior thigh midline.
  - Vertical extension TUG, including the trilobed TUG.[4]
  - Diagonal upper gracilis (DUG) flap to improve donor site morbidity.
  - Coning of the TUG flap and use of cartilage graft for nipple reconstruction.

39.5 Preoperative Considerations

While abdominally based free flaps remain the accepted standard for most breast reconstruction patients, the TUG flap has emerged as popular alternative especially in patients with a slender body habitus with insufficient abdominal tissue. It should still be noted that TUG flaps have less volume than abdominal flaps and should be limited to small-to-moderate-sized breast reconstruction unless incorporated as a secondary flap or two TUG flaps are stacked for unilateral breast reconstruction.

Additionally, in patients with less vertical laxity of the thigh, consideration should be given to performing the gracilis myocutaneous flap with a vertical skin paddle (VUG) as this may potentially avert some of the donor site complications of a transverse skin paddle.

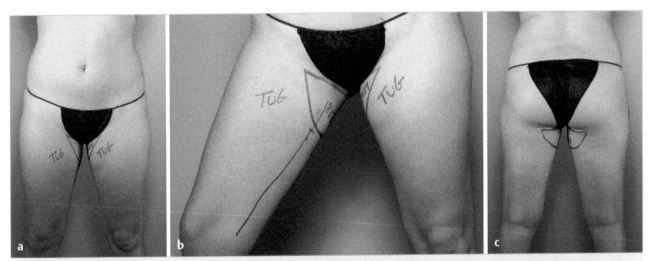

Fig. 39.3 (a-c) Preoperative markings. Skin paddle is typically marked as an ellipse or horizontal crescent. The anterior margin should not extend to the inguinal crease. Posteriorly, the markings may extend to the gluteal crease. Pinch test is useful to determine the width of the flap with adequate laxity for direct closure.

39.6 Positioning and Skin Markings

For most applications of the TUG flap, lithotomy or supine positioning with lower extremities frog-legged can be used for harvest. The skin paddle is usually marked in a horizontal crescent or ellipse. The superior marking for the TUG flap typically resides within the groin crease but should ideally be no closer than 4 cm to the midline (introitus). A pinch test can be used to assess width of the flap to determine the inferior marking. Usually the flap is no wider than 9 to 10 cm in order to allow for direct closure. Anteriorly, the flap should not cross the inguinal crease as this can potentially disrupt the lymphatic system and cause iatrogenic lower extremity lymphedema. Posteriorly, the flap may extend into the gluteal crease. Other variations of the gracilis myocutaneous flap include skin paddles such as a lazy S shape, vertical upper gracilis, and fleur-de-lis pattern (▶ **Fig. 39.3**).

39.7 Operative Technique

Perforators of the medial circumflex artery arise most commonly 10 cm distal to the pubic tubercle. A Doppler is beneficial in identifying these perforators and including them when planning the skin paddle. Dissection should be avoided over the femoral triangle for reasons previously discussed.

Initial incision is made along the superior border and dissection is carried down to the muscle. This is done in order to determine exact flap vertical height for safe donor site closure as well as to quickly identify the septum between the adductor longus and gracilis. The fascia overlying the adductor longus is elevated from anterior to posterior and this allows increased blood supply into the TUG flap by preserving all fascial perforators. This maneuver also exposed the pedicle to the flap, allowing for easy adjustment of the skin paddle to center it appropriately. Pinch test is once again used to confirm how wide the flap can be taken. The inferior incision is then made and carried down through muscular fascia. Once the gracilis is encountered, dissection may proceed superficial to

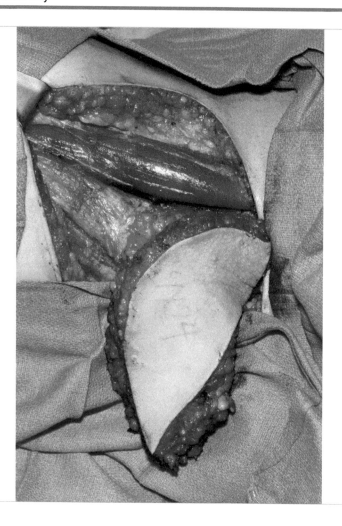

Fig. 39.4 Operative view of elevated TUG flap. Note that this flap is raised from superior to inferior and pinch test is performed to ensure adequate laxity for direct closure. This flap can be taken as a perforator flap or with muscle for a myocutaneous flap.

muscle should a perforator flap be attempted or, more commonly, the muscle may be dissected out as a myocutaneous flap.

Once ensured that the perforators are within the muscle to be harvested, the muscle can be segmentally harvested and the flap can then be raised distal to proximal. Anterior dissection of the flap is harvested only in the subcutaneous plane until posterior to the femoral triangle after which the plane of dissection is carried deeper down to the adductor fascia. Posteriorly, dissection is carried down to the muscular fascia of the semimembranosus muscle which may be included with the flap. Once the flap is harvested to the medial circumflex femoral pedicle, it is then skeletonized all the way to the profunda femoris (▶ Fig. 39.4).

39.8 Donor Site Closure

Closure of the donor site is similar to that of a medial thigh lift (▶ Fig. 39.5). Undermining should be relatively limited so as to avoid injury to lymphatics. The superficial fascia of the lower edge of the wound is typically secured to Colles' fascia superiorly in order to help prevent significant scar migration and traction on the labia.

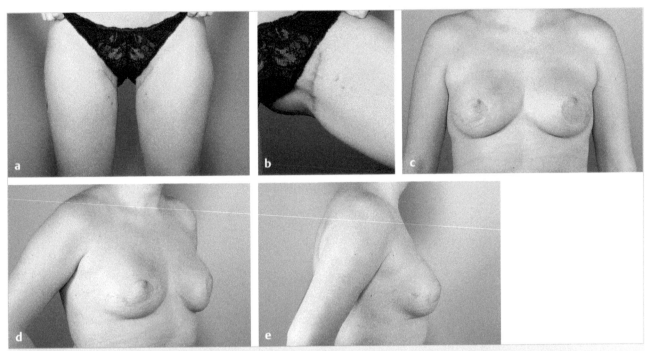

Fig. 39.5 (a,b) Postoperative donor site. The donor site scar is easily concealed in the groin crease. Intraoperatively, the superficial fascia of the lower edge of the wound is typically secured to Colles' fascia superiorly to prevent scar migration and widening. (c-e) Postoperative reconstructed breasts. The TUG flap is an excellent option for the slender patients with little abdominal tissue and can be used for reconstruction of small-to-medium-sized breasts.

39.9 Pearls and Pitfalls

- The flap may be coned to increase projection or included with another flap to increase volume.
- Care should be taken in planning and dissecting the flap to avoid risk of lymphedema and labial spreading.
- The distal third of the thigh should not be included in the flap as blood supply becomes more tenuous.

References

[1] Yousif NJ, Matloub HS, Kolachalam R, Grunert BK, Sanger JR. The transverse gracilis musculocutaneous flap. Ann Plast Surg 1992;29(6):482–490

[2] Park JE, Alkureishi LW, Song DH. TUGs into VUGs and friendly BUGs: transforming the gracilis territory into the best secondary breast reconstructive option. Plast Reconstr Surg 2015;136(3):447–454

[3] Peek A, Müller M, Ackermann G, Exner K, Baumeister S. The free gracilis perforator flap: anatomical study and clinical refinements of a new perforator flap. Plast Reconstr Surg 2009;123(2):578–588

[4] Saint-Cyr M, Wong C, Oni G, et al. Modifications to extend the transverse upper gracilis flap in breast reconstruction: clinical series and results. Plast Reconstr Surg 2012;129(1):24e–36e

40 Profunda Artery Perforator Flap

Mark Schaverien

Abstract

The profunda artery perforator is utilized predominantly as a free flap for reconstruction of the breast, head, and neck and is a secondary option for free flap reconstruction of the breast in women with insufficient abdominal tissues. In selected patients, there is an abundance of soft and pliable medial and posterior thigh adipose tissue that is ideal for breast reconstruction and can be coned to create an aesthetically pleasing breast mound. The profunda artery perforator flap has the advantages over the transverse upper gracilis myocutaneous flap of being able to recruit the more abundant soft-tissue volume lateral to midline of the posterior thigh region, resulting in a more posterior scar location, while avoiding dissection in the femoral triangle and therefore any risk of causing lower extremity lymphedema. Other advantages over the transverse upper gracilis flap include a longer pedicle and reduced donor site morbidity by preservation of the gracilis muscle. The main disadvantage is the anatomical variation in the vascular pedicle and, therefore, potential variability in the location of the skin paddle in relation to the groin and gluteal creases. This chapter details all the issues involved in reconstructive surgery involving the profunda artery perforator flap, from typical indications, to anatomy, to preoperative considerations, to the operative technique. Two variations are discussed, and advice is given on donor site closure.

Keywords: adductor magnus muscle, profunda femoris artery, semimembranosus muscle, posterior femoral cutaneous nerve

40.1 Introduction

The profunda artery perforator (PAP) flap, first described in 2001 by Angrigiani et al, is utilized predominantly as a free flap for reconstruction of the breast and head and neck.[1] It is a secondary option for free flap reconstruction of the breast in women with insufficient abdominal tissues.[2] In selected patients there is an abundance of soft and pliable medial and posterior thigh adipose tissue that is ideal for breast reconstruction and which can be coned to create an aesthetically pleasing breast mound. The flap is harvested with a transverse skin paddle that leaves a scar in the region of the medial thigh groin crease and posterior gluteal crease that can be well-hidden by clothing. It has the advantages over the transverse upper gracilis (TUG) myocutaneous flap of being able to recruit the more abundant soft-tissue volume lateral to midline of the posterior thigh region, resulting in a more posterior scar location and avoiding dissection in the femoral triangle and therefore any risk of causing lymphedema. Other advantages over the TUG flap include a longer pedicle and reduced donor site morbidity by preservation of the gracilis muscle. The main disadvantage is anatomical variation in the vascular pedicle and, therefore, potential variability in the location of the skin paddle in relation to the groin and gluteal creases. The PAP flap may be a primary option in women with significant soft-tissue excess of the medial and posterior thigh, or in women with insufficient abdominal soft-tissue volume for bilateral breast reconstruction. The flap weight is usually similar to that of the mastectomy, typically 300 to 400 g (range: 150–900 g).

For head and neck reconstruction, the flap is typically harvested with a vertically oriented skin paddle that provides thinner soft-tissue thickness when compared with the anterolateral thigh (ALT) flap, with greater pliability that is ideal for partial glossectomy reconstruction.[3] The vertical skin paddle potentially enables all of the PAPs to be evaluated and the largest to be selected. Where muscle is required, a chimeric flap with a portion of adductor magnus muscle can be designed. The vertical free flap has also been described for lower extremity reconstruction as an alternative to the ALT flap.[4]

The flap can also be used for reconstruction of the perineal region as a pedicled flap. The flap can be designed as either a V–Y or propeller flap.

40.2 Typical Indications

- Breast reconstruction (free flap).
- Partial glossectomy reconstruction (free flap).
- Perineal reconstruction (pedicled flap).

40.3 Anatomy

The most common perforator location is the medial posterior thigh posterior to the **gracilis muscle** in the region of the **adductor magnus muscle** (▶Fig. 40.1). This is most commonly located 5 cm caudal to the gluteal fold and approximately 4 cm posterior to the midline of the medial thigh, with a sizeable perforator found in 85% of thighs. The next most common perforator location is lateral to the midline arising in the vicinity of the biceps femoris and vastus lateralis muscles.[5] At least two perforators arise from the **profunda femoris artery** (range: 2–5), and, in approximately 25% of cases, the perforators arise from a common trunk off the profunda. Perforators predominantly take a septocutaneous course arising between the **adductor magnus** and **semimembranosus muscles**, but sometimes take a short intramuscular course through the

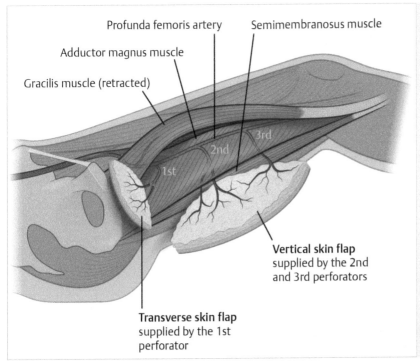

Profunda femoris artery   Semimembranosus muscle

Adductor magnus muscle

Gracilis muscle (retracted)

3rd

2nd

1st

Vertical skin flap
supplied by the 2nd and 3rd perforators

Transverse skin flap
supplied by the 1st perforator

Fig. 40.1 Anatomy of the profunda artery perforator (PAP) flap. The flap can be harvested with either a proximal transverse skin paddle for use in breast reconstruction or a vertical skin paddle for head and neck reconstruction. The most proximal PAP arises in the region of the adductor magnus muscle posterior to the gracilis muscle, approximately 4 cm posterior to the midline of the medial thigh and 5 cm inferior to the gluteal fold. The majority of perforators have a septocutaneous course.

adductor magnus muscle. The average artery diameter at the profunda femoris artery is 2.2 mm and the mean vein diameter of 2.8 mm, with a pedicle length of approximately 10 cm (range: 7–13 cm). Sensory innervation of the flap is via a branch of **posterior femoral cutaneous nerve**.

40.4 Variations

- Skin paddle can be designed as a vertical, horizontal, or fleur-de-lis pattern.
- Flap can be harvested as a myocutaneous flap incorporating a portion of the adductor magnus muscle.

40.5 Preoperative Considerations

Preoperative imaging with CT or MR angiography can be performed for breast reconstruction using a transverse skin paddle to aid in design of the skin paddle (▶ Fig. 40.2). A hand-held Doppler probe is used to identify the location of the profunda perforators preoperatively with the patient positioned as for surgery. The skin paddle is then designed based on the perforator locations. The medial perforator, entering posterior to the gracilis muscle, is the most common and is typically chosen to facilitate harvest in the supine position and reduce operation duration. The internal mammary vessels or their perforators are used as recipients due to the relatively short pedicle length.

When the flap is being harvested for head and neck defect reconstruction, caution should be exercised in patients with high BMI where the flap may be excessively thick and this should be evaluated preoperatively.

40.6 Positioning and Skin Markings

For breast reconstruction, the transverse skin paddle may be harvested with the patient prone, particularly for bilateral breast reconstruction; however, this potentially results in a long ischemic time. Ipsilateral flap harvest is preferred. More commonly, the patient is positioned supine with the leg either frog-legged

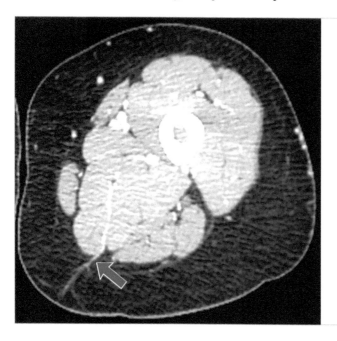

Fig. 40.2 Preoperative imaging using CT or MR angiography is utilized for breast reconstruction to identify the position of the most proximal profunda perforator. If the perforator is not located within a proximal flap design, then either a TUG flap can be planned or the skin island designed in a more caudal location.

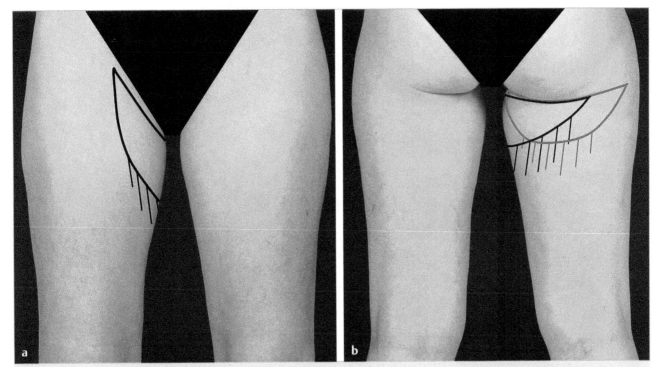

Fig. 40.3 Skin markings for the PAP flap. The black marking illustrates the skin paddle for the flap harvested in the supine frog-legged or lithotomy position with posterior to anterior harvest technique allowing conversion to a TUG flap if the PAPs are found to be unsuitable, medially marked 1 to 2 cm from the groin crease, and posteriorly marked in the gluteal crease, then once the PAP is confirmed to be adequate the medial aspect can be revised to begin around the gracilis muscle. The blue marking illustrates the skin paddle design for flap harvested in the prone position with the superior flap border marked in the gluteal crease taking care not to go beyond the lateral aspect of the gluteal fold. The superior marking can be moved onto the lower part of the buttock to increase the flap volume. The lower incision is made approximately 7 cm below this. The subcutaneous fat under the Scarpa's fascia is harvested with the flap caudal to the inferior flap border. Injury to the posterior femoral cutaneous nerve located in the midline of the posterior thigh must be avoided to prevent paresthesia of the posterior thigh.

or placed in the lithotomy position. The flap can then either be harvested from anterior to posterior or posterior to anterior. The advantage of the posterior-to-anterior approach is that the profunda perforators can be explored, and if found to be unsuitable, then a TUG flap can be harvested instead. The vertical skin paddle is harvested with the leg in a supine frog-legged position.

The superior marking is at the gluteal fold. The inferior marking is marked depending on pinch and individual patient factors, but is typically marked approximately 7 cm below the superior marking. The superior border of the flap may be sited above the gluteal fold to recruit more tissue depending on the perforator location. The flap is designed as an ellipse of approximately 27 cm in width (▶ Fig. 40.3).

40.7 Operative Technique

Refer to Video 40.1 for an example of the operative technique for the profunda artery perforator flap. When in the preferred supine position, the patient's legs are placed in a frog-leg position. Incisions are made along the flap markings down to the subcutaneous fat, and continuing through the Scarpa's fascia. Caudally, as much fat as possible under the Scarpa's fascia is then included with the flap, but at the cephalad aspect the incision is straight down through the muscle fascia. The flap is then raised from posterior to anterior until the profunda artery perforator(s) are found posterior to the gracilis muscle (►Fig. 40.4a). If the perforator is appreciated to be adequate, then a PAP flap is raised, but if not,

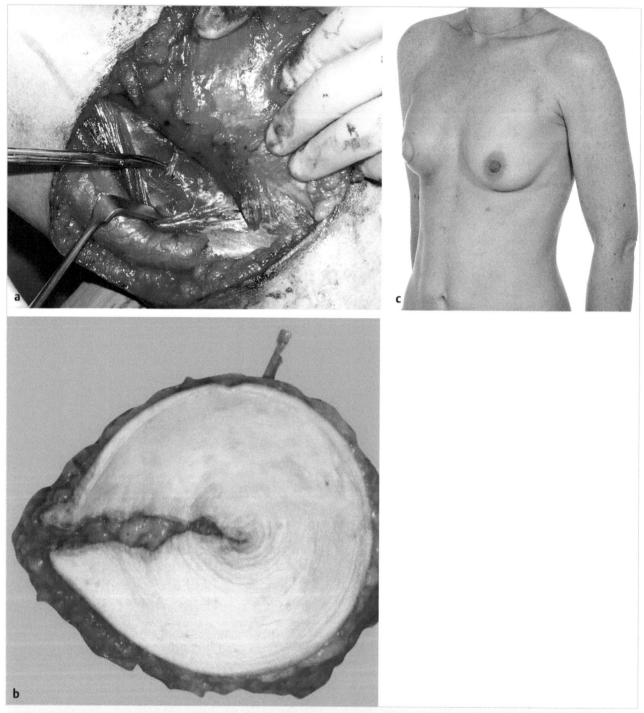

Fig. 40.4 **(a)** In the supine frog-leg position the transverse skin paddle is raised from posterior to anterior until the medial profunda perforator arising posterior to the gracilis muscle in the region of the adductor magnus muscle is identified. If it is of suitable caliber, then a PAP flap is raised, otherwise flap harvest proceeds as for a TUG flap. **(b)** For immediate breast reconstruction, the flap can be coned. Immediate nipple reconstruction can be performed in the setting of skin-sparing mastectomy at the apex of the cone. **(c)** Postoperative photograph at 6 weeks following right skin-sparing mastectomy and immediate breast reconstruction.

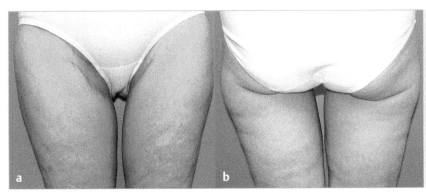

Fig. 40.5 (a,b) Typical scar location following PAP flap harvest with a transverse skin paddle in the supine position. Dissection in the femoral triangle is avoided to prevent lymphedema in the donor limb.

then the flap is harvested as a standard TUG flap. Once the flap is raised, then for immediate breast reconstruction, it can be coned to form a breast mound (▶Fig. 40.4b), and a nipple reconstruction may also be performed at the apex of the cone (▶Fig. 40.4c).

A vertically designed skin paddle is harvested from anterior to posterior as there is no specific bailout flap, and all perforators are appraised before deciding which to include in the flap. After identifying the perforator, standard perforator dissection proceeds toward the profunda femoris artery with ligation of side branches to the adductor magnus muscle until the desired pedicle length and vessel diameter is achieved. If the perforator takes an intramuscular course, then the muscle is spread without division of the fibers. The branches to the adductor magnus muscle can be used to harvest a portion of muscle with the flap if required.

40.8 Donor Site Closure

It is important to directly approximate the Scarpa's fascia to reduce the risk of donor site dehiscence and scar widening. The remainder of the wound is closed in layers, followed by a running subcuticular absorbable suture to close the skin (▶Fig. 40.5). Dressings are difficult to apply and adhere in this area and the incision is best dressed with surgical glue or an adhesive skin closure system.

40.9 Pearls and Pitfalls

- The short pedicle length requires the use of the internal mammary vessels in breast reconstruction for medial positioning of the flap.
- When used for breast reconstruction, the flap is best indicated in immediate reconstruction as it can be coned to give an aesthetically pleasing breast mound. It is also possible in the setting of immediate reconstruction to perform a nipple reconstruction where the cone is formed.
- When a transverse skin paddle is used, the scar may need to be located caudally from the groin crease in a more conspicuous position depending on the position of the proximal perforator. This can be revised in a secondary procedure to raise the scar so that it is camouflaged in the medial groin crease and gluteal fold.
- In transverse flap designs injury to the posterior cutaneous nerve of the thigh should be avoided. This can lead to significant donor site morbidity from paresthesia of the posterior thigh.

References

[1] Angrigiani C, Grilli D, Thorne CH. The adductor flap: a new method for transferring posterior and medial thigh skin. Plast Reconstr Surg 2001;107(7):1725–1731

[2] Allen RJ, Haddock NT, Ahn CY, Sadeghi A. Breast reconstruction with the profunda artery perforator flap. Plast Reconstr Surg 2012;129(1):16e–23e

[3] Scaglioni MF, Kuo YR, Yang JC, Chen YC. The posteromedial thigh flap for head and neck reconstruction: anatomical basis, surgical technique, and clinical applications. Plast Reconstr Surg 2015;136(2):363–375

[4] Mayo JL, Canizares O, Torabi R, Allen RJ Sr, St Hilaire H. Expanding the applications of the profunda artery perforator flap. Plast Reconstr Surg 2016;137(2):663–669

[5] Haddock NT, Greaney P, Otterburn D, Levine S, Allen RJ. Predicting perforator location on preoperative imaging for the profunda artery perforator flap. Microsurgery 2012;32(7):507–511

41 Posterior Thigh Flap

Jeffrey H. Kozlow

Abstract

The posterior thigh flap is a fasciocutaneous flap based on the descending branch of the inferior gluteal artery. It is frequently called a gluteal thigh flap; however, a gluteal thigh flap is generally a flap that extends proximally to the inferior gluteal vessels. The posterior thigh flap is a workhorse flap for reconstruction in the region of the ischial tuberosity or perineum. Common usage in the perineum includes vulvar, perianal, or posterior vaginal reconstructions. The harvest is simple and can be done in a variety of positions, which makes the flap of great utility to the reconstructive surgeon. It can also contain the posterior cutaneous nerves of the thigh allowing for a sensate flap. Although technically possible, it has rarely been used as a free flap. In this chapter, the author guides the surgeon through every step of the procedure, beginning with typical indications, then a discussion of the relevant anatomy, followed by preoperative considerations, a discussion of the operative technique, and concluding with donor site closure. Four variations are also cited.

Keywords: descending branch of the inferior gluteal artery, gluteus maximus muscle, biceps femoris muscle, semitendinosus muscle, posterior femoral cutaneous nerve of the thigh

41.1 Introduction

The posterior thigh flap is a fasciocutaneous flap based on the **descending branch of the inferior gluteal artery**. It is frequently also called a gluteal thigh flap; however, a gluteal thigh flap is generally a flap that is extended proximally to the inferior gluteal vessels. Initially popularized by Hurwitz in 1980, it is a common workhorse flap for reconstruction in the region of the ischial tuberosity or perineum.[1] Common usage in the perineum includes vulvar, perianal, or posterior vaginal reconstructions.[2] The harvest is simple and can be done in a variety of positions making the flap of great utility to the reconstructive surgeon. It can also contain the posterior cutaneous nerves of the thigh allowing for a sensate flap. Although technically possible, it has rarely been used as a free flap.

41.2 Typical Indications

- Ischial pressure sore reconstruction.
- Perineum reconstruction.
- Vulvar reconstruction.
- Posterior or lateral vaginal wall reconstruction.
- Sacral reconstruction.
- Lateral thigh/hip reconstruction.

41.3 Anatomy

The posterior thigh flap is an axially designed, fasciocutaneous flap based on the descending branch of the inferior gluteal artery. The inferior gluteal artery

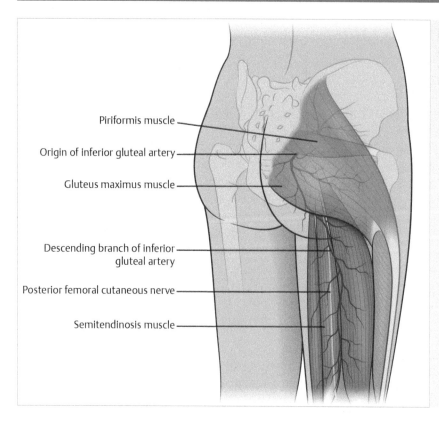

Piriformis muscle

Origin of inferior gluteal artery

Gluteus maximus muscle

Descending branch of inferior gluteal artery

Posterior femoral cutaneous nerve

Semitendinosis muscle

Fig. 41.1 Vascular anatomy of inferior gluteal artery and descending branch in relation to regional muscles.

leaves the deep muscular pelvis below the piriformis muscle and then runs below the **gluteus maximus muscle**. The descending branch typically originates from the inferior gluteal artery and also runs deep to the gluteus maximus. It then exits into the posterior thigh at the midpoint of the inferior gluteal border. It courses subfascially down the middle of the posterior thigh to the knee. The descending branch vessels stay above and between the **biceps femoris and semitendinosus muscles**. Multiple cutaneous perforators are found along the course of the vessel, which supply the overlying skin and subcutaneous tissue.

Multiple flap designs have been described including V–Y advancement flaps, broad-based transposition flaps, and island-based flaps. Perforator-based propeller flaps can also be performed for local defects near the descending branch of the inferior gluteal artery.

The **posterior femoral cutaneous nerve of the thigh** is within the same connective tissue sheath as the main vasculature approximately 72% of the time making a sensate flap easy (▶ **Fig. 41.1**).[2]

41.4 Variations

- Less than 10% of the time, the descending branch arises from the **profunda femoris, medial circumflex femoral, or lateral circumflex femoral** (less critical for flap harvest).
- An additional superficial plexus of vessels to the posterior thigh also exists from the gluteal artery perforators, although this is not typically used for flap harvest.
- Can include portion of gluteus maximus as well (care needed in ambulatory patients).
- Additional pedicle length can be obtained by following the pedicle further proximal with inclusion of the **inferior gluteal artery** (gluteal thigh flap).[3]

41.5 Preoperative Considerations

Preoperative considerations are similar to other reconstructive procedures. Patient risk factors for delayed wound healing, such as tobacco use and poorly controlled diabetes mellitus, should be optimized when possible. Obesity increases the thickness of the flap and makes rotation of the flap more difficult without skeletonization of the pedicle. Given the utilization of this flap in ischial pressure sore reconstruction, many patients will have associated paraplegia or tetraplegia. It is critical that wheelchair mapping be performed before allowing for increased amounts of sitting or direct pressure on the flap reconstruction. Previous flaps harvested from the area should be noted preoperatively. Specifically, patients who have previously undergone a large gluteus maximus rotation flap or an inferior gluteal artery perforator flap may have had transection of the descending branch during the previous flap harvest.

41.6 Positioning and Skin Markings

Marking for the flap includes first identifying the midpoint between the greater trochanter and the ischial tuberosity as the location of where the descending branch exits underneath the gluteus maximus. A Doppler device can be helpful to identify the artery in the posterior thigh. The axis of the flap is then designed centered over the posterior thigh by connecting the exit point of the pedicle with the center of the popliteal fossa. A flap can be designed up to 15 cm wide and extended to just above the popliteal fossa. However, from a practical standpoint, the widest flap that allows for primary closure of the donor is typically approximately 10 to 12 cm wide depending on the patient's body habitus. Wider flaps generally require a graft for closure. The flap is often left attached through the skin/subcutaneous tissues proximally (▶ Fig. 41.2), although a true

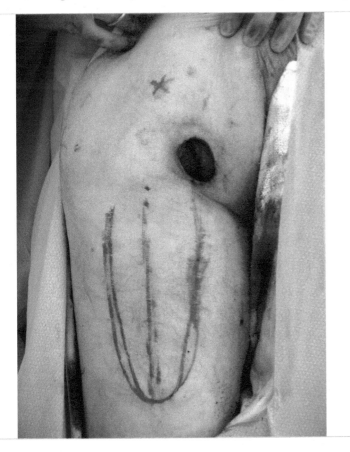

Fig. 41.2 Preoperative markings for a posterior thigh flap while leaving the skin/subcutaneous base of the flap intact.

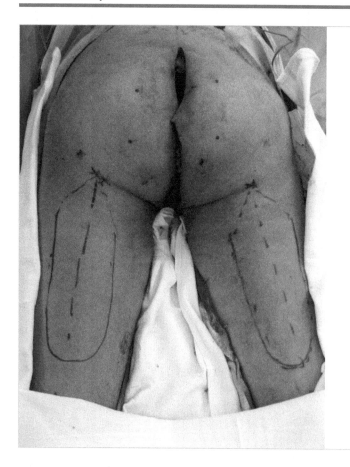

Fig. 41.3 Preoperative markings for bilateral posterior thigh flaps as island flaps.

island pedicle flap can be designed or the proximal tissue can be deepithelialized to help with rotation (►**Fig. 41.3**). This flap can be harvested with the patient either in the prone or lithotomy positions. However, the initial markings are easiest with the patient prone or standing in the pre-op area.

41.7 Operative Technique

The flap is typically harvested starting distally and then elevating it proximally. The incision is made through the distal skin, subcutaneous tissues, and deep fascia. The flap is then elevated from distal to proximal in this plane with care taken to avoid dissection in between the hamstring musculature (►**Fig. 41.4**). The pedicle can often be visualized in the mid- and distal third of the thigh. Further flap modifications can then be made if necessary to include the descending branch pedicle as one moves proximally. The standard dissection is carried up to the inferior margin of the gluteus maximus (►**Fig. 41.5**). A medial or lateral skin bridge can also be left to enhance venous drainage. If an island pedicle flap is required, an incision can be made proximally below the gluteal crease. Leaving a wide subcutaneous pedicle can be advantageous, although full dissection of the pedicle can be performed. For additional pedicle length to reach a sacral defect, one can divide the gluteus maximus muscle and continue to follow the descending branch from its origin from the inferior gluteal artery. More than minor release of the gluteus maximus is not recommended in ambulatory patients.

After elevation, the flap can then be transposed into the defect and inset with standard technique (►**Fig. 41.6**). In ischial pressure sore reconstruction, the

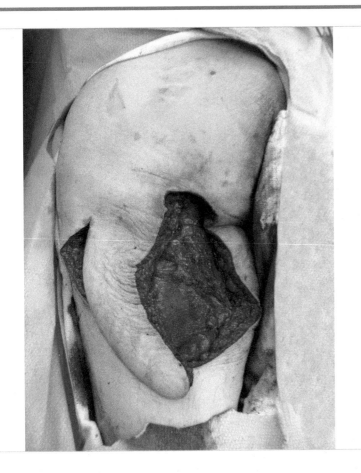

Fig. 41.4 The posterior thigh flap has been elevated from distal to proximal. The medial incision was extended into the ischial pressure sore defect to allow for rotation and preservation of the dermal–cutaneous base of the proximal flap.

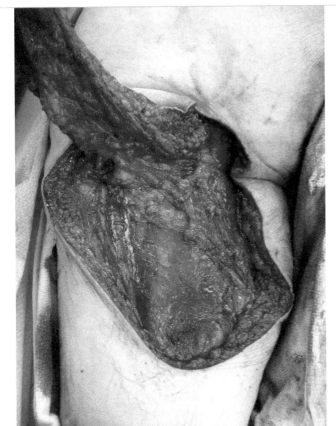

Fig. 41.5 The posterior flap has been elevated to the margin of the gluteus maximus muscle. The length and mobility of the flap will allow for easy transposition.

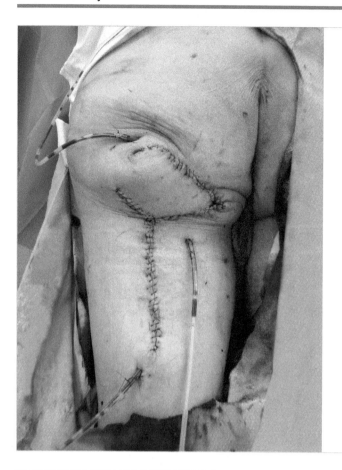

Fig. 41.6 The flap is then inset into the ischial pressure ulcer. The distal flap was deepithelialized to provide additional soft-tissue bulk. The donor site was closed primarily.

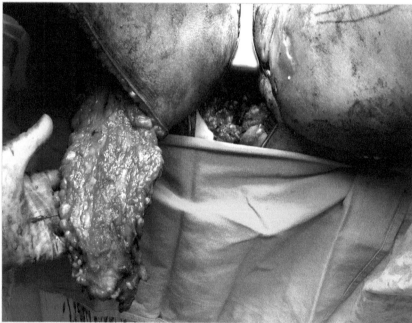

Fig. 41.7 A perineal defect following an abdominal perineal resection. A posterior thigh flap has been harvested from the right thigh in the lithotomy position.

distal flap can be deepithelialized to help fill the underlying dead space and provide additional soft-tissue padding for sitting. Given the typical defect size, drains are often left beneath the flap closure.

For perineal reconstruction, the flap can be tunneled subcutaneously through the thigh in order to reach the defect. In this example, the patient has undergone an abdominal perineal resection for Crohn's disease. A posterior thigh flap was harvested in the lithotomy position (▶**Fig. 41.7**). A subcutaneous tunnel

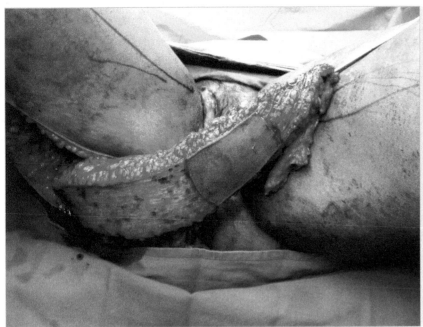

Fig. 41.8 The proximal and distal ends of the flap have been deepithelialized. The proximal portion was deepithelialized to allow for subcutaneous transposition. The distal flap was used to fil the pelvic outlet.

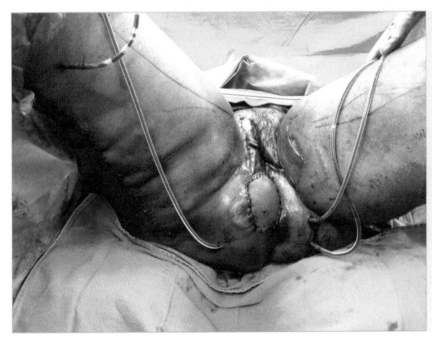

Fig. 41.9 Final inset of the flap with primary closure of the right thigh donor site.

was created between the thigh and the perineum. The proximal end of the flap was deepithelialized for transposition. An island flap could have also been performed, but it was elected to leave a broader base for venous drainage. The distal end of the flap was also deepithelialized to fill the pelvic outlet (▶Fig. 41.8). The flap was then inset to reconstruct the defect with primary closure of the donor site (▶Fig. 41.9).

41.8 Donor Site Closure

Donor site closure for this flap is typically simple assuming that an appropriate width flap has been harvested. Suprafascial undermining can be performed both medially and laterally if needed. A layered, linear closure of the posterior thigh is then performed generally over a drain. Typically, the most challenging part of the closure of the area is where the donor site scar meets the rotated flap.

41.9 Pearls and Pitfalls

- Dissection of the flap is easiest and safest when below the deep fascia. Suprafascial dissection can place the pedicled flap at risk of injury.
- Elevation of the flap is best done from distal to proximal. A hand-held Doppler can be used to identify the pedicled flap on the deep site to ensure that the proximal dissection includes the descending branch of the inferior gluteal artery.

References

[1] Hurwitz DJ, Walton RL. Closure of chronic wounds of the perineal and sacral regions using the gluteal thigh flap. Ann Plast Surg 1982;8(5):375–386
[2] Friedman JD, Reece GR, Eldor L. The utility of the posterior thigh flap for complex pelvic and perineal reconstruction. Plast Reconstr Surg 2010;126(1):146–155
[3] Windhofer C, Brenner E, Moriggl B, Papp C. Relationship between the descending branch of the inferior gluteal artery and the posterior femoral cutaneous nerve applicable to flap surgery. Surg Radiol Anat 2002;24(5):253–257

42 Soleus Muscle Flap

Eric I-Yun Chang

Abstract

The soleus muscle flap has been used primarily for reconstruction of defects within the middle third of the leg, whereas a distally based soleus flap may be employed for defects of the lower third of the leg and ankle. The skin over the soleus muscle has also been utilized as a free perforator flap for head and neck reconstruction where thin, pliable tissue is necessary. The donor site morbidity from harvest of a hemisoleus or full soleus muscle flap is minimal. This chapter covers all the relevant steps in reconstruction using the soleus muscle flap, from typical indications, to anatomy, to preoperative considerations, to surgical technique, to donor site closure, as well as mentioned three variations.

Keywords: popliteal artery, peroneal artery, posterior tibial artery, pedicles

42.1 Introduction

The soleus muscle flap has been used primarily for reconstruction of defects within the middle third of the leg while a distally based soleus flap may be employed for defects of the lower third of the leg and ankle.[1,2] Recently, the skin over the soleus muscle has also been utilized as a free perforator flap for head and neck reconstruction where thin, pliable tissue is necessary.[3] There is minimal donor site morbidity from harvest of a hemisoleus or full soleus muscle flap.

42.2 Typical Indications

- Soft-tissue defects within the middle third of the lower extremity.
- Soft-tissue defects within the distal third of the lower extremity.

42.3 Anatomy

The soleus muscle is a bipennate muscle with medial and lateral components that are separated by a central intermuscular septum. It is located deep to the gastrocnemius muscle and the plantaris muscle. This median raphe allows the soleus muscle to be split longitudinally so that harvest of half of the muscle (hemisoleus) preserves foot plantar flexion by the remaining muscle belly. The origin of the soleus muscle is the posterior surface of the proximal third of the fibula (lateral soleus) as well as the proximal half of the medial border of the tibia (medial soleus) and the insertion joins with the gastrocnemius tendon to form the Achilles tendon which attaches to the calcaneus and functions to plantar flex the foot at the ankle joint (▶ **Fig. 42.1**).[4]

The soleus muscle has a segmental blood supply that is divided into three distinct regions: the upper, middle, and lower thirds. It is a Mathes and Nahai type II muscle, containing dominant pedicles from the **popliteal, peroneal**, and **posterior tibial arteries** and minor pedicles from the **posterior tibial artery**. The proximal portion is supplied by a consistent branch from the popliteal artery. One or two branches of the peroneal artery or the tibioperoneal trunk supplies the middle third of the lateral soleus muscle, while branches from the posterior

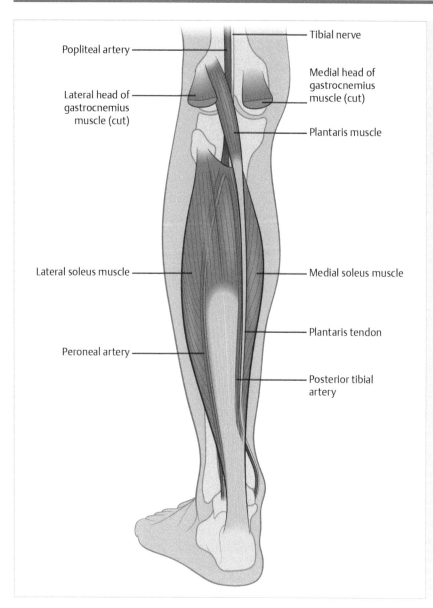

Popliteal artery

Lateral head of gastrocnemius muscle (cut)

Lateral soleus muscle

Peroneal artery

Tibial nerve

Medial head of gastrocnemius muscle (cut)

Plantaris muscle

Medial soleus muscle

Plantaris tendon

Posterior tibial artery

Fig. 42.1 Anatomy of soleus muscle.

tibial artery supply the middle third of the medial soleus muscle. The distal portion receives the blood supply from branches of the peroneal and/or posterior tibial vessels and is considered an accessory to the pedicles of the proximal and middle portions of the muscle. These accessory branches most commonly arise from the distal posterior tibial vessels just above the level of the medial malleolus and provide the basis for distally based soleus flaps.[2,5] Occasionally, distal perforators to the soleus are absent, making the distally based soleus muscle flap less reliable than the proximally based soleus muscle flap.

The motor innervation to the soleus muscle arises from the **medial popliteal and posterior tibial nerves**. The nerves accompany the blood vessels with the medial popliteal nerve supplying the proximal muscle and the posterior tibial nerve branches innervating the middle and distal regions.[5]

42.4 Variations

- Distally based medial soleus muscle flap, which may be rotated 90 to 180 degrees to cover defects of the lower third of the leg and ankle.

- Composite free fibula and soleus muscle flap (not covered here).
- Free soleus myocutaneous perforator flap used to reconstruct intraoral defects of the tongue, buccal mucosa, and palate (not covered here).

42.5 Preoperative Considerations

If there is a question regarding the vascular inflow to the lower extremity, preoperative radiographic evaluation with angiography is recommended to confirm patency of the vessels as well as to identify the location of the perforators. The soleus flap is usually harvested as a muscle flap and covered with a skin graft. A skin paddle can be included with the soleus or lateral soleus muscle, supplied by musculocutaneous perforators in the upper third of the lateral aspect of the leg. Larger skin islands can be harvested if septocutaneous branches from the peroneal artery (same perforators included in the fibula osteocutaneous flap) are included.

42.6 Positioning and Skin Markings

The patient is placed in the supine position with certain variations based on the location of the defect. If the defect is located within the middle third of the lower extremity, the leg is flexed at the knee and hip and propped at the ankle in order to maintain this position to allow for exposure and elevation of the lateral soleus or full soleus muscle flap (▶ Fig. 42.2). A skin incision is planned longitudinally 2 cm posterior to the posterior border of the fibula from 5 cm below the fibular head to just above the lateral malleolus. If a skin paddle is to be included with the upper two-thirds of the soleus muscle, a Doppler ultrasound is used to design the skin markings. In many cases, the lateral approach is reserved for harvest of the soleus muscle with the fibula bone.

For medial hemisoleus muscle flap harvest, a "frog-leg" position is used. An incision is planned from the proximal leg to just above the medial malleolus, parallel and about 2 cm posterior to the medial border of the tibia.

If the defect is located along the distal third of the lower extremity, a distally based medial hemisoleus flap may be harvested without flexing the knee or hip. A frog-leg position is often employed for a distally based soleus flap along the medial aspect of the lower extremity.

42.7 Operative Technique

42.7.1 Lateral Hemisoleus or Full Soleus Muscle Flap (Lateral Approach)

The pedicled soleus muscle flap is most reliable for coverage of defects along the middle third of the lower extremity (▶ Fig. 42.3a). If a wound in this region is present, the incision is extended from the wound proximally and distally and debrided of all nonviable tissue (▶ Fig. 42.3b). Otherwise, the incision is made as described above. The lateral origins of the soleus muscle are divided from the fibula, providing exposure of the peroneal vessels. The dissection proceeds to release the soleus muscle from the overlying gastrocnemius muscle as well as the insertion onto the Achilles tendon. Dissection proceeds from distal to proximal, ligating blood vessels as needed to provide adequate rotation of the flap and sparing the larger, more proximal blood vessels coming from the peroneal artery. The entire soleus muscle or a hemisoleus flap may be rotated based on the extent of the defect that requires coverage. Harvest of a hemisoleus flap

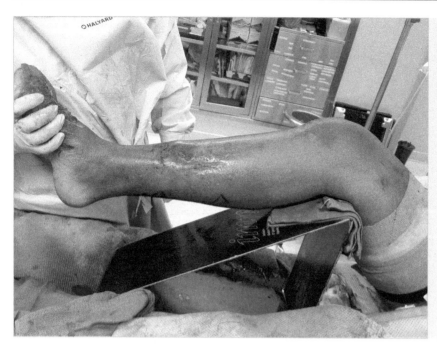

Fig. 42.2 Preoperative positioning of the right lower extremity with flexion of the knee and hip to allow exposure for elevation of a hemisoleus flap.

enables a greater arc of rotation (▶ **Fig. 42.3c**). The soleus muscle is secured to the surrounding soft tissues for reconstruction of the defect and a skin graft is utilized for coverage of the soleus muscle.

42.7.2 Medial Hemisoleus or Full Soleus Muscle Flap (Medial Approach)

For the medial soleus muscle flap, care is taken not to damage the greater saphenous vein and the saphenous nerve during the exposure. As with the lateral approach, the muscle is separated from the gastrocnemius muscle and Achilles tendon. The medial origins of the muscle from the tibia are divided, exposing the flexor digitorum longus muscle, posterior tibial artery and nerve (the neurovascular bundle lies between the soleus and flexor digitorum muscles), posterior tibial muscle, and the flexor hallucis longus muscle. The muscle is divided distally at the level of the malleolus. If a hemisoleus muscle is planned, the muscle is split along the median raphe. Dissection proceeds from distal to proximal, ligating minor segmental blood vessels as needed to obtain adequate rotation, and preserving major blood vessels from the posterior tibial artery and peroneal artery.

42.7.3 Distally Based Medial Hemisoleus Flap

The distally based hemisoleus flap is elevated by making a longitudinal incision along the soleus muscle anterior to the Achilles tendon and parallel to the tibia. The incision may be extended from the proximal portion of the open wound in order to prevent tunneling the flap under a skin bridge. The skin is retracted laterally and a Doppler probe is used to identify the location of the distal perforators from the posterior tibial artery. Once the distal perforators are identified, dissection proceeds proximally to identify the next cephalad perforator which enters the soleus muscle at the point where the gastrocnemius muscle inserts onto the Achilles tendon. The soleus muscle is divided 2 to 3 cm above this proximal perforator and then dissected off the Achilles tendon. The raphe

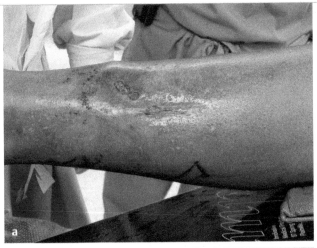

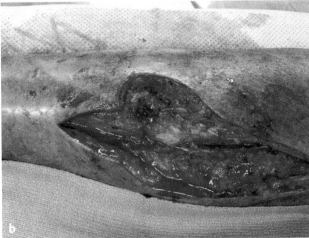

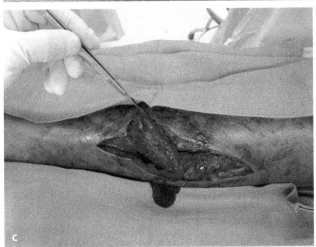

Fig. 42.3 **(a)** Chronic wound and osteomyelitis with draining sinus after traumatic tibia fracture along the middle third of the right lower extremity. **(b)** Radical debridement of surrounding soft tissue and sinus tract with exposure of the tibia. **(c)** Elevation of a medial hemisoleus flap for soft tissue coverage of the exposed tibia. The distal aspect of the soleus muscle has been dissected from the Achilles tendon and the intermuscular raphe has been divided to preserve the lateral hemisoleus.

between the two heads of the soleus muscle is incised along the longitudinal axis to the level of the distal perforators which serves as the pivot point for the hemisoleus flap.

42.8 Donor Site Closure

The donor site incision is closed primarily with minimal undermining. However, the soleus muscle that has been mobilized and transposed for reconstruction of the lower extremity defect will require a skin graft for coverage.

42.9 Pearls and Pitfalls

- Viability of the distally based medial hemisoleus flap should be confirmed by vascular examination, Doppler ultrasound, and healthy bleeding from the cut edge of the muscle belly.
- Harvest a portion of the muscle surrounding the dominant perforators for a free soleus flap during proximal dissection to the source vessel to protect the perforators.

References

[1] Tobin GR. Hemisoleus and reversed hemisoleus flaps. Plast Reconstr Surg 1985;76(1):87–96
[2] Schierle CF, Rawlani V, Galiano RD, Kim JY, Dumanian GA. Improving outcomes of the distally based hemisoleus flap: principles of angiosomes in flap design. Plast Reconstr Surg 2009;123(6):1748–1754
[3] Wolff KD, Hölzle F, Kolk A, Hohlweg-Majert B, Kesting MR. Suitability of the anterolateral thigh perforator flap and the soleus perforator flap for intraoral reconstruction: a retrospective study. J Reconstr Microsurg 2011;27(4):225–232
[4] Beck JB, Stile F, Lineaweaver W. Reconsidering the soleus muscle flap for coverage of wounds of the distal third of the leg. Ann Plast Surg 2003;50(6):631–635
[5] Pelissier P, Casoli V, Demiri E, Martin D, Baudet J. Soleus-fibula free transfer in lower limb reconstruction. Plast Reconstr Surg 2000;105(2):567–573

43 Gastrocnemius Muscle Flap

Alexander F. Mericli, David M. Adelman, and Kevin Hagan

Abstract

The gastrocnemius muscle is a workhorse flap for lower extremity reconstruction. Based proximally, the muscle can be rotated to effectively resurface defects involving the knee and superior third of the tibia. The muscle has both a medial and lateral head. The medial head is used most commonly due to its larger size, greater arc of rotation and reach, and because, unlike the lateral head, it is not possible to injure the common peroneal nerve during its dissection. Both heads of the gastrocnemius muscle may be needed to cover large defects of the knee or upper leg. The soleus muscle should be left intact in these cases to preserve plantar flexion of the ankle joint. This flap is most often designed as a muscle-only flap, but it can also be used as a myocutaneous flap. The gastrocnemius muscle flap is relatively straightforward to perform and represents a durable and reliable method of reconstruction. In this chapter the authors walk surgeons through each phase of the procedure, beginning with typical indications, followed by anatomy, then by preoperative considerations, then to the surgical technique itself, concluding with donor site closure. Two variations are included in the discussion.

Keywords: sural nerve, lesser saphenous vein, medial artery, lateral sural artery, popliteal artery, medial nerve, lateral sural motor nerve, tibial nerve, common peroneal nerve

43.1 Introduction

The gastrocnemius muscle is a workhorse flap for lower extremity reconstruction. Based proximally, the muscle can be rotated to effectively resurface defects involving the knee and superior third of the tibia.[1,2,3] The muscle has both a medial and lateral head and either can serve as a flap independently; the medial head is used most commonly due to its larger size, greater arc of rotation and reach, and because, unlike the lateral head, it is not possible to injure the common peroneal nerve during its dissection. Both heads of the gastrocnemius muscle may be needed to cover large defects of the knee or upper leg. The soleus muscle should be left intact in these cases to preserve plantar flexion of the ankle joint. The flap is most often designed as a muscle-only flap; however, it can also be employed as a myocutaneous flap. The gastrocnemius muscle flap is relatively straightforward to perform and represents a durable and reliable method of reconstruction.

43.2 Typical Indications

- Knee wound coverage.
- Wounds of the superior third of the leg.
- Wounds of the popliteal fossa.

43.3 Anatomy

The gastrocnemius muscle has a medial and a lateral head (▶ Fig. 43.1). The medial head originates from the posterior surface of the femur, superior to the

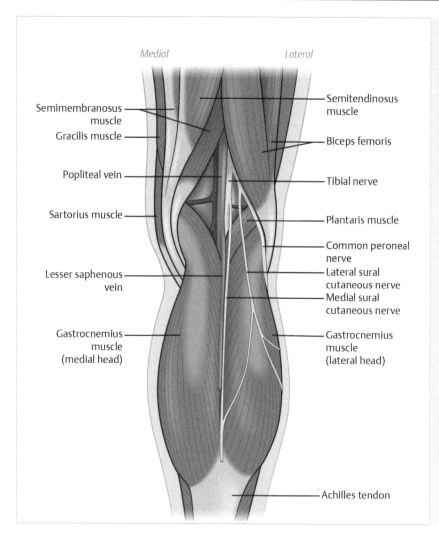

Medial   Lateral

Semimembranosus muscle

Gracilis muscle

Popliteal vein

Sartorius muscle

Lesser saphenous vein

Gastrocnemius muscle (medial head)

Semitendinosus muscle

Biceps femoris

Tibial nerve

Plantaris muscle

Common peroneal nerve

Lateral sural cutaneous nerve

Medial sural cutaneous nerve

Gastrocnemius muscle (lateral head)

Achilles tendon

Fig. 43.1 Anatomy of the posterior leg, demonstrating the medial and lateral heads of the gastrocnemius muscle.

medial condyle. The lateral head originates along the lateral epicondyle of the femur. Both heads insert into the Achilles tendon. The muscle bellies extend from the popliteal fossa to the middle third of the leg. The medial head is about 15 cm long and the lateral head is about 12 cm long, on average. The plantaris muscle and tendon lie between the gastrocnemius and soleus and is a key landmark during dissection. The **sural nerve** and **lesser saphenous vein** travels in the septum between the medial and lateral heads. The gastrocnemius functions to both flex the knee and plantar flex the ankle.

The vascular supply is type I according to Mathes and Nahai classification, with each head independently supplied by a single dominant vascular pedicle, **the medial and lateral sural arteries**. The **popliteal artery** gives off the medial and lateral sural arteries while traveling through the popliteal fossa (▶ **Fig. 43.2**). The medial sural artery is 5.1 cm in length on average and the lateral sural artery is 4.8 cm in length on average. Both the medial and lateral heads do have minor vascular supplies. The medial gastrocnemius muscle is also supplied by small perforating branches of the lateral sural artery and posterior tibial artery. The lateral gastrocnemius muscle's minor pedicle is the medial sural artery. The skin over the gastrocnemius muscle is supplied by musculocutaneous perforators, which are concentrated in the proximal part of the muscle.

The muscle is innervated by the **medial and lateral sural motor nerves**, which are branches of the **tibial nerve**. The nerves are about 5 cm in length and

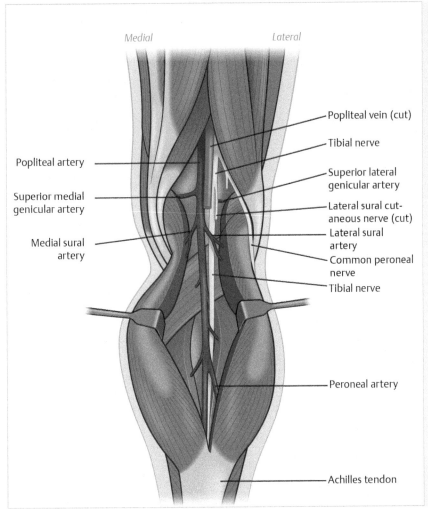

Fig. 43.2 Associated neurovascular anatomy of the gastrocnemius flap.

Medial   Lateral

Popliteal artery

Superior medial
genicular artery

Medial sural
artery

Popliteal vein (cut)

Tibial nerve

Superior lateral
genicular artery

Lateral sural cut-
aneous nerve (cut)

Lateral sural
artery

Common peroneal
nerve

Tibial nerve

Peroneal artery

Achilles tendon

enter muscle on its deep surface, with the sural vascular pedicle. The nerve can be cut when raising a pedicled flap to prevent undesirable contraction.

Knowledge of the **common peroneal nerve** anatomy is of utmost importance when elevating a lateral gastrocnemius muscle flap (▶ **Fig. 43.2**). The common peroneal nerve follows the posterior and medial aspect of the biceps tendon. It crosses over the lateral gastrocnemius muscle head distal to the muscle's origin. The nerve restricts the arc of rotation and can become strangulated if the muscle flap is rotated and inset on slight tension.

43.4 Variations

- Gastrocnemius muscle or myocutaneous free flap (rarely used due to the availability of other options with superior pedicle length and caliber).
- Medial sural artery perforator flap based on musculocutaneous perforators from the medial sural artery (not covered).

43.5 Preoperative Considerations

Although not typically performed, a CT angiogram, conventional angiogram, or MR angiogram may be obtained preoperatively in patients with peripheral vascular disease, or in those with suspicion of injury to the popliteal vessels or its branches, such as in trauma reconstruction. The contour of the muscle and arc of rotation can be assessed and estimated preoperatively through physical examination. Generally, the surface contour of the muscle can be visualized and inspected, and can be emphasized by asking the patient to plantar flex the ankle against resistance.

43.6 Positioning and Skin Markings

Both the medial and lateral gastrocnemius muscle flaps can be harvested in a variety of positions. The most common position is supine, with the knee flexed. The hip is then abducted for the medial gastrocnemius, and adducted for the lateral gastrocnemius. The flap can also be harvested with the patient prone or in the decubitus position.

A transverse line is marked in the knee flexion crease in the popliteal fossa; this marks the location of where the medial and lateral sural arteries emerge from the popliteal artery. The midline of the muscle, between the medial and lateral heads, should also be marked. In most instances, the flap is being used as a muscle-only flap in order to reconstruct an already present wound. In this scenario, either the medial or lateral gastrocnemius muscle can be harvested through an incision extending radially out from the wound to be reconstructed. If the flap is to be a myocutaneous flap, then the skin overlying the entire muscle, extending from popliteal crease to the proximal extent of the Achilles tendon, can be included with the flap if necessary. However, the skin paddle generally should be less than 6 cm in width in order to allow primary closure of the donor site. The skin paddle should not extend into the popliteal crease.

43.7 Operative Technique

43.7.1 Medial Gastrocnemius Flap

A longitudinal incision is made in the middle third of the leg, 2 cm posterior to the medial border of the tibia, and curves proximally to reach the popliteal fossa. If the popliteal fossa must be crossed in order to facilitate a more proximal pedicle dissection, then the cutaneous incision should be angulated at the popliteal crease. Dissection should proceed through the subcutaneous tissue and crural fascia overlying the muscle, which are elevated off the muscle up to the decussation of the medial and lateral heads. Care should be taken to avoid dividing the lesser saphenous vein and sural nerve, structures that travel in the aponeurotic sheet between the two muscle heads. The two muscle bellies are separated from one another along their entire length. The muscle is dissected as far proximally as is necessary to facilitate rotation and a tension-free inset. Visualization of the vascular pedicle is not required. Before disinserting the hemigastrocnemius from the Achilles tendon, the plane between the soleus and gastrocnemius muscle is identified and developed bluntly. The plantaris tendon should also be identified in this plane. The muscle is then divided from its contribution to the Achilles tendon, leaving a 1 cm cuff of tendon on the muscle flap (▶Fig. 43.3a). The arc of rotation is then tested (▶Fig. 43.3b,c); if mobilization is inadequate, the muscle is dissected more proximally. The proximal insertion can also be transected in order to advance the flap distally. Once the vascular pedicle is visualized, it can be protected and the muscle origin divided for optimal rotation/advancement. The fascia of the deep surface of the muscle can also be scored for additional advancement and coverage of the defect (▶Fig. 43.3d).

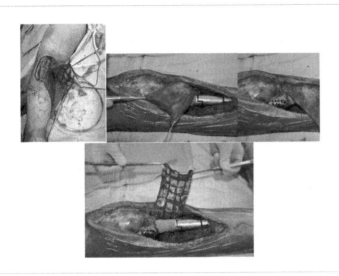

Fig. 43.3 (a) Elevated medial gastrocnemius muscle flap. Note the distal 1-cm cuff of Achilles tendon; this is useful to incorporate into the flap as an aid to inset. (b,c) The gastrocnemius muscle has a wide arc of rotation. It can typically be elevated and rotated to the knee superiorly, the popliteal fossa posteriorly, of the middle third of the tibia anteriorly. (d) The fascia along the deep and superficial surfaces of the muscle can be scored to increase the surface area of the flap and to provide for additional advancement.

Lateral Gastrocnemius Flap

The lateral belly is exposed through a longitudinal incision along the proximal middle third of the leg directly overlying the muscle, or through a radial incision extending out from the knee or proximal tibial wound. The crural fascia is incised and subcutaneous tissues elevated off the surface of the muscle. The lesser saphenous vein and sural nerve are identified and protected. The lateral gastrocnemius is separated from the underlying soleus muscle and disinserted from the Achilles, leaving a 1 cm cuff of tendon in continuity with the muscle flap. The raphe between the medial and lateral bellies is divided, creating a hemigastrocnemius muscle flap. During lateral dissection, care must be taken to avoid injury of the common peroneal or superficial peroneal nerves. Injury can occur from inadvertent transection, overzealous retraction, or extrinsic pressure from flap positioning. The muscle can be passed beneath the common peroneal nerve for greater reach, but risks stretch injury to the nerve. Similar to the medial variant, the arc of rotation can be increased by dividing the muscle belly's origin after visualization and protection of the vascular pedicle.

Myocutaneous Gastrocnemius Flap

Although the skin overlying either of the muscle bellies can be included with the flap, the donor site can rarely be closed primarily unless the skin paddle is very small (< 6 cm width). This necessitates skin grafting for closure, which is less aesthetic. Thus, it is preferable to transfer the muscle as a muscle-only flap with skin graft for coverage, thus allowing primary closure of the donor site.

43.8 Donor Site Closure

For muscle flaps, the donor site is closed primarily. If a myocutaneous flap is performed, a skin graft may be required for closure if the skin paddle is wider than about 6 cm, depending on the individual patient's skin laxity. Closed suction drainage of the donor site is recommended.

43.9 Pearls and Pitfalls

- Utilize the 1-cm cuff of Achilles tendon on the distal flap to aid insetting and to offset tension from the muscle fibers.

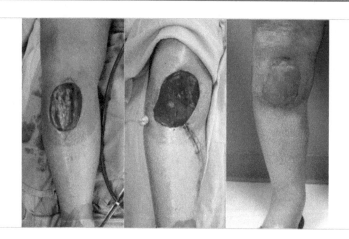

Fig. 43.4 A 10 × 7 cm defect of the anterior superior leg with wound base of denuded tibia after sarcoma excision. The patient's leg was irradiated preoperatively; note the hyperpigmentation. A medial gastrocnemius muscle flap was elevated and rotated to reconstruct the defect. Final result at 2 months postoperative; note the acceptable aesthetics and color match with a muscle flap with skin graft.

- Scoring the deep and superficial fascia overlying the gastrocnemius muscle will allow for expansion of the muscle to cover a greater surface area. This maneuver also helps improve skin graft revascularization.
- The medial head of the gastrocnemius muscle is generally preferred due to its greater arc of rotation, larger size, and avoidance of the peroneal nerve.
- A muscle flap and skin graft are usually preferred over a myocutaneous flap due to the donor site morbidity associated with skin paddle harvest. A skin-grafted muscle flap usually heals well and provides a durable reconstruction with acceptable aesthetics (▶ **Fig. 43.4**).

References

[1] Arnold PG, Mixter RC. Making the most of the gastrocnemius muscles. Plast Reconstr Surg 1983;72(1):38–48

[2] Feldman JJ, Cohen BE, May JW Jr. The medial gastrocnemius myocutaneous flap. Plast Reconstr Surg 1978;61(4):531–539

[3] McCraw JB, Fishman JH, Sharzer LA. The versatile gastrocnemius myocutaneous flap. Plast Reconstr Surg 1978;62(1):15–23

44 Medial Sural Artery Perforator Flap

Edward I. Chang

Abstract

The medial sural artery perforator flap is a cutaneous flap that is a refinement of the medial gastrocnemius flap. There have been a number of studies delineating the perforator anatomy over the years, and while the precise dimensions and measurements vary, there are generally a plethora of perforators arising from either the medial or lateral branch of the medial sural artery supplying the overlying skin. This flap provides relatively thin, pliable tissue compared to other donor sites and has the advantage of allowing primary closure of the donor site in most cases. This chapter includes all the information needed for a successful surgical outcome, beginning with typical indications, a discussion of relevant anatomy, preoperative considerations, operative technique, and donor site closure. Three variations are included in the discussion.

Keywords: medial gastrocnemius flap, popliteal artery, lateral sural artery, gastrocnemius muscle, medial sural artery, posterior cutaneous nerve of the thigh

44.1 Introduction

The medial sural artery perforator (MSAP) flap is a cutaneous flap that is a refinement of the **medial gastrocnemius flap**, which was first described at the turn of the century.[1,2,3] There have been a number of studies delineating the perforator anatomy over the years, and while the precise dimensions and measurements vary, there are generally a plethora of perforators arising from either the medial or lateral branch of the medial sural artery supplying the overlying skin. The flap provides relatively thin, pliable tissue compared to other donor sites and also has the advantage of allowing primary closure of the donor site in most cases.

44.1.1 Typical Indications

- Pedicle flap for coverage of knee defects or defects in proximal third of lower leg.
- Free flap coverage and resurfacing of extremity wounds for both the upper and lower extremity.
- Free fasciocutaneous flap for complex head and neck reconstruction including pharyngeal reconstruction, glossectomy defects, and defects of the intraoral lining.

44.2 Anatomy

The main artery for the MSAP flap is the medial sural artery, which is a branch off the **popliteal artery** that arises at about the same level as the **lateral sural artery**. Together, the medial and lateral sural arteries supply the **gastrocnemius muscle** and overlying skin. The other branches of the popliteal artery include the medial and lateral superior geniculate arteries (superior to the sural arteries) and the medial and lateral inferior geniculate arteries (inferior to the sural arteries). The medial sural artery often has a **medial and a lateral branch** both of which travel through the medial belly of the gastrocnemius muscle. The perforators supplying the MSAP flap can arise from either the medial or the lateral branch; however, studies have shown that the larger perforators often arise from the lateral branch, which is more posterior and closer to the midline raphe of the medial and lateral gastrocnemius muscles.[4,5] There are also perforators that arise from the lateral sural artery and pass through the lateral gastrocnemius muscle, making the lateral sural artery perforator flap an alternative; however, these are less reliable than the perforators arising from the medial sural artery making the MSAP flap much more reliable. The **posterior cutaneous nerve of the thigh** can be included when a sensate flap is needed.

The location of the perforators is quite variable depending on which study one reads, but generally they emerge approximately 8 to 12 cm distal to the popliteal crease, about 4.5 cm from the midline.[4,5] The precise number of perforators is also variable, with most authors reporting two to four, but they are almost always musculocutaneous perforators and therefore an extensive intramuscular dissection is needed in order to obtain a pedicle that is of adequate length and caliber to use for free tissue transfer. For a pedicled flap, dissection proceeds as proximally as is necessary to obtain the sufficient length needed to mobilize and rotate the flap into the defect without tension or compromising the pedicle.

The anatomic landmarks and axis for the MSAP flap are based on the midpoint of the popliteal crease and the medial malleolus. The perforator territory is skin of the medial half of the upper third of the posterior calf, typically yielding an area of about 8 × 12 cm. With an extensive intramuscular dissection that is required for the harvest of this flap, the average pedicle length ranges from 10.2 to 12.7 cm. The average diameters of the artery and vein reported in the literature are 2.2 and 2.6 mm, respectively. While the flap thickness clearly varies based on body habitus, the skin overlying the calf region is often thinner than other donor sites with an average thickness ranging from 4.8 to 8.4 mm.[5,6]

44.3 Variations

- The flap can be harvested as a pedicle flap or a free flap and can also be harvested as a chimeric flap including portions of the medial gastrocnemius muscle if additional bulk is needed.
- The location of the perforators is quite variable, and a freestyle approach should be considered when harvesting the flap.
- If multiple perforators are encountered, the flap can be divided into two separate skin paddles for resurfacing adjacent digits or for complex head and neck reconstruction.

44.4 Preoperative Considerations

The patient selection should be based on surgeon experience and patient body habitus. For most patients, the skin is considerably thinner compared to other donor sites such as the anterolateral thigh (ALT) flap or lateral arm flap. Therefore, for patients who have prohibitively thick subcutaneous tissue in the thighs or upper arm, the MSAP represents an attractive alternative. However, the MSAP flap is not typically thinner or more pliable than a forearm-based flap, which should also be considered when deciding which donor site to use. The benefit of using a MSAP flap compared to a forearm-based flap is the donor site of a flap 6 to 7 cm in width can be closed primarily without the need for a

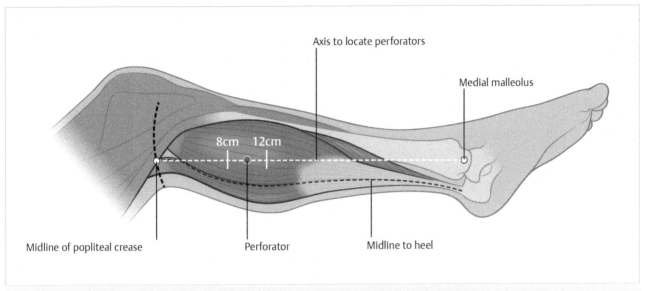

Axis to locate perforators

Medial malleolus

8cm   12cm

Midline of popliteal crease

Perforator

Midline to heel

Fig. 44.1 Surgical landmarks for medial sural artery perforator (MSAP) flap design.

skin graft. While this has not been studied extensively, there is a potential for concern in patients with peripheral vascular disease where atherosclerosis can have an impact on the flap pedicle. Therefore, in patients with severe peripheral vascular disease, diabetes, claudication, or an abnormal peripheral pulse examination, consideration should be given to an alternate donor site.

44.5 Positioning and Skin Markings

The standard markings used for designing the medial sural artery perforator flap are based on the popliteal crease and the medial malleolus. The patient should be marked in the standing position to minimize any distortion of the line when the patient is supine in the frog-leg position. The line from the midpoint of the popliteal crease to the medial malleolus is the axis for the MSAP flap, and the greatest density of the perforators is located approximately 8 to 12 cm from the popliteal crease and there are rarely any perforators within 6 cm of the popliteal crease or beyond 18 cm from the crease (▶ Fig. 44.1). One may still wish to use a hand-held Doppler to help localize the perforators prior to making the skin incision, which is reminiscent of the freestyle perforator flap approach. Alternatively, a generous strategic incision can be made in order to gain proper exposure to explore both anteriorly and posteriorly that still allows harvest of the flap regardless of whether the perforator is found anterior or posterior to the axis.

44.6 Operative Technique

Refer to Video 44.1 for an example of the operative technique for the medial sural artery perforator flap. The patient is typically marked as described and ideally in the standing position in order to have the most accurate axis marking the midpoint of the popliteal crease to the medial malleolus. While this line is a reasonable guide for the location of the perforators, more often than not, the perforators are located posterior to this axis. The greatest cluster of perforators are found within 8 to 12 cm from the popliteal crease, and a hand-held Doppler may be used in order to localiz any perforators to help guide the initial skin incision.

The patient needs to be flexed at the hips and externally rotated in order to have access to the medial calf region (frog-leg position). Alternatively, the patient can be placed in lithotomy position in order to have the surgeon stand or sit in between the patient's legs, which will certainly facilitate the MSAP flap harvest. Dissection is easiest in the prone position; however, flap harvest can be safely performed with the patient in the supine frog-leg position, on a standard operating table, from either side of the patient regardless of the handedness of the surgeon.

The anterior skin incision is made first centering the skin island either where a Doppler signal has been identified or to the above-mentioned axis of the flap if no signal is found (▶ Fig. 44.2). Once the skin incision is completed, dissection proceeds through the subcutaneous tissue until the fascia overlying the gastrocnemius muscle is encountered. The fascia is then incised and a subfascial dissection is performed elevating posteriorly until a perforator is encountered.

Once a perforator is identified, the perforator dissection begins from the level of the fascia through the gastrocnemius muscle as proximally as possible to allow for the greatest caliber and length of the MSAP flap pedicle. The intramuscular dissection is quite tedious as there are a number of muscular branches arising from the pedicle that should be carefully ligated. It is prudent not to skeletonize the pedicle, and leaving a small cuff of muscle around the pedicle will minimize inadvertent injury to the pedicle. The MSAP flap perforators can arise from either the medial or lateral branch of the medial sural artery rather than a single trunk, as mentioned above. Care should be taken to spare the motor nerve to the medial belly of the gastrocnemius muscle.

Once the pedicle has been dissected, the posterior incision is made centering the flap on the perforator (▶ Fig. 44.3). The pedicle is then dissected as proximally as possible in order to obtain an adequate size and length of the artery and vein to perform a microvascular anastomosis, or to obtain adequate reach when being harvested as a pedicled flap (▶ Fig. 44.4).

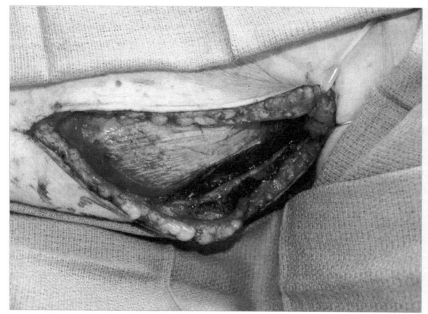

Fig. 44.2 The anterior incision is made in order to identify the perforator in a subfascial plane. The perforator is dissected through an intramuscular course as proximal as possible to obtain the needed length and diameter of the vessels. The right calf is shown.

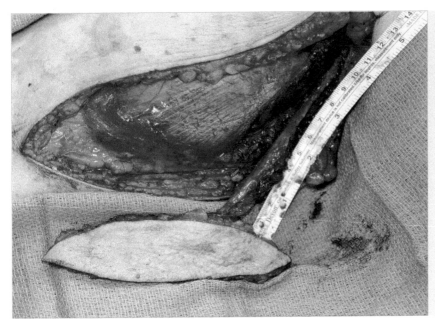

Fig. 44.3 The pedicle is typically on average approximately 10 cm in length, although it can be shorter depending on the location of the perforator.

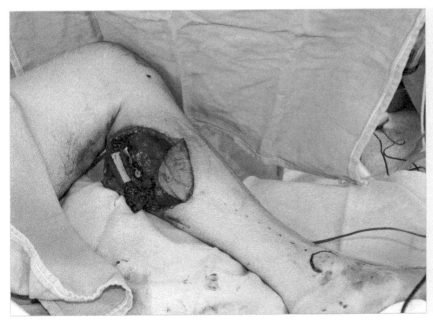

Fig. 44.4 Elevated medial sural artery perforator (MSAP) flap demonstrating the markings of the axis from the midpoint of the popliteal crease to the medial malleolus.

44.7 Donor Site Closure

The donor site for the medial sural artery perforator flap can generally be closed primarily. The laxity of the overlying skin in the medial calf region will dictate the amount of skin that can be removed that can still allow for primary closure. For most patients, flaps that are less than 6 to 7 cm in width can be closed without difficulty, although there is variability in the pliability of the skin in the gastrocnemius region. In the setting that the donor site cannot be closed without tension, the underlying medial gastrocnemius muscle provides a healthy bed of tissue to support a skin graft. A closed suction drain should be placed in the donor site.

44.8 Pearls and Pitfalls

- The patient should be marked in the standing position in order to draw an accurate axis for the design of the flap.
- The perforators are often more posterior than anticipated. Subfascial dissection is easier than suprafascial dissection, and facilitates perforator identification.
- The perforator location is quite variable, and the flap design is more reminiscent of a freestyle perforator dissection through the gastrocnemius muscle, which can be quite tedious.
- The main pedicle may not necessarily be the main medial sural artery but rather the medial or lateral branch. Dissecting the branches proximally to the takeoff will provide larger-caliber vessels and longer pedicle length.

References

[1] Cavadas PC, Sanz-Giménez-Rico JR, Gutierrez-de la Cámara A, Navarro-Monzonís A, Soler-Nomdedeu S, Martínez-Soriano F. The medial sural artery perforator free flap. Plast Reconstr Surg 2001;108(6):1609–1615, discussion 1616–1617

[2] Kim HH, Jeong JH, Seul JH, Cho BC. New design and identification of the medial sural perforator flap: an anatomical study and its clinical applications. Plast Reconstr Surg 2006;117(5):1609–1618

[3] Hupkens P, Westland PB, Schijns W, van Abeelen MHA, Kloeters O, Ulrich DJO. Medial lower leg perforators: An anatomical study of their distribution and characteristics. Microsurgery 2017;37(4):319–326

[4] Molina AR, Citron I, Chinaka F, Cascarini L, Townley WA. Calf perforator flaps: a freestyle solution for oral cavity reconstruction. Plast Reconstr Surg 2017;139(2):459–465

[5] Kao HK, Chang KP, Chen YA, Wei FC, Cheng MH. Anatomical basis and versatile application of the free medial sural artery perforator flap for head and neck reconstruction. Plast Reconstr Surg 2010;125(4):1135–1145

[6] Song X, Wu H, Zhang W, et al. Medial sural artery perforator flap for postsurgical reconstruction of head and neck cancer. J Reconstr Microsurg 2015;31(4):319–326

45 Reverse Sural Artery Flap

Jon Ver Halen

Abstract
Reliable pedicled flap options for reconstruction of the distal third of the lower leg are limited, but the neurocutaneous sural flap had been used for reconstruction of soft-tissue defects of the distal third of the leg. The reversed sural flap, which is a distally based version of the sural flap, is most commonly used as a reliable soft-tissue reconstructive option for moderate-size defects around the heel and perimalleolar regions. This flap can also be used in cases involving simultaneous bone injury, chronic osteomyelitis, and when there is a need for sensate coverage, especially when free flap reconstruction carries a high risk. In this chapter, every salient feature of this reconstructive procedure is covered, beginning with typical indications and anatomy, to preoperative considerations and operative technique, concluding with donor site closure. A citing of eight variations is included.

Keywords: sural artery, saphenous vein, popliteal artery, popliteal vein, medial sural cutaneous nerve, tibial nerve

45.1 Introduction

Reliable pedicled flap options for reconstruction of the distal third of the lower leg are limited. In 1992, Masquelet et al described the use of the neurocutaneous sural flap for reconstruction of soft-tissue defects of the distal third of the leg.[1] The reversed sural flap, which is a distally based version of the sural flap, is most commonly used to provide a reliable soft-tissue reconstructive option for moderate-size defects around the heel and perimalleolar regions.[2,3] This flap can also be used in cases involving simultaneous bone injury, chronic osteomyelitis, and a need for sensate coverage, especially when free flap reconstruction carries relatively high risk.

45.2 Typical Indications

- Soft-tissue defects of distal third of the leg, specifically the heel, or medial or lateral malleolus.

45.3 Anatomy

The flap is located between the popliteal fossa and the midportion of the leg, centered over the midline raphe between the medial and lateral heads of the gastrocnemius muscle.

The proximally based sural artery flap is a fasciocutaneous, Mathes and Nahai type I flap (one dominant pedicle). It is based on a direct cutaneous artery (i.e., the **sural artery**) and lesser **saphenous vein**, emanating from the **popliteal artery and vein**.[4] This pedicle branch descends from the popliteal fossa between the heads of the gastrocnemius muscle in the deep fascial layer, and courses inferiorly superficial to the gastrocnemius muscle. The medial sural artery pedicle is approximately 4 to 6 cm in length, and 1.4 mm in diameter. The

medial sural cutaneous nerve (S1–S2), a branch of the **tibial nerve** within the popliteal fossa, courses with the lesser saphenous vein and cutaneous artery. The nerve and vascular pedicle enter the skin at the midposterior leg. The skin flap is designed between the popliteal fossa and the midposterior leg, centered over the median raphe between the medial and lateral heads of the gastrocnemius muscle. Maximal dimensions are 15 × 6 cm, with a typical need to skin graft the flap donor site.

The reversed sural artery flap has a similarly designed skin paddle and perforator blood supply, but is distally based. The distal blood supply is provided from perforators from the peroneal artery, which anastomose with axially oriented vessels and choke vessels in the flap pedicle, and which travel along with the sural nerve. Similarly, venous drainage occurs retrograde through the lesser saphenous vein, and relies on valvular incompetence and venous tributaries to ensure adequate venous drainage.

45.4 Variations

- Free flap: microvascular transplantation based on the medial sural artery perforator, or peroneal perforator-based sural neurofasciocutaneous flap.[5]
- Tissue expanded flap: this expansion can increase flap dimensions prior to flap elevation.
- Neurosensory flap: the flap includes the sural nerve and may be used as a sensate flap.[6]
- Delayed flap: recommended in patients with multiple comorbidities, including age more than 70 years, history of smoking, obesity, diabetes, or peripheral arterial disease.[7]
- Distally based superficial sural artery flap: excluding the sural nerve.
- Adipofascial flap: used in patients with multiple comorbidities.[8]
- Perforator/island flap: possible to narrow flap pedicle from a wide neurofasciocutaneous pedicle, to narrow perforator-based flap.[9]
- Musculocutaneous flap: gastrocnemius muscle cuff harvested for cases of osteomyelitis.

45.5 Preoperative Considerations

Since the flap is ultimately perfused through perforators of the peroneal artery, vascular studies may be warranted in patients in whom vessel patency is in question. General criteria for limb salvage surgery should be met (e.g., patient has a sensate, mobile, and durable foot). The flap has mainly been described as a reversed flap for reconstructing defects of the lower third of the leg, heel, and medial and lateral malleoli, and, therefore, the discussion of the operative technique will be restricted to this variant of the flap.[10] Significant lower extremity edema can increase the difficulty of flap harvest and mobilization, and increase risks of wound dehiscence, infection, and flap failure. In patients with vascular disease, smoking history, edema, or other risk factors, surgical delay is recommended.

45.6 Positioning and Skin Markings

Prone positioning with adequate padding is usually used. However, supine position with the extremity free, or lateral position has been described. A tourniquet can be used to create a bloodless field, but is not necessary.

The flap is supplied by the superficial sural artery that accompanies the sural nerve (▶Fig. 45.1). The artery gives off small branches to the skin in the lower two-thirds of the leg. In the lower part of the tibiofibular space, the superficial sural artery anastomoses with septocutaneous branches from the peroneal artery. Venous drainage is provided from retrograde flow through the lesser saphenous vein.

A line connecting the midpopliteal point, and the midpoint between the lateral malleolus and the lateral border of the Achilles tendon marks the vascular axis of the flap. The proximal extent of the flap should be limited to 5 cm distal to the popliteal crease. The entire width of the calf skin can be harvested. Distally, skin can be harvested up to 5 cm proximal to the lateral malleolus. The pivot point is placed 5 cm proximal to the tip of the lateral malleolus. A skin island can be designed according to a previously prepared template of the recipient defect (▶Fig. 45.2).

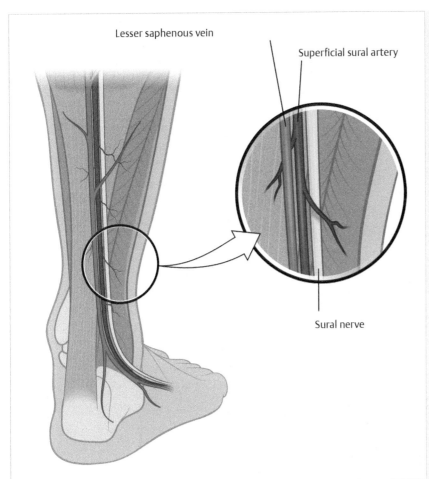

Lesser saphenous vein

Superficial sural artery

Sural nerve

Fig. 45.1 The flap is supplied by the superficial sural artery that accompanies the sural nerve. The artery gives off small branches to the skin in the lower two-thirds of the leg. In the lower part of the tibiofibular space, the superficial sural artery anastomoses with septocutaneous branches from the peroneal artery. Venous drainage is provided from retrograde flow through the lesser saphenous vein.

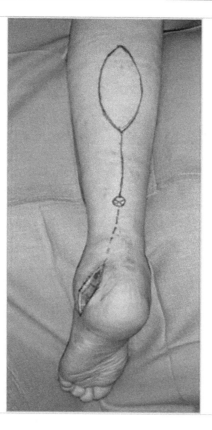

Fig. 45.2 A line connecting the midpopliteal point, and the midpoint between the lateral malleolus and the lateral border of the Achilles tendon marks the vascular axis of the flap. The proximal extent of the flap should be limited to 5 cm distal to the popliteal crease. The entire width of the calf skin can be harvested. Distally, skin can be harvested up to 5 cm proximal to the lateral malleolus. The pivot point is placed 5 cm proximal to the tip of the lateral malleolus. A skin island can be designed according to a previously prepared template of the recipient defect.

45.7 Operative Technique

The reverse sural fasciocutaneous flap is made up of skin and subcutaneous fat, the superficial and deep fascia of the posterior part of the leg, sural nerve, the sural vein, the superficial sural artery, and the lesser saphenous vein. Arterial perfusion is provided through the superficial sural artery, which runs parallel to the sural nerve. Flap blood supply is accomplished by distal reverse flow of the superficial sural artery, and is dependent on perforators of the peroneal arterial system. There are numerous anastomoses between the peroneal artery and the vascular axis of the flap. The most distal perforator, which is the pivot point of the flap and must be preserved, is usually found at a distance of 4 to 5 cm above the tip of lateral malleolus. The pedicle (4–5 cm in width) consists of subcutaneous tissue, deep fascia, the lesser saphenous vein, the sural nerve, and accompanying arteries.

The skin incision is begun along the line in which the fascial pedicle will be taken.[11] The subdermal layer is dissected to expose the sural nerve, accompanying superficial sural vessels, and lesser saphenous vein (▶ **Fig. 45.3**). If necessary, the skin paddle can then be reoriented to be properly centered over the course of the sural nerve, artery, and lesser saphenous vein. The skin paddle is then incised. The proximal border of the flap is explored, and the lesser saphenous vein, the sural nerve, and accompanying vessels are ligated and cut. At this point, the skin incisions can then be closed if a delay procedure is required.

If a single-stage procedure is being performed, the skin island is next elevated with the deep fascia (▶ **Fig. 45.4**). If a very thin adipofascial flap is preferred, the deep fascia without a skin island can be elevated safely (and then skin grafted, if necessary). The subcutaneous fascial pedicle is then elevated, with a width of 2 to 3 cm on either side of the nerve and the vessels. The flap is then rotated

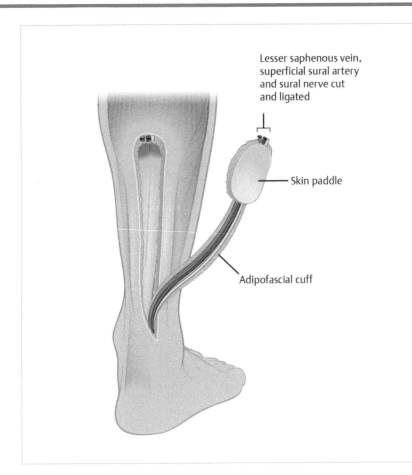

Lesser saphenous vein, superficial sural artery and sural nerve cut and ligated

Skin paddle

Adipofascial cuff

Fig. 45.3 Skin incision is begun along the line in which the fascial pedicle will be taken. The subdermal layer is dissected to expose the sural nerve, accompanying superficial sural vessels, and lesser saphenous vein. In general, an adipofascial cuff of 2 to 3 cm is included on each side of the nerve/artery/vein pedicle. If necessary, the skin paddle can be reoriented to be properly centered over the course of the sural nerve, artery, and lesser saphenous vein. The skin paddle is then incised. The proximal border of the flap is explored, and the lesser saphenous vein, the sural nerve, and accompanying vessels are ligated and cut. At this point, the skin incisions can then be closed if a delay procedure is required.

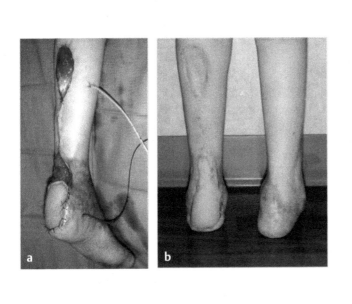

Fig. 45.4 (a,b) If flap elevation is continued, the skin island is elevated with the deep fascia. If a thin flap is preferred, the deep fascia without a skin island can be elevated safely (and then skin grafted, if necessary). The subcutaneous fascial pedicle is then elevated, with a width of 2 to 3 cm on either side of the nerve and the vessels. The flap is then rotated over its pedicle up to 180 degrees, and adapted to the defect. The skin bridge is usually closed over the pedicle. In instances where the subcutaneous tunnel is constricted, the skin bridge can be left open and the pedicle base can be skin grafted. The donor site can be closed primarily, or skin grafted.

over its pedicle up to 180 degrees, and adapted to the defect. The skin bridge is usually closed over the pedicle. In instances where the subcutaneous tunnel is constricted, the skin bridge can be left open and the pedicle base can be skin grafted.

45.8 Donor Site Closure

In general, the donor site defect can be closed primarily when the flap is less than 3-cm wide. Larger donor site defects should be covered with a split-thickness skin graft.

The pedicle skin bridge is usually closed over the flap pedicle. In instances where the subcutaneous tunnel is constricted, the skin bridge is left open and the pedicle base is skin grafted.

Postoperatively, strict elevation of the extremity is encouraged for 5 days, after which patients are allowed to ambulate with compressive stockings while still elevating the extremity most of the day. After 10 days, normal activities are resumed. Compressive stockings are discontinued after 6 weeks.

45.9 Pearls and Pitfalls

- Flap delay procedure should be used in patients at high risk for flap complications. These include age more than 70 years, history of smoking, obesity, diabetes, or peripheral arterial disease.
- Most flap complications are secondary to impaired venous drainage. Delay procedures or modification of pedicle design to augment venous drainage may improve flap success.

References

[1] Masquelet AC, Romana MC, Wolf G. Skin island flaps supplied by the vascular axis of the sensitive superficial nerves: anatomic study and clinical experience in the leg. Plast Reconstr Surg 1992;89(6):1115–1121

[2] Hasegawa M, Torii S, Katoh H, Esaki S. The distally based superficial sural artery flap. Plast Reconstr Surg 1994;93(5):1012–1020

[3] Schmidt K, Jakubietz M, Djalek S, Harenberg PS, Zeplin PH, Jakubietz R. The distally based adipofascial sural artery flap: faster, safer, and easier? A long-term comparison of the fasciocutaneous and adipofascial method in a multimorbid patient population. Plast Reconstr Surg 2012;130(2):360–368

[4] Wang CY, Chai YM, Wen G, et al. The free peroneal perforator-based sural neurofasciocutaneous flap: a novel tool for reconstruction of large soft-tissue defects in the upper limb. Plast Reconstr Surg 2011;127(1):293–302

[5] Mojallal A, Wong C, Shipkov C, et al. Vascular supply of the distally based superficial sural artery flap: surgical safe zones based on component analysis using three-dimensional computed tomographic angiography. Plast Reconstr Surg 2010;126(4):1240–1252

[6] Akita S, Mitsukawa N, Rikihisa N, et al. Descending branch of the perforating branch of the peroneal artery perforator-based island flap for reconstruction of the lateral malleolus with minimal invasion. Plast Reconstr Surg 2013;132(2):461–469

[7] Parrett BM, Pribaz JJ, Matros E, Przylecki W, Sampson CE, Orgill DP. Risk analysis for the reverse sural fasciocutaneous flap in distal leg reconstruction. Plast Reconstr Surg 2009;123(5):1499–1504

[8] Coşkunfirat OK, Velidedeoğlu HV, Sahin U, Demir Z. Reverse neurofasciocutaneous flaps for soft-tissue coverage of the lower leg. Ann Plast Surg 1999;43(1):14–20

[9] Jeng SF, Wei FC, Kuo YR. Salvage of the distal foot using the distally based sural island flap. Ann Plast Surg 1999;43(5):499–505

[10] Price MF, Capizzi PJ, Watterson PA, Lettieri S. Reverse sural artery flap: caveats for success. Ann Plast Surg 2002;48(5):496–504

[11] Ríos-Luna A, Villanueva-Martínez M, Fahandezh-Saddi H, Villanueva-Lopez F, del Cerro-Gutiérrez M. Versatility of the sural fasciocutaneous flap in coverage defects of the lower limb. Injury 2007;38(7):824–831

46 Fibula Osteocutaneous Free Flap

Geoffroy C. Sisk and Patrick B. Garvey

Abstract

The free fibula bone flap, based on the peroneal artery, is used to reconstruct defects in the long bones of the extremities. This flap can be used as a free fibula osseous flap for mandible reconstruction and can be dissected in a way that allows a skin paddle to be included with the bone flap by capturing osteoseptocutaneous perforators originating from the peroneal artery. The inclusion of a skin paddle expands the flap's applicability to defects involving both bone and soft tissue. The flap has also been used for reconstruction of the mandible after oncologic resection and is the most commonly utilized method of reconstruction for defects requiring vascularized bone replacement. Its osteocutaneous variant is a favored method of reconstruction for composite defects of the mandible and midfacial skeleton. The authors of this chapter carefully cover each step in the use of the fibula osteocutaneous free flap, beginning with typical indications, then anatomy, then preoperative considerations, then the surgical technique, and concluding with donor site closure. Three variations are touched upon in the discussion.

Keywords: skin paddle, mandible, osteomyocutaneous, osseous, fibula flap harvest

46.1 Introduction

The free fibula bone flap, based on the peroneal artery, was first described by Ian Taylor in 1975 to reconstruct defects in the long bones of the extremities.[1] In 1979, Arthur Adamo described his experience with using the free fibula osseous flap for mandible reconstruction.[2] In the early 1980s, Chen and Wei described a flap dissection technique that allowed a skin paddle to be included with the bone flap by capturing osteoseptocutaneous perforators originating from the peroneal artery.[3,4] The inclusion of a skin paddle expanded the flap's applicability to defects involving both bone and soft tissue. In 1989, Hidalgo described the use of the fibula free osteocutaneous flap for reconstruction of the mandible after oncologic resection.[5] Today, the fibula free flap is the most commonly utilized method of reconstruction for defects requiring vascularized bone replacement, and its osteocutaneous variant is a favored method of reconstruction for composite defects of the mandible and midfacial skeleton.[6]

46.2 Typical Indications

- Composite defects of the mandible with skin paddle for replacement of mucosa and/or skin.
- Maxillectomy defects requiring replacement of bone for orbital support or alveolus reconstruction and placement of osseointegrated dental implants.
- Defects of the long bones of the extremities, particularly radius, tibia, and femur (with or without a skin paddle).
- Bone defects of the spine and pelvic ring (with or without a skin paddle).

46.3 Anatomy

The lower leg is divided into four muscular compartments: anterior (containing tibialis anterior, extensor digitorum longus, and extensor hallucis longus), lateral (peroneus muscles), deep posterior (flexor digitorum longus, flexor hallucis longus, and tibialis posterior), and superficial posterior (soleus and gastrocnemius). The fibula borders all four of these muscular compartments, and an understanding of the flap dissection relies heavily on an appreciation of the bone's anatomical relationship with the compartments, their contents, and the soft-tissue structures that divide them (▶ Fig. 46.1).[7]

The tibia and fibula comprise the bony lower leg, articulating with one another at proximal and distal tibiofibular joints and joined in between by a fibrous interosseous membrane which divides the anterior and deep posterior muscular compartments. The dominant blood supply of the fibula is the peroneal artery, one of three arteries that supply the distal lower extremity.[8] After passing behind the tibial plateau, the popliteal artery divides into the anterior tibial artery and tibioperoneal trunk. The anterior tibial artery then crosses the interosseous membrane from the deep posterior compartment into the anterior compartment. The tibioperoneal trunk then divides into the posterior tibial artery and the peroneal artery. The peroneal artery courses posterior to interosseous membrane within the deep posterior compartment, sending osseous branches directly into the posterior–medial aspect of the fibula. On the lateral surface of the fibula, the lateral muscular compartment is separated from the anterior and superficial posterior compartment by the anterior and posterior intermuscular crural septae, respectively; it is within the posterior crural septum that the osteoseptocutaneous perforators travel. These perforators originate

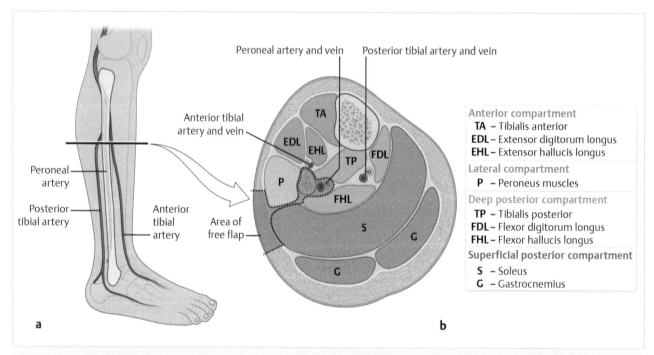

Fig. 46.1 **(a)** Vascular anatomy of the lower leg in relation to the tibia and fibula bones and **(b)** cross-sectional anatomy of the lower leg. The fibula osteocutaneous free flap includes the fibula bone, peroneal artery and vein, and perforating blood vessels to the skin paddle that travel along the posterior surface of the posterior intermuscular septum, as indicated by the dashed lines on cross section.

from the peroneal artery and arborize to supply the skin at or slightly posterior to the posterior margin of the fibula bone.

The peroneal artery also provides the dominant blood supply to a number of nearby muscular structures that may be considered when designing flaps for three-dimensionally or anatomically complex defects. In the deep posterior compartment, the flexor hallucis longus is supplied by direct muscular perforators and can be included with the flap distally. In addition, the proximal portion of the soleus is also supplied by peroneal artery branches and can be incorporated if flap design considerations require muscle in the proximal portion of the flap.

The lateral sural cutaneous nerve (LSCN) is generally considered to be the dominant source of sensory innervation to the lateral calf, but there is evidence that other small cutaneous nerves may provide sensory innervation to an overlapping neurosomal territory.[9,10] The LSCN originates from the common peroneal nerve near the fibular head and most commonly courses inferiorly along the superficial surface of the soleus muscle, parallel to the posterior intermuscular septum. Innervation of the flap is not routinely performed, but harvest of sensate flaps using the LSCN has been described and may be particularly useful for some operative indications such as creation of a neophallus.

46.4 Variations

- Osteomyocutaneous incorporating flexor hallucis longus or soleus muscle.
- Osseous.
- Multiple skin paddles.

46.5 Preoperative Considerations

Computed tomography angiography (CTA): peroneus magnus; vascular insufficiency if weak or absent pulses. Rare for skin paddle to be too bulky.

46.6 Positioning and Skin Markings

The patient is positioned in the supine position. A padded heel support is secured to the operating room table and positioned to keep the leg from which the fibula is to be harvested in an internally rotated, near 90-degree, bent position. The most prominent palpable points of the fibula head and the lateral malleolus are marked. A paper ruler is stretched between these two points, and the anterior and posterior borders of the lateral surface of the fibula are marked by drawing two longitudinal, parallel lines along the anterior and posterior edges of the paper ruler (▶Fig. 46.2). A horizontal line is drawn 5 cm from the fibular head representing the approximate future location of the proximal fibula osteotomy. A second horizontal line is drawn 7 cm proximal to the lateral malleolus, representing the approximate future location of the distal fibula osteotomy. In a lean patient, the longitudinal attachment of the posterior crural septum to the subcutaneous investing fascia of the lower leg can be appreciated as a slightly depressed longitudinal line about 1 to 2 cm posterior to the fibula. This line should be marked, as it represents the line along which the cutaneous perforasomes of the peroneal artery septocutaneous perforators will be centered. Two-thirds the distance along this line between the fibular head and lateral malleolus is marked as the point around

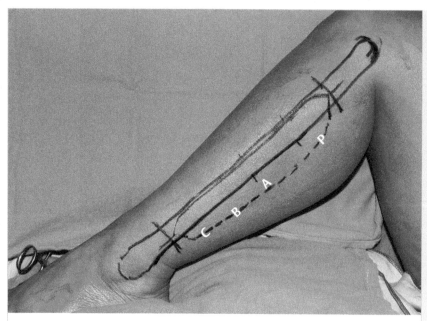

Fig. 46.2 Skin markings for the fibula osteocutaneous free flap. Osteotomies are planned 5 cm inferior to the fibular head and 7 cm superior to the lateral malleolus. The skin paddle is centered over the posterior border of the fibula. While a proximal perforator (*marked "P"*) is usually present about one-third of the distance between the fibular head and lateral malleolus, the fibula osteocutaneous free flap skin paddle is usually designed to incorporate one to three distal perforators (*marked "A," "B," and "C"*), most commonly arising about 0.5, 0.6, and 0.75 the distance between the fibular head and lateral malleolus, respectively, in order to maximize pedicle length.

which the majority of the septocutaneous peroneal artery perforators will be found.[4,8,11,12,13,14] A hand-held Doppler can more specifically localize the perforators along the posterior crural septum. The anterior incision for the skin island is marked along the previously drawn anterior border of the fibula, at least 2 to 3 cm anterior to the perforator.[6] This anterior incision is marked along the anterior border of the fibula for 8 cm in longitudinal length, centered on the perforator. Superior and inferior to this, the incisional line is curved posteriorly to run up the middle of the fibula until ending 1 cm beyond the marks for the distal and proximal osteotomies.

If the surgical plan calls for a second skin island to be harvested to create a double-skin island free fibula flap, the approximate location of the proximal perforator is marked along the posterior crural septum at one-third the length between the fibular head and lateral malleolus.[8,14,15] The location of this perforator can be confirmed with a hand-held Doppler. Understand that a proximal perforator originating from the peroneal artery is not always available in all patients, so surgeons intending to raise a double-skin island free fibula flap should have a backup plan in case no reliable proximal perforator exists.

The lower leg is circumferentially prepped and draped in a sterile fashion. A well-padded, sterile tourniquet is applied to the patient's distal thigh, just above the knee. The tourniquet should not be positioned at midthigh because this increases the chances of creating a venous tourniquet whereby the tourniquet compresses the femoral vein but not the femoral artery. A venous tourniquet results in increased, rather than decreased, bleeding during the dissection on tourniquet.

46.7 Operative Technique

Refer to Video 46.1 for an example of the operative technique for the fibula osteocutaneous free flap. The patient's leg is elevated and wrapped tightly from toes to above the knee with an Esmarch soft rubber bandage to expel venous blood from the limb (i.e., exsanguinate the lower leg).[6] With the Esmarch applied and the leg elevated, the tourniquet is inflated to 250 mm Hg for 120 minutes.

The Esmarch is then removed and the leg is returned to the heel support, so that it is again flexed at the knee and slightly internally rotated at the hip.

A longitudinal incision is made along the prior markings. Dissection is taken down through the subcutaneous fat to the deep crural fascia of the lateral leg overlying the lateral fascial compartment of the leg. The deep fascia is incised to enter the lateral compartment in the proximal third of the leg. Proper location of the fascial incision may be confirmed by passing a curved dissecting forceps anteriorly to feel the anterior crural septum. The tendon of the peroneus longus muscle is identified to also confirm that the lateral compartment has been entered. The deep fascia is then longitudinally incised along the entire length of the lateral compartment, taking care to identify and avoid injury to the superficial peroneal nerve in the distal lateral compartment. Although some surgeons favor a suprafascial dissection to the posterior crural septum before entering the lateral compartment in an effort to minimize donor morbidity of the fibula flap harvest, it is the author's preference to harvest the skin island with a subfascial dissection technique in order to avoid chance injury to the arborization of the septocutaneous perforator and thereby optimize perfusion of the overlying skin island (▶Fig. 46.3).

The peroneus longus and brevis muscles are then dissected anteriorly from the posterior crural septum (▶Fig. 46.4). The septocutaneous peroneal artery perforators are identified running up the posterior crural septum from the fibula to the overlying skin of the lateral lower leg. The peroneus longus and brevis muscles are then dissected from the lateral surface of the fibula from posterior to anterior. Care is taken to identify and avoid injury to the superficial peroneal nerve running in the lateral compartment. Dissection of the peroneus longus and brevis muscles from the lateral surface of the fibula continues from posterior to anterior along the length of the fibula until exposing the entire length of the anterior crural septum.

Dissection then continues along the superficial peroneal nerve until clearly identifying its proximal origin from the common peroneal nerve. At this origin from the common peroneal nerve, the deep peroneal nerve can be seen running with the anterior tibial vessels. The anterior tibial vessels and deep peroneal nerve traverse the interosseous membrane from the deep posterior fascial

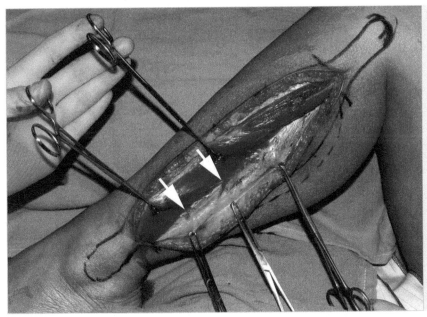

Fig. 46.3 The anterior border of the skin paddle is incised first and the posterior intermuscular septum is identified. Septocutaneous perforators are seen through the septum (*arrows*).

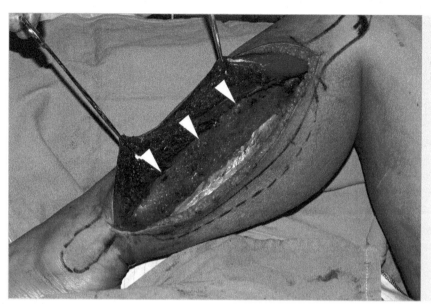

Fig. 46.4 The peroneus longus and brevis muscles are dissected off the fibula, exposing the anterior intermuscular septum (*arrowheads*).

compartment to the anterior fascial compartment.[6] Given that the popliteal artery first divides below the tibial plateau into the anterior tibial artery and tibioperoneal trunk, identifying the point at which the anterior tibial artery crosses the interosseous membrane marks the point just distal to which the proximal fibula osteotomy should be performed. Indeed, following this strategy guarantees maximal exposure of the origin of the peroneal artery and maximal length of the peroneal artery pedicle to the fibula flap. Placing the osteotomy just distal to the origin of the anterior tibial vessels exposes the tibioperoneal artery before it bifurcates laterally to the peroneal artery and medially to the posterior tibial artery. At this point in the dissection, a large right angle dissector is passed through the interosseous membrane and around the proximal fibula followed by a narrow copper malleable retractor to protect the underlying neurovascular structures when performing the proximal osteotomy.[6] Distally, a right angle is also passed through the interosseous membrane and around the fibula followed by a second narrow copper malleable just proximal to the strong, fibrotic, anterior tibiofibular ligament attaching the distal fibula to the fibular notch of the distal, lateral tibia (▶ **Fig. 46.5**).

The anterior crural septum is longitudinally divided to enter the anterior fascial compartment, exercising care as this structure is divided to not injure the anterior tibial vessels or deep peroneal nerve (▶ **Fig. 46.6**). The extensor digitorum and extensor hallucis muscles in the anterior compartment are the first muscles encountered in the anterior compartment and are dissected off the anterior surface of the fibula to expose the interosseous membrane. Now the distal and proximal osteotomies are performed with a sagittal oscillating saw or a Gigli flexible wire saw. The interosseous membrane, a structure that passes between the medial surface of the fibula and the lateral surface of the tibia, is then longitudinally divided to enter the deep posterior compartment. Dividing the interosseous membrane allows lateral traction on the fibula bone so that exposure of the remaining dissection of the medial and posterior attachments of the fibula is improved.

The first structure visualized deep to the interosseous membrane in the deep posterior compartment is the tibialis posterior muscle, characterized by its feather-like, bipennate muscle fibers organized along a medial raphe.[6] The peroneal artery lies lateral to this median raphe of the tibialis posterior muscle

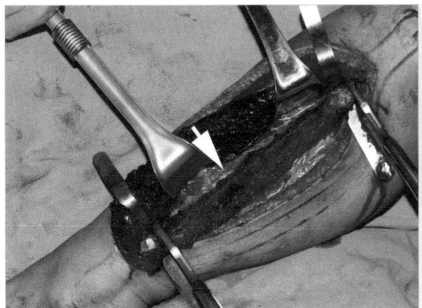

Fig. 46.5 After incising the anterior intermuscular septum, the extensor digitorum longus and extensor hallucis longus muscles are dissected off the fibula exposing the interosseous membrane (*arrow*). Malleable retractors are placed around the fibula bone in the locations of the planned superior and inferior osteotomies. The anterior tibial blood vessels are partially seen between the two large retractors holding the lateral and anterior compartment muscles.

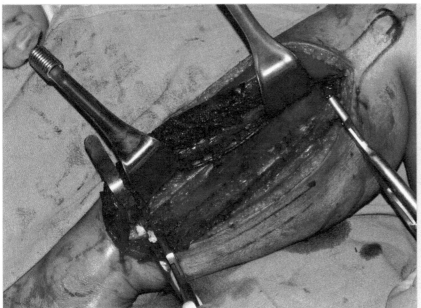

Fig. 46.6 After superior and inferior osteotomies are made, lateral traction is provided with bone clamps and the interosseous membrane is incised longitudinally. The tibialis posterior muscle is dissected from the fibula bone, exposing peroneal blood vessels. The distal peroneal blood vessels are ligated and divided.

and the posterior tibial artery lies medial to the median raphe. The peroneal artery also lies dorsal to the tibialis posterior muscle and ventral to the flexor hallucis longus muscle like the meat between two slices of bread. The tibialis posterior muscle is then dissected from distal to proximal along the leg off the peroneal artery and venae comitantes, with the line of dissection placed just medial to the vessels. Upon initiating this dissection, the peroneal artery is identified just distal to the distal fibular osteotomy, where it is ligated and divided. There are many muscular branches of the peroneal artery to the tibialis posterior muscle and flexor hallucis muscle, all of which should be meticulously ligated and divided, particularly in head and neck reconstructions, for any branch that is not controlled in the leg may later lead to a compressive, postoperative hematoma in the neck that can cause flap compromise.

Once the dorsal fascia of the tibialis posterior is divided, the peroneal artery is clearly visible in the deep posterior compartment, ventral to the flexor hallucis longus. The flexor hallucis longus is shorter than the tibialis posterior muscle, as it originates from the fibula around the proximal and middle thirds of the fibula. From the anterior approach, the flexor hallucis muscle can be completely dissected off the fibula if care is taken to stay ventral to the thin transverse intermuscular septum that divides the deep posterior compartment from the superficial posterior compartment.[6] The septocutaneous perforators originate from the peroneal artery just dorsal to the transverse intermuscular septum before wrapping posteriorly and then laterally to travel up the posterior crural septum to the lateral skin of the leg. To dissect the flexor hallucis longus off the posterior–medial surface of the fibula, the distal muscle fibers of this muscle are divided until reaching the avascular plane ventral to the transverse intermuscular septum. In this plane, a finger or curved dissector can be safely passed deep to the flexor hallucis muscle and the muscle divided, taking care to ligate and divide any muscular branches of the peroneal artery.[6]

The final stages of the fibula flap harvest involve detaching the proximal attachments of the soleus muscle from the proximal fibula and completing the skin island of the fibula flap. The posterior crural septum is longitudinally divided proximal to the septocutaneous perforator. The soleus muscle origins from the proximal fibula are divided, taking care to ligate and divide any muscle branches from the peroneal artery to the soleus muscle. Distally, the origin of the septocutaneous perforator is identified on the posterior medial fibula just dorsal (i.e., below) the transverse intermuscular septum.[6] The transverse intermuscular septum is then longitudinally divided to enter the superficial posterior compartment. Along the medial surface of the fibula, the septocutaneous perforators of the peroneal artery give off several small, delicate muscle branches to the lateral soleus muscle. These branches should be ligated and divided as close as possible to the point at which they enter the soleus muscle so as to avoid injury to the perforator itself.[6] The remainder of the lateral soleus is then dissected away from the fibula so that the undersurface of the deep fascia of the leg is visible. At this point the arborization of the septocutaneous peroneal artery perforator can be seen along the undersurface of the deep fascia of the leg.[6] Bone wax is applied to the distal and proximal cut surfaces of the fibula to facilitate hemostasis and the tourniquet is deflated. With experience, this entire dissection up to this point can be completed in less than 2 hours.

Now, all that remains to complete the harvest of the flap is to make the posterior skin incision, which requires completion of the recipient site resection (▶ Fig. 46.7). Once the recipient site resection is completed, a template of the skin island is made with a piece of the Esmarch tourniquet bandage and transferred to the fibula harvest site. A 5–0 polypropylene suture marks the skin location of the cutaneous Doppler signal overlying the peroneal artery septocutaneous perforator. The location of the perforator arborization on the undersurface of the deep fascia of the leg is transferred to the skin surrounding the 5–0 polypropylene marking the Doppler signal so as to capture as much of the perforasome as possible. The longitudinal incision on the lateral leg is then temporarily coapted with staples. The Esmarch template is centered over the cutaneous Doppler signal and marked borders of the perforasome. The posterior skin incision is then made to create the skin island of the fibula flap. The deep fascia is incised posteriorly and dissection proceeds deep to the fascia from posterior to anterior toward the posterior crural septum. The sural nerve and lesser saphenous vein should be identified, and every effort should be made to avoid injuring these structures when possible. Nevertheless, if these structures run through the middle of the skin island such that sparing them

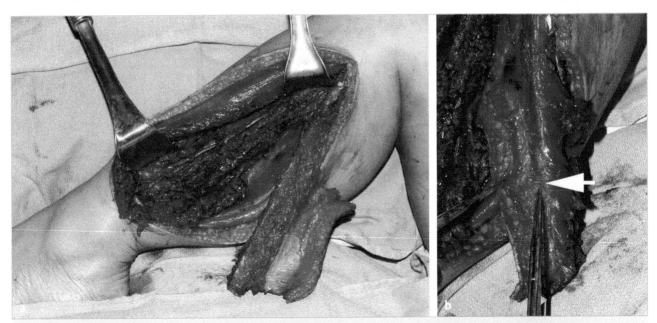

Fig. 46.7 Completed dissection. **(a)** The posterior tibial blood vessels are visible within the wound bed, medial to the cut edge of the flexor hallucis longus muscle. **(b)** The cutaneous perforating blood vessels are visible on the posterior surface of the posterior intermuscular septum seen in the close-up view (*arrow*).

might compromise the perfusion of the skin island, the author recommends sacrificing the sural nerve and lesser saphenous vein. Once the subfascial dissection of the skin island is completed, the flap is now entirely isolated on its vascular pedicle.

46.8 Donor Site Closure

The donor site is closed by placing a closed suction drain in the deep posterior compartment. The cut edge of the muscles of the lateral compartment are coapted to the cut edge of the muscles of the anterior compartment with interrupted absorbable sutures. The deep fascia of the leg is closed primarily proximal to the harvest site of the fibula skin island. The cut fascial edges surrounding the skin island donor site are circumferentially secured with absorbable suture to the superficial surface of the lateral compartment muscles. A split-thickness skin graft is harvested with a dermatome from the proximal lateral thigh (▶Fig. 46.8). The skin graft can be fenestrated and secured over the fibula flap skin island donor site with staples or sutures. A bolster is placed over the skin island to prevent shearing of the graft. The lower leg is then wrapped with soft sterile gauze followed by ACE wraps. The drain is placed to bulb suction. The leg is placed into a fixed-ankle fracture walking boot to minimize donor site pain in the immediate postoperative period and thereby encourage early patient mobilization.

46.9 Pearls and Pitfalls

- For mandible reconstruction, use the contralateral fibula to the mandibulectomy defect in order to place the skin island in the floor of the mouth, the vascular pedicle posteriorly, and the lateral surface of the fibula laterally for plating.

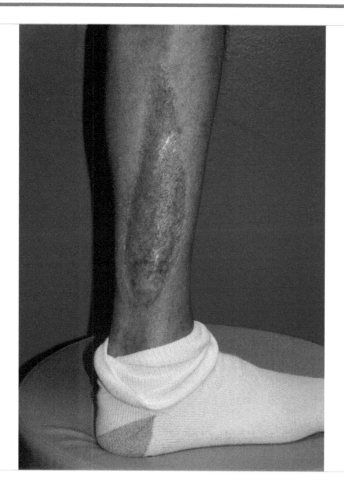

Fig. 46.8 Donor site appearance following osteocutaneous free flap harvest and donor site reconstruction with a split-thickness skin graft.

- For maxilla reconstruction, use the ipsilateral fibula to place the skin island intraorally for palatal resurfacing, the lateral surface of the fibula anteriorly for plating, and the pedicle posteriorly.
- Make your initial skin incision around the perforator at least 2 to 3 cm anterior to the posterior border of the fibula and the skin crease of the posterior crural septum to ensure capturing the perforasome, avoid injuring the septocutaneous perforator, and optimize perfusion of the skin island.
- Surgeons without sufficient experience in harvesting fibula flaps are discouraged from harvesting the skin island in the suprafascial plane. Until proficiency with fibula flap harvest is achieved, surgeons are encouraged to harvest the skin island in the subfascial plane.
- Trace the superficial peroneal nerve proximally to its origin from the common peroneal nerve. Clearly identifying these structures decreases the chances of inadvertently injuring them during flap harvest.
- Find the origin of the superficial peroneal nerve in order to clearly identify the deep peroneal nerve. The deep peroneal nerve runs with the anterior tibial vessels.
- Identify the point at which the anterior tibial vessels and deep peroneal nerve cross the interosseous membrane from the deep posterior compartment to the anterior compartment. This marks the location just distal to which the proximal fibula osteotomy should be placed. Doing this ensures maximal exposure of the peroneal artery origin from the tibioperoneal trunk and maximal flap pedicle length.

- The peroneal artery runs along the posterior–medial surface of the fibula, between the tibialis posterior muscle and the flexor hallucis muscle, like the meat between two slices of bread in a sandwich.
- Most of the fibula can be harvested on tourniquet from the anterior approach. This facilitates clear identification of the medial origin of the peroneal artery septocutaneous perforator in the superficial posterior compartment as it wraps around the fibula. Following this strategy makes injury to the perforator and problems with skin island perfusion very unlikely.
- Harvesting the majority of the fibula from the anterior approach improves the efficiency of the fibula flap harvest, as with experience the harvest can be completed in less than 2 hours on tourniquet. Thus, once the recipient site resection has been completed, there is little flap dissection left to complete other than the posterior skin incision of the skin island, allowing the entire reconstruction to be completed in a reasonable amount of time.
- Identify the arborization of the peroneal artery on the undersurface of the deep fascia of the leg from the superficial posterior compartment while still on tourniquet. Then transfer the limits of the visible perforasome to the overlying skin. This allows for optimal centering of the skin island over the perforasome and optimal perfusion of the fibula flap skin island.

References

[1] Taylor GIMG, Miller GD, Ham FJ. The free vascularized bone graft. A clinical extension of microvascular techniques. Plast Reconstr Surg 1975;55(5):533–544

[2] Adamo AK Sr, Szal RL. Timing, results, and complications of mandibular reconstructive surgery: report of 32 cases. J Oral Surg 1979;37(10):755–763

[3] Chen ZWYW, Yan W. The study and clinical application of the osteocutaneous flap of fibula. Microsurgery 1983;4(1):11–16

[4] Wei FCCH, Chen HC, Chuang CC, Noordhoff MS. Fibular osteoseptocutaneous flap: anatomic study and clinical application. Plast Reconstr Surg 1986;78(2):191–200

[5] Hidalgo DA. Fibula free flap: a new method of mandible reconstruction. Plast Reconstr Surg 1989;84(1):71–79

[6] Largo RDGP, Garvey PB. Updates in head and neck reconstruction. Plast Reconstr Surg 2018;141(2):271e–285e

[7] Chang EICM, Clemens MW, Garvey PB, Skoracki RJ, Hanasono MM. Cephalometric analysis for microvascular head and neck reconstruction. Head Neck 2012;34(11):1607–1614

[8] Garvey PBCE, Chang EI, Selber JC, et al. A prospective study of preoperative computed tomographic angiographic mapping of free fibula osteocutaneous flaps for head and neck reconstruction. Plast Reconstr Surg 2012;130(4):541e–549e

[9] Boyd JBCA, Caton AM, Mulholland RS, Tong L, Granzow JW. The sensate fibula osteocutaneous flap: neurosomal anatomy. J Plast Reconstr Aesthet Surg 2013;66(12):1688–1694

[10] Boyd JBCA, Caton AM, Mulholland RS, Granzow JW. The sensate fibular osteoneurocutaneous flap in oromandibular reconstruction: clinical outcomes in 31 cases. J Plast Reconstr Aesthet Surg 2013;66(12):1695–1701

[11] Anthony JPRE, Ritter EF, Young DM, Singer MI. Enhancing fibula free flap skin island reliability and versatility for mandibular reconstruction. Ann Plast Surg 1993;31(2):106–111

[12] Ribuffo D, Atzeni M, Saba L, et al. Clinical study of peroneal artery perforators with computed tomographic angiography: implications for fibular flap harvest. Surg Radiol Anat 2010;32(4):329–334

[13] Lykoudis EGKM, Koutsouris M, Lykissas MG. Vascular anatomy of the integument of the lateral lower leg: an anatomical study focused on cutaneous perforators and their clinical importance. Plast Reconstr Surg 2011;128(1):188–198

[14] Yu P, Chang EI, Hanasono MM. Design of a reliable skin paddle for the fibula osteocutaneous flap: perforator anatomy revisited. Plast Reconstr Surg 2011;128(2):440–446

[15] Winters HA, de Jongh GJ. Reliability of the proximal skin paddle of the osteocutaneous free fibula flap: a prospective clinical study. Plast Reconstr Surg 1999;103(3):846–849

47 Medial Plantar Artery Flap

Edward I. Chang

Abstract

The medial plantar artery perforator flap is an excellent option for reconstruction of plantar defects of the foot, but it has also been used as a free flap for more distant defects, including the contralateral foot or for replacing toe and finger pulp. The benefit of this flap is that it provides glabrous skin that is ideally suited for reconstruction of weight-bearing portions of the foot, such as the heel. In addition, the medial plantar artery flap also provides sensate skin that can provide protective sensation to the reconstructed area. Each step of the procedure involving the medial plantar artery flap is reviewed in this chapter, including typical indications, anatomy, preoperative considerations, operative technique, and donor site closure.

Keywords: medial plantar artery, posterior tibial artery, flexor digitorum brevis, abductor hallucis muscles, medial plantar nerve

47.1 Introduction

The medial plantar artery perforator flap is an excellent option for reconstruction of plantar defects of the foot, but it has also been described as a free flap for more distant defects including the contralateral foot or for replacement of toe and finger pulp. The benefit of the medial plantar artery flap is that the flap provides glabrous skin that is ideally suited for reconstruction of weight-bearing portions of the foot such as the heel. In addition, the medial plantar artery flap also provides sensate skin that can provide protective sensation to the reconstructed area.[1,2]

47.2 Typical Indications

- Heel defects resulting from trauma, oncologic resection, or ulcers can easily be reconstructed with the medial plantar artery flap, but requires skin grafting to the donor site unless the defect is 2 cm or less in width.
- The medial plantar artery perforator flap can be harvested as a free flap to provide glabrous skin for reconstruction of defects of the foot, toes, hands, or fingers.

47.3 Anatomy

The skin flap is supplied by the **medial plantar artery**, a branch of the **posterior tibial artery**, which is one of the two terminal branches of the tibial–peroneal trunk. The medial plantar artery arises between the **flexor digitorum brevis** and **abductor hallucis muscles** and is typically smaller than the lateral plantar artery (▶ **Fig. 47.1**).[3,4] The artery is accompanied by small venae comitantes. Additionally, cutaneous veins may also drain the flap and may be of larger diameter than the venae comitantes and could be used instead when the flap is utilized as a free flap. The **medial plantar nerve**, which provides sensation to the flap, travels with the artery and is one of the distal branches of the posterior tibial nerve. The medial plantar nerve divides distally into branches supplying the great toe.[5]

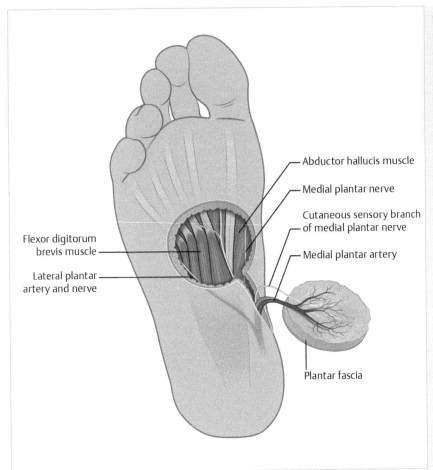

Fig. 47.1 Anatomical depiction of the plantar aspect of the foot demonstrating the medial plantar artery arises between the flexor digitorum brevis and abductor hallucis muscles.

Abductor hallucis muscle

Medial plantar nerve

Cutaneous sensory branch of medial plantar nerve

Medial plantar artery

Flexor digitorum brevis muscle

Lateral plantar artery and nerve

Plantar fascia

47.4 Variations

The use of a distally based medial plantar artery flap has also been described as this is supplied by retrograde blood flow through the medial plantar artery.

47.5 Preoperative Considerations

All patients should undergo a thorough vascular examination prior to considering a medial plantar flap paying particular attention to the runoff to the foot. Vascular studies such as an ankle–brachial index, Doppler and ultrasound flow studies, and potentially an angiogram may be warranted. Defects that result from trauma may often warrant an angiogram to evaluate the vasculature and perfusion to the foot. The medial plantar artery is a branch of the posterior tibial artery, so injury to the posterior tibial artery precludes the use of the medial plantar flap as a reconstructive option. Similarly, for diabetic and vascular ulcers, a diseased posterior tibial artery would also be a contraindication to a medial plantar artery flap.

47.6 Positioning and Skin Markings

The medial plantar artery flap is elevated without the use of a tourniquet so that the cutaneous perforator can be identified and the perfusion of the flap can be assessed during the flap elevation. It is helpful to have a pillow to elevate the heel and foot paying careful attention to avoid any pressure to the leg.

A hand-held Doppler is used in order to identify the perforator from the medial plantar artery, and the flap should be centered along the axis of the perforator.

The metatarsal head of the great toe should be marked as this is a weight-bearing surface and the flap should not extend to the metatarsal head. Ideally, the distal margin of the flap should not extend beyond one centimeter proximal to the metatarsal head. The medial aspect of the flap should not extend onto the dorsum of the foot and is generally defined by the plane of the navicular bone. The lateral/plantar margin of the flap is defined by the midline of the foot. While the flap can extend beyond the midline, this becomes more a random pattern flap because lateral plantar artery supplies the skin lateral to the midline.

47.7 Operative Technique

After the patient is prepped, a hand-held Doppler is used to identify the main perforator of the medial plantar artery supplying the flap. The flap is designed within the instep of the foot centered over the main perforator. The lateral/plantar margin of the flap is incised first, and the dissection proceeds in a subfascial plane. The perforator can be identified arising from between the flexor digitorum brevis and abductor hallucis muscles. The perforator can be traced to the main pedicle, which is in turn dissected proximally between the muscles in order to gain more length on the pedicle. The abductor hallucis muscle may be quite diminutive and can be sacrificed in order to maximize the pedicle length. The medial/dorsal flap incision is made once the perforator has been isolated, and dissection again proceeds down through the fascia. If a substantial cutaneous vein is encountered, it may be preserved if it does not limit the arc of rotation to improve venous drainage of the flap, since the venae comitantes are quite small. As mentioned above, a cutaneous vein may be larger and easier to use as the draining vein when the medial plantar artery flap is used as a free flap. The remaining margins of the flap are incised, and the flap is then elevated from distal to proximal (▶ Fig. 47.2).

47.8 Donor Site Closure

The donor site is along the instep of the foot, which is a nonweight-bearing surface of the foot. The donor site defect is easily resurfaced with a full- or split-thickness skin graft that can be harvested if primary closure is not achievable (▶ Fig. 47.3). The leg should be kept elevated and the patient should be maintained in a nonweight-bearing status until the skin graft has had adequate time to heal. A dangling protocol is recommended before the patient is mobilized and allowed to ambulate.

47.9 Pearls and Pitfalls

- The distal extent of the medial plantar flap should never extend onto the weight-bearing surface of the foot, so the dissection should never proceed to within 1 cm of the metatarsal head.
- A hand-held Doppler ultrasound is useful to identify the location of the perforator so the flap can be centered over the flap. The abductor hallucis muscle can be divided in order to increase the arc rotation of the flap.

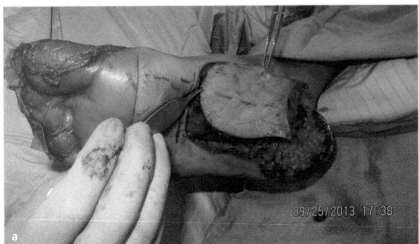

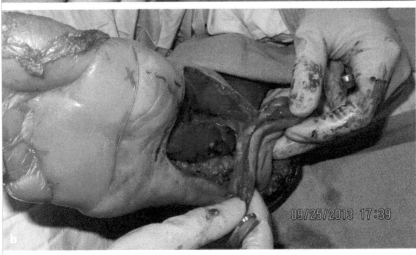

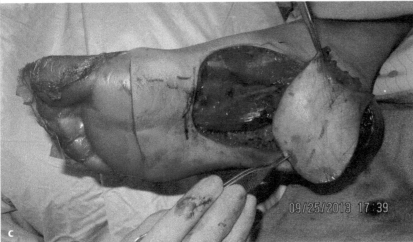

Fig. 47.2 **(a)** Medial plantar artery perforator flap elevated based on medial plantar artery, which is a branch of the posterior tibial artery. A hand-held Doppler ultrasound is helpful in localizing the perforator. **(b)** The pedicle is visualized arising between the flexor digitorum brevis and abductor hallucis muscles. **(c)** Flap inset following rotation of the flap also demonstrating the donor site that will be skin grafted.

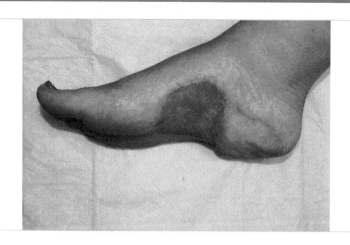

Fig. 47.3 Postoperative photo with skin graft to the donor site and excellent contour of the flap.

References

[1] Shanahan RE, Gingrass RP. Medial plantar sensory flap for coverage of heel defects. Plast Reconstr Surg 1979;64(3):295–298

[2] Yang D, Yang JF, Morris SF, Tang M, Nie C. Medial plantar artery perforator flap for soft-tissue reconstruction of the heel. Ann Plast Surg 2011;67(3):294–298

[3] Koshima I, Narushima M, Mihara M, et al. Island medial plantar artery perforator flap for reconstruction of plantar defects. Ann Plast Surg 2007;59(5):558–562

[4] Duman H, Er E, Işík S, et al. Versatility of the medial plantar flap: our clinical experience. Plast Reconstr Surg 2002;109(3):1007–1012

[5] Baker GL, Newton ED, Franklin JD. Fasciocutaneous island flap based on the medial plantar artery: clinical applications for leg, ankle, and forefoot. Plast Reconstr Surg 1990;85(1):47–58, discussion 59–60

Part 8

Lymphedema

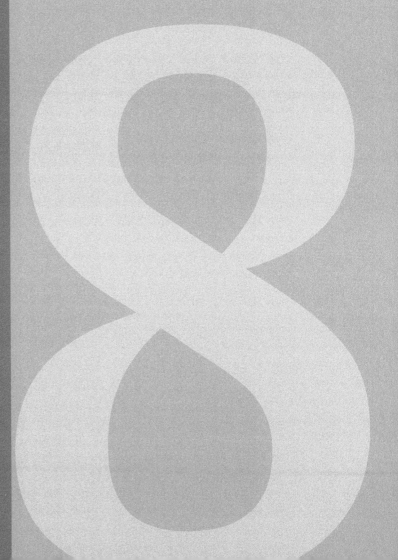

48 Supraclavicular Lymph Node Transfer

Martin J. Carney and Suhail K. Kanchwala

Abstract

Lymphedema following oncologic surgery can be a debilitating condition for patients. Often, the upper or lower extremities will be affected, thus creating a daily functional hindrance. Some sequelae of secondary lymphedema include predisposition for infection, pain, swelling, pitting edema, and chronic skin changes. Conservative means of treatment include garment compression and decompressive massage, which must occur each day. Vascularized lymph node transfer represents a potential cure for iatrogenic lymphedema. The reconstruction consists of a free flap harvested with lymph nodes connected to a known vascular outflow, which is then transferred to the affected limb using a microsurgical technique. An ideal vascularized lymph node transfer flap should be accessible with a low risk of donor site morbidity, have sufficient pedicle length, and a donor site scar that can be easily hidden. The supraclavicular lymph node flap may meet all of these functional requirements. This flap consists of vascularized tissue containing cervical lymph nodes. A worthy consideration for any use of this flap is the status of the donor site following removal of lymph tissue. Groin tissue appears to have higher counts of lymph nodes, but they hold a much greater risk of secondary lymphedema or lymphorrhea at the site of harvest. The supraclavicular lymph node transfer flap remains a workhorse flap for vascularized lymph node transfer. It consists of a readily concealable donor site and most likely has the lowest risk of secondary lymphedema at the donor site when compared to the other flaps currently in practice. Its consistent anatomy has clear nodal tissue and can be offered to moderately obese patients with reasonable outcomes. This chapter reviews each step of the reconstructive procedure. Typical indications are listed, followed by a discussion of anatomy, the preoperative considerations, the surgical technique, and finally, donor site closure. Two variations to the procedure are mention.

Keywords: vascularized lymph node transfer, supraclavicular lymph node flap, subclavian vein, accessory thoracic duct, thoracic duct, transverse cervical artery, supraclavicular sensory nerves

48.1 Introduction

Lymphedema following oncologic surgery can be a debilitating disease state for patients. Often the upper or lower extremities will be affected creating a daily functional hindrance. Some sequelae of secondary lymphedema include predisposition for infection, pain, swelling, pitting edema, and chronic skin changes. Conservative means of treatment include garment compression and decompressive massage which must occur each day. **Vascularized lymph node transfer** (VLNT) represents a potential cure for iatrogenic lymphedema. VLNT consists of a free flap harvested with lymph nodes connected to a known vascular outflow, which is then transferred to the affected limb using a microsurgical technique. An ideal VLNT flap should be accessible with low risk of donor site morbidity, have sufficient pedicle length, and a donor site scar that can be easily hidden. The **supraclavicular lymph node** flap (SCL) might meet all of these functional requirements. SCL was first described in 2012 by Becker et al and consisted of vascularized tissue containing cervical lymph nodes.[1] A worthy consideration for any area of VLNT is the status of the donor site following removal of lymph tissue. Groin tissue appears to have higher counts of lymph nodes, but hold a much greater risk of secondary lymphedema or **lymphorrhea** at the site of harvest. The SCL remains a workhorse flap for VLNT, consists of a readily concealable donor site, and most likely has the lowest risk of secondary lymphedema at the donor site when compared to the other flaps currently in practice.[2] In our experience, the SCL maintains consistent anatomy, has clear nodal tissue, and can be offered to moderately obese patients with reasonable outcomes.

48.2 Typical Indications

- Secondary lymphedema of the extremities after oncologic procedures (lymph node dissection or lymphadenectomy).

48.3 Anatomy

The target pocket of lymph nodes lies in the subcutaneous fatty tissue which overlies important neurovascular structures in the supraclavicular region. Lymph nodes in this area belong to the cervical grouping and primarily drain the thyroid, lung, esophagus, and breast tissue. Outflow of lymphatics coalesces into either the **subclavian vein** through the **accessory thoracic duct** (right) or the **thoracic duct** (left) (▶ **Fig. 48.1**).[3] This proximity and connection to the thoracic duct make the right SCL preferable to harvest in all scenarios except for right upper extremity lymphedema.

The dominant blood supply of the SCL comes from a dominant perforating vessel arising from the **transverse cervical artery** (TCA). This arterial supply most often originates from the thyrocervical trunk (▶ **Fig. 48.2**). Variant TCA can originate in different areas, however, including at the subclavian artery, which can be seen in up to 25% of patients. The perforating artery usually resides at the medial portion of the clavicle and in between the sternocleidomastoid muscle and the external jugular vein (EJV). This flap can be harvested with or without overlying skin paddle depending on the soft tissue needs of the recipient site. The transverse cervical vein accompanies the artery and is one of two drainage sources used for the flap. Our experience preferentially selects two venous outflows to maximize lymphovenous output from the SCL in the affected area.

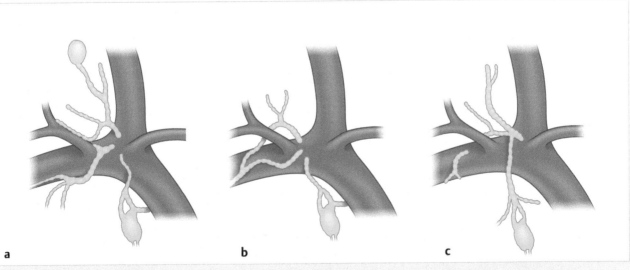

Fig. 48.1 (a-c) Variations in the cervical lymph node anatomy in the supraclavicular flap.

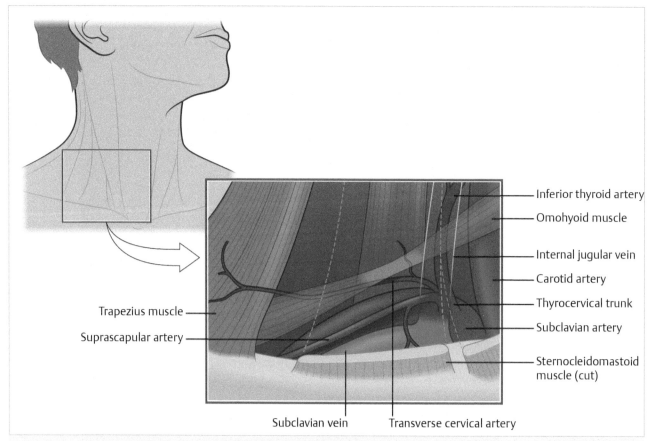

Fig. 48.2 Vascular anatomy of the supraclavicular lymph node flap and overlying skin.

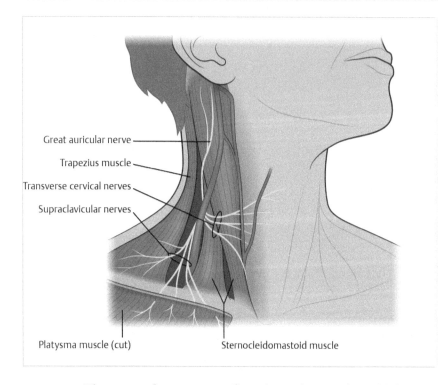

Fig. 48.3 Superficial nerves of the supraclavicular lymph node flap which must be sacrificed during dissection and may result in numbness and paresthesia.

The second venous outflow is to the EJV, in which the inferior portion creates a second viable output.

Cervical nerves arising from C3 and C4 are present directly below the platysma and are known as **supraclavicular sensory nerves** (▶Fig. 48.3). This structure can be sacrificed in order to continue dissection deep toward pedicle exposure. Just below the critical vascular structures and flap lie the phrenic nerve, spinal accessory nerve, and nerves of the brachial plexus within fascial investment. These vital structures should not be damaged or exposed prior to donor site closure.

48.4 Variations

- Supraclavicular lymph node flap with skin island.
- Supraclavicular lymph node flap without skin island.

48.5 Preoperative Considerations

Establishing guidelines for operative candidates is important in the surgical management of lymphedema. Patients must be diagnosed with secondary lymphedema, a known origin, and have been cancer free for at least 3 to 5 years. Additionally, 6 months of conservative therapy should be employed to attempt circumference reduction of the affected extremity. Surgical management should be considered if therapy has plateaued or failed. Patient history should be focused on discerning the origin of secondary lymphedema and also take into account the location of the problem currently. The side of harvest is dependent on previous head and neck surgery as well as, if upper extremity, which arm is affected. Physical examination of the area should note important anatomical landmarks such as the clavicle, sternocleidomastoid, and EJV. No imaging for preoperative evaluation of the donor site is necessary.[4] **Lymphoscintigraphy** of the affected limb as well as intraoperative **indocyanine green** (ICG) can be used to assess the lymphatic channels and accurately plan for the most effective recipient site.

48.6 Positioning and Skin Markings

The SCL harvest is done with the patient in the supine position and head tilted away from the operative site. This head positioning allows for greater exposure of the harvest area. The lateral aspect of the sternocleidomastoid muscle and the EJV are marked prior to planning the flap size. Next, a transversely oriented skin paddle (~ 7 × 3 cm) is drawn superior to the clavicle (▶ Fig. 48.4). The sternocleidomastoid is overlapped and the skin paddle should be centered over the EJV tracings.[5] The lymph nodes harvested are contained within the fat pockets deep to these tracings and the exact bundle location densities are still not agreed upon. In our experience, the tissue in the lateral portion of these

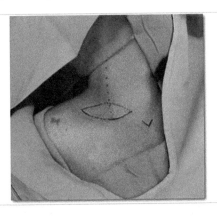

Fig. 48.4 Preoperative markings of the supraclavicular lymph node flap.

tracings holds the highest node density and we have now changed our dissection pattern from the traditional lateral approach to now starting medially and working laterally.

48.7 Operative Technique

Descriptions have historically begun the dissection from a lateral approach; however, we now begin by moving the skin paddle slightly more medially and dissect laterally. We believe the majority of nodes are lateral to the TCA and reversing the dissection plane might help preserve vasculature to the target nodes. First an inferior and medial incision is created along the lines previously marked. The goal at the onset is to remove all nodes en bloc and cause the least amount of disturbance to the vascular and lymphatic channels. Next, the platysma is carefully transected. The incision is then taken down through the subcutaneous fatty tissue located above the clavicle, which helps to elevate and reflect the flap superiorly while identifying the pedicle. A superficial vein can be identified at this tissue plane and should be preserved if possible. The flap is raised medially through the platysma and will eventually expose the lateral portion of the sternocleidomastoid. Once through the platysma, the supraclavicular sensory nerves are seen and divided. Some descriptions note that these nerve ends can be buried separately and deep in the harvested pocket in order to prevent neuroma formation. Next, the lateral sternocleidomastoid is retracted away or divided with a small portion left on the flap and increasing operative exposure. The **omohyoid muscle** crosses the field in a transverse fashion and can then be elevated superiorly and divided. This division allows for even further exposure underneath the elevated flap.

At this point, the TCA and transverse cervical vein should be carefully dissected out. These vessels run transversely and can be traced back to the thyrocervical trunk as well as the internal jugular vein (►Fig. 48.5). If the TCA is very small, the surgeon must optimize the pedicle length by ligating other branches off the thyrocervical trunk such as the ascending cervical and inferior thyroid vessels. The vasculature overlies the anterior scalene muscle and should be bluntly raised off of this plane. After completed elevation, vital neurovascular structures including the phrenic nerve, spinal accessory nerves, and superior portion of the brachial plexus should be notably intact and undamaged. The incision can be completed on the superior portion of the flap and the EJV is dissected out to be harvested as well. The EJV can be clipped superiorly and prepared for

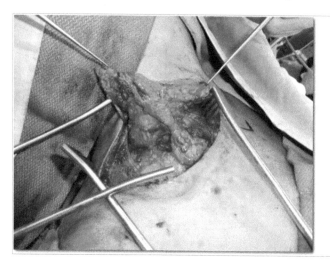

Fig. 48.5 Superior elevation of the supraclavicular lymph node flap exposing the underlying vasculature.

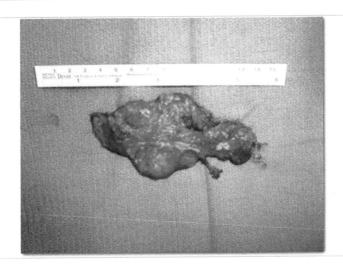

Fig. 48.6 Supraclavicular lymph node flap harvest completed and entire flap removed prior to implantation within the affected limb.

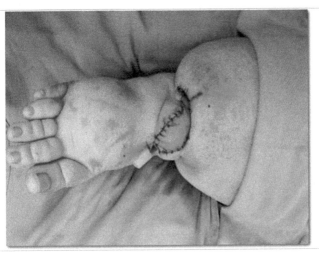

Fig. 48.7 Supraclavicular lymph node flap inset with end-to-end anastomosis of transverse cervical artery to dorsalis pedis artery. The venous anastomoses consisted of transverse cervical vein to the dorsalis pedis vena comitantes and external jugular vein to a local superficial vein both in an end-to-end manner.

anastomosis on the inferior end. The TCA pedicle should be followed laterally back to the thyrocervical trunk where it can then be divided. All of the fat in the 3- to 4-cm radius should be taken with the EJV and transverse cervical vein in order to cause minimal disruption to the target nodes (▶ Fig. 48.6).

Medial-to-lateral dissection and en bloc fat pocket harvest have decreased operative time at our institution. Two venous anastomoses at the affected site are often preferred for greater extrusion of interstitial fluid. Upper extremity patients can have the flap placed in the axilla, elbow, or wrist. Similarly, for lower extremity patients the flap can be inset in the groin, popliteal fossa, or dorsum of the ankle (▶ Fig. 48.7).

48.8 Donor Site Closure

With meticulous dissection, the donor site should be ready for immediate primary closure. A drain can be placed laterally in the dissected plan and exit that in the same direction. Care should be taken to avoid proximity of the drain to vital structures. Next, the platysma can be approximated with absorbable interrupted sutures and the skin closed with a running subcuticular suture. Donor site lymphedema following the operation should be minimal and standard microvascular postoperative procedure should ensue. The scar should be well hidden within relaxed skin tension lines running through the supraclavicular fossa.

References

[1] Becker C, Vasile JV, Levine JL, et al. Microlymphatic surgery for the treatment of iatrogenic lymphedema. Clin Plast Surg 2012;39(4):385–398

[2] Steinbacher J, Tinhofer IE, Meng S, et al. The surgical anatomy of the supraclavicular lymph node flap: a basis for the free vascularized lymph node transfer. J Surg Oncol 2017;115(1):60–62

[3] Mardonado AA, Chen R, Chang DW. The use of supraclavicular free flap with vascularized lymph node transfer for treatment of lymphedema: a prospective study of 100 consecutive cases. J Surg Oncol 2017;115(1):68–71

[4] Ooi AS, Chang DW. 5-step harvest of supraclavicular lymph nodes as vascularized free tissue transfer for treatment of lymphedema. J Surg Oncol 2017;115(1):63–67

[5] Gerety PA, Pannucci CJ, Basta MN, et al. Lymph node content of supraclavicular and thoracodorsal-based axillary flaps for vascularized lymph node transfer. J Vasc Surg Venous Lymphat Disord 2016;4(1):80–87

49 Inguinal Lymph Node Transfer

Deana Shenaq and David W. Chang

Abstract

The most recent development in the treatment of lymphedema is the free tissue transfer of vascularized lymph nodes, which has been shown to have a greater degree of improvement in lymphedema than nonvascularized grafting. In this procedure, healthy lymph nodes are harvested from one region and transferred to another—either to the original site of injury (i.e., axilla or groin) or within a lymphedematous limb (e.g., wrist or ankle). One theory postulates that orthotopically transplanted lymph nodes act as a sponge to absorb lymph fluid and direct it into the vascular network, whereas another theory believes the transfer of vascularized lymph nodes induces angiogenesis. Lymph node donor sites include the groin, thorax, submental or supraclavicular areas, omentum, and mesentery. Vascularized lymph node transfer utilizing inguinal lymph nodes can be combined with microvascular breast reconstruction or be performed alone for the treatment of lymphedema. In this chapter, the authors set forth the critical steps in this reconstructive procedure, beginning with typical indications, anatomy, preoperative considerations, surgical technique, and ending with donor site closure. Two variations to the procedure are cited.

Keywords: superficial circumflex iliac artery, superficial inferior epigastric artery

49.1 Introduction

The most recent development in the treatment of lymphedema is the free tissue transfer of vascularized lymph nodes, which has been shown to have a greater degree of improvement in lymphedema than nonvascularized grafting. Vascularized lymph node transfer (VLNT) was first pioneered successfully in an animal model in 1979 and used clinically for a patient by Clodius et al in 1982.[1] In this procedure, healthy lymph nodes are harvested from one region and transferred to another, either to the original site of injury (i.e., axilla or groin) or within a lymphedematous limb (e.g., wrist or ankle). Becker et al presented one of the first series of vascularized groin lymph node free flaps for the treatment of upper extremity lymphedema.[2] One theory postulates that orthotopically transplanted lymph nodes act as a sponge to absorb lymph fluid and direct it into the vascular network, while another theory hypothesizes that transfer of vascularized lymph nodes induces angiogenesis. Lymph node donor sites described include the groin, thorax, submental or supraclavicular areas, omentum, and mesentery. VLNT utilizing inguinal lymph nodes can be combined with microvascular breast reconstruction or performed alone for the treatment of lymphedema.

49.2 Typical Indications

- Lymphedema of upper and lower extremity.
- Upper extremity lymphedema in combination with breast reconstruction.

49.3 Anatomy

The lower anterior abdominal free flap blood supply is derived from the deep inferior epigastric artery (DIEA) originating from the external iliac artery. The groin is one of the most popular donor sites for the harvest of vascularized lymph nodes, and anatomical studies have shown that their blood supply is reliably based on the **superficial circumflex iliac artery**, and the **superficial inferior epigastric artery**, both of which are branches of the femoral artery.

Inguinal lymph nodes are found in five different regions: central (saphenofemoral junction), superomedial, superolateral, inferomedial, and inferolateral. The nodes that drain the lower limb are located medially and centrally, and therefore, harvesting the laterally based nodes that drain the suprailiac region (superolateral region) is advisable to avoid ipsilateral donor site lymphedema. Although some debate persists regarding the safety for harvesting medial nodes, there is a general consensus that preserving the deeper lymphatics and nodes inferior to the inguinal ligament is paramount (▶ **Fig. 49.1**).

49.4 Variations

- Vascularized lymph node transfer in conjunction with autologous breast reconstruction with an abdominally based free flap for upper extremity lymphedema.
- Vascularized inguinal lymph node transfer alone for either upper or lower extremity lymphedema.

49.5 Preoperative Considerations

The ideal candidate for free lymph node transfer is one with moderate secondary lymphedema who is compliant with physical therapy and is committed to continued extremity wrapping or garment wearing postoperatively. Overweight patients are encouraged to lose weight so that their preoperative BMI is at least less than 35. The authors advocate for patients to be out of bed and ambulating on postoperative day 1, and thus, those patients who are nonambulatory preoperatively are often not considered surgical candidates.

During the initial consultation, based on a patient's clinical stage of lymphedema stage, a recommendation is made to proceed with surgery the following options of lymphovenous bypass (LVB) alone, VLNT, or combination of both. LVB alone is usually reserved for those patients with mild lymphedema. For severe lymphedema, debulking may be necessary (▶ **Table 49.1**). If a patient is undergoing VLNT in conjunction with autologous breast reconstruction, we do not perform LVB concurrently to avoid a lengthy surgery, but instead, usually complete this at a secondary procedure as early as 3 months later.

Preoperatively, each patient is evaluated by a lymphedema therapist, who performs a quantitative volumetric and qualitative analysis of the limb and symptoms. Patients are then also evaluated at 3, 6, and 12 months postoperatively for signs of improvement. Typically, preoperative lymphoscintigraphy studies are not performed on patients with secondary lymphedema from a known cause. Patients who present with primary lymphedema always undergo confirmatory lymphoscintigraphy preoperatively to document lymphatic dysfunction.

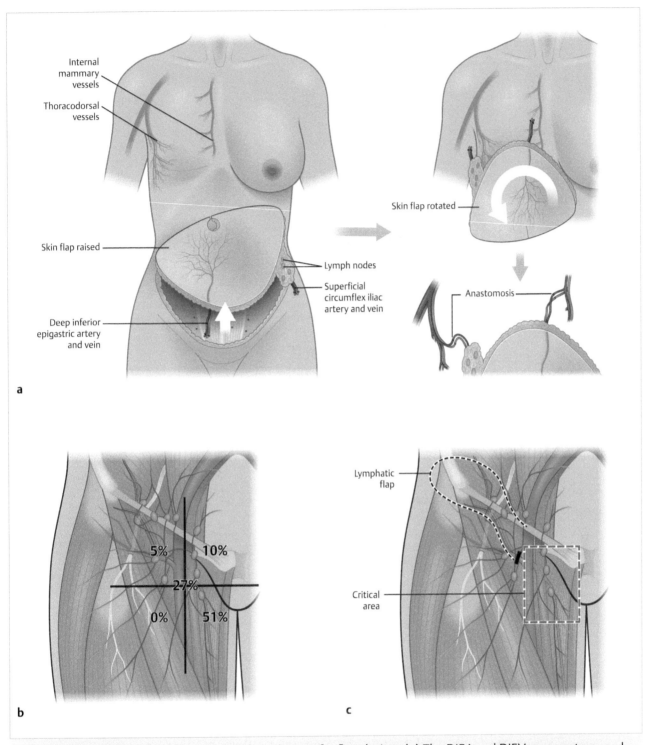

Fig. 49.1 Contralateral vascularized lymph node transfer flap design. **(a)** The DIEA and DIEV are anastomosed to the IMA and IMV, whereas the lymph nodes are placed in the axilla and anastomosed to available vessels in the axilla. **(b)** These drawings depict methods of preserving the lymphatic vascular function of the lower limb. Location of the sentinel lymph nodes draining the lower limb by van der Ploeg et al. **(c)** Recommended lymphatic flap design.

Table 49.1 Surgical recommendations for the treatment of lymphedema based on clinical stage

Clinical stage	Surgical recommendations
I (mild)	LVB alone
II (mild–moderate)	VLNT alone or VLNT + LVB
III (moderate)	VLNT + LVB
IV (severe)	Charles' procedure Debulking

Abbreviations: LVB, lymphovenous bypass; VLNT, vascularized lymph node transfer.

49.6 Positioning and Skin Markings

The patient is positioned supine and prepped from the supraclavicular region down to the mons. The lymphedematous limb, including the axilla if targeting upper extremity lymphedema, is also prepped into the field. If performing inguinal lymph node transfer in conjunction with breast reconstruction, typically the patient's abdomen is marked in the preoperative area to assess the amount of abdominal tissue that can be safely harvested to ensure adequate primary donor site closure. The transverse abdominal incision is located slightly lower than the normal DIEP/MS-TRAM (deep inferior epigastric pedicle/muscle-sparing transverse rectus myocutaneous) flap incision to capture inguinal lymph nodes with the abdominal flap. In the chest, the prior mastectomy incision is utilized to gain access to the internal mammary vessels, which will serve as recipient vessels. The incision is widened in order to adequately expose the axilla and completely resect any fibrotic scar resulting from prior surgeries or radiation.

49.7 Operative Technique

For postmastectomy patients with lymphedema, a low transverse abdominal flap containing lymph nodes and lymphatic vessels is a convenient option for simultaneous breast reconstruction and lymphedema treatment.[3,4] The blood supply is based on the DIEP, and lymph nodes are harvested en bloc with the abdominal flap along the superficial circumflex iliac or superficial inferior epigastric vessels.

In general, for patients undergoing unilateral breast reconstruction in conjunction with VLNT, an ipsilateral abdominal flap is preferred with the lymph node flap oriented contralateral to the mastectomy defect. The VLNT is perfused via the abdominal flap pedicle (AFP) and an additional arterial anastomosis is unnecessary; however, an extra venous anastomosis is always performed in the axilla. The lateral thoracic, serratus branch or circumflex scapular vessels are excellent options for VLNT recipient veins. The AFP flap is oriented ipsilateral to the mastectomy defect, and the breast flap is rotated 180 degrees to be anastomosed to the internal mammary vessels so that the VLNT can be placed in the axilla.

Abdominal flap dissection begins in the typical fashion with a low transverse incision and preparation of lymphatic tissue from the groin. Care should be taken not to violate the deep inguinal lymphatic system and the inguinal ligament in order to prevent lymphatic dysfunction at the donor limb. To avoid precipitating donor site lymphedema, we routinely employ reverse mapping to identify the sentinel lymph nodes critical for lower extremity drainage, which is similar to the mapping technique used by breast surgeons to identify sentinel nodes during axillary node dissections.[5] Preoperatively, technetium is injected into the first and second webspaces of the foot on the side of planned inguinal donor site. The technetium ideally travels to the sentinel draining nodes in the groin. An intraoperative gamma probe/Geiger counter is used to detect the sentinel inguinal lymph node(s) to avoid removing them with the abdominal flap (►Fig. 49.2). To further target nodes for harvest, Dayan et al inject 0.2 mL of indocyanine green intradermally in four locations along a line 5 cm superior and parallel to the inguinal ligament.[5] Utilizing the SPY Elite (LifeCell Corp., Branchburg, NJ) near-infrared fluorescence technology, they perform lymphangiography to simultaneously identify draining truncal nodes, targeted for harvest or inclusion with the abdominal flap. One potential pitfall of harvesting any lymph node flap is the development of donor site seroma or lymph leak. In order to avoid this, careful surgical dissection with loupe magnification is needed, with meticulous clipping of lymphatic vessels feeding the donor lymph nodes. We have found that clipping the lymphatic vessels rather than indiscriminate use of electrocautery leads to fewer issues with postoperative lymph leaks or seromas.

Once the lymph node bundle to be transplanted is identified, dissection continues until the superficial inferior epigastric and circumflex iliac veins (SIEV and SCIV) are reached. These nodes are surrounded by and identified within fatty tissue and found within the superficial inguinal basin, located lateral to the SIEV and superior to the inguinal ligament. The groin flap is elevated from lateral to the medial at the level of the muscular aponeurosis and is connected to the DIEP/MS-TRAM flap at the level of the superficial epigastric vessel pedicle. The superficial circumflex iliac or epigastric veins should be dissected circumferentially and ligated at their origin to ensure adequate pedicle length (►Fig. 49.3). The abdominal flap is then elevated per routine.

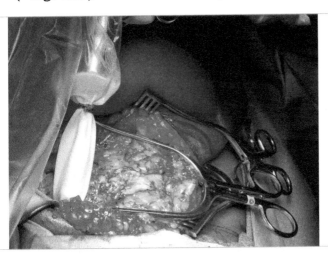

Fig. 49.2 An intraoperative gamma probe/Geiger meter counter is used to detect the sentinel inguinal lymph node(s) to avoid removing them with the abdominal flap.

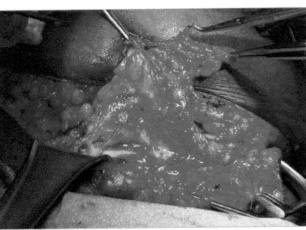

Fig. 49.3 The inguinal lymph nodes after they have been harvested with the superficial circumflex iliac vein. This patient underwent VLNT in conjunction with free flap breast reconstruction.

A two-team approach is used for simultaneous recipient site preparation. This begins with extensive axillary scar resection and release, which is widely agreed upon as an important component to ensuring successful lymph node transfer and subsequent symptom alleviation. Wide excision is performed to remove all fibrotic scar until healthy adipose tissue is reached, typically at the level of the axillary or thoracodorsal vessels. Lysis of the scar and adhesions in the axilla is necessary also for identification of a recipient vein for the vascularized lymph nodes. The thoracodorsal, serratus, or lateral thoracic veins are used if available. We prefer to couple the recipient vein with the SCIV or SIEV on the abdominal flap if possible; otherwise, the veins are handsewn.

Microanastomosis between the inferior epigastric and internal mammary vessels is usually performed prior to venous anastomosis in the axilla. Dissection of the internal mammary vessels is typically performed in the third intercostal space with removal of a segment of the rib cartilage if necessary, but we typically use a rib-sparing approach.

49.8 Donor Site Closure

The abdominal donor site is closed as in any standard DIEP or MS-TRAM flap. Typically, two drains are placed in the abdomen, and one is tunneled adjacent to the area where the inguinal flap was taken in order to close off dead space in this area. Care must be taken to avoid creating a volume deficit in the groin where the lymph nodes were taken, by ensuring that subcutaneous fat from upper abdominal flap and surrounding areas fills in this region.

49.9 Pearls and Pitfalls

- In order to avoid precipitating donor site lymphedema, take care to harvest only the superficial inguinal lymph nodes located medial to the SIEV and superior to the inguinal ligament. Reverse lymph node mapping of the inguinal region can aid with identifying the sentinel draining nodes of the lower limb to avoid removing them with the groin flap.
- During dissection of the inguinal lymph node flap, clip any lymphatic vessels, rather than cauterize, in order to avoid lymphatic damage and lymph leaks in the groin.
- When combined with breast reconstruction, the vascularized lymph nodes can survive off the deep inferior epigastric pedicle, but we recommend additional venous drainage based on the superficial system with anastomosis to the thoracodorsal vein, or a branch thereof, in the axilla.
- Extensive recipient site scar resection and release is necessary to ensure an adequate recipient bed and facilitate the identification of recipient vessels.
- In order to maximize results, patients must remain compliant with lymphedema therapy postoperatively, including continued wear of compression garments.

References

[1] Clodius L, Smith PJ, Bruna J, Serafin D. The lymphatics of the groin flap. Ann Plast Surg 1982;9(6):447–458

[2] Becker C, Assouad J, Riquet M, Hidden G. Postmastectomy lymphedema: long-term results following microsurgical lymph node transplantation. Ann Surg 2006;243(3):313–315

[3] Saaristo AM, Niemi TS, Viitanen TP, Tervala TV, Hartiala P, Suominen EA. Microvascular breast reconstruction and lymph node transfer for postmastectomy lymphedema patients. Ann Surg 2012;255(3):468–473

[4] Nguyen AT, Chang EI, Suami H, Chang DW. An algorithmic approach to simultaneous vascularized lymph node transfer with microvascular breast reconstruction. Ann Surg Oncol 2015;22(9):2919–2924

[5] Dayan JH, Dayan E, Smith ML. Reverse lymphatic mapping: a new technique for maximizing safety in vascularized lymph node transfer. Plast Reconstr Surg 2015;135(1):277–285

50 Lymphoyenous Anastomosis

Edward I. Chang

Abstract

Lymphedema is a chronic, debilitating condition that can result from a variety of etiologies or, in some cases, as an inherited congenital form where the drainage of lymphatic fluid, typically from an extremity, has been compromised. In the Western world, the most common cause of lymphedema arises from cancer treatment where lymph node dissections and adjuvant therapies, such as radiation and chemotherapy, have impaired the lymphatic drainage from a limb. Historically, patients were treated with reductive procedures aimed to remove the excess volume and fibrotic tissue; however, novel approaches have emerged to address the underlying pathology. The lymphovenous anastomosis, also known as the lymphovenous bypass operation, aims to improve the drainage from the affected limb by creating a shunt from the obstructed lymphatic system to the systemic circulation. Patients undergoing a lymphovenous anastomosis have a significant subjective improvement in their symptoms and a reduced dependency on conservative management. However, fewer patients demonstrate an objective decrease in volume, and even fewer have a complete response. This chapter details each step in this procedure, from typical indications, to anatomy, to preoperative considerations, to surgical technique, and to donor site closure.

Keywords: indocyanine green, lymphazurin blue, lymphoscintigraphy, magnetic resonance lymphangiograms

50.1 Introduction

Lymphedema is a chronic debilitating condition that can result from a variety of etiologies or in some cases as an inherited congenital form where the drainage of lymphatic fluid, typically from an extremity, has been compromised. In the Western world, the most common cause of lymphedema arises from cancer treatment where lymph node dissections and adjuvant therapies such as radiation and chemotherapy have impaired the lymphatic drainage from a limb.[1,2] Historically, patients were treated with reductive procedures aimed to remove the excess volume and fibrotic tissue; however, novel approaches have emerged to address the underlying pathology. The lymphovenous anastomosis (LVA), also known as lymphovenous bypass, operation aims to improve the drainage from the affected limb by creating a shunt from the obstructed lymphatic system to the systemic circulation. Patients undergoing an LVA have a significant subjective improvement in their symptoms and greatly decreased dependency on conservative management including compression garments, pneumatic compression pumps, massage, and decongestive therapy; however, fewer patients demonstrate an objective decrease in volume and even fewer have a complete response.

50.2 Typical Indications

- LVA can be effective for treatment of early-stage lymphedema where the existing lymphatic structures and architecture have been preserved and are still present. Advanced-stage lymphedema occurs when the lymphatic channels have become fibrotic and scarred and therefore are no longer available to perform an anastomosis to a vein.

50.3 Anatomy

The location of the lymphatic channels is quite variable and can run very superficially just deep to the dermis, or they can be in the deep fat, beneath the fascia that is analogous to Scarpa's fascia. The ability to localize patent lymphatic channels has been revolutionized with the use of **indocyanine green** (ICG) lymphangiography. The fluorescent dye binds to proteins that are absorbed into the lymphatic system when injected subcutaneously and will therefore identify channels that are amenable to a bypass procedure. The overwhelming majority of patent channels are identified below the level of the elbow for the upper extremity and the knee for the lower extremity. For the upper extremity, most patent channels are identified on the dorsum of the hand and forearm rather than the volar side of the upper extremity. The ability to perform the anastomosis is obviously also dependent on the ability to identify an adjacent vein to serve as a recipient for the anastomosis. Once the appropriate targets have been identified using ICG fluorescent imaging, the use of **lymphazurin blue**, a dye that is also absorbed into the lymphatic system, is helpful in visualizing the lymphatic channels within the subcutaneous fat, once the skin incision has been made. However, new technologies are emerging frequently to aid in the visualization of veins as well as lymphatic channels.[3]

The field of lymphedema surgery has ushered in the new term "supermicrosurgery" as the lymphatic channel and the vein are typically 0.8 mm in diameter or less. At present, the current limit for completing a successful LVA is approximately 0.3 mm due to limitations of optics and magnification, supermicrosurgical instruments, microvascular needle and suture size, and human capability. However, as the field is rapidly evolving, there is a possibility that these limits may not persist in the future.

50.4 Variations

- The lymphatic channel may not contain lymphazurin dye and therefore careful dissection and identification of lymphatic vessels is crucial to successful outcomes and to avoid inadvertently cutting channels without the blue dye.
- Occasionally, a vein may not be present adjacent to the lymphatic vessel and an anastomosis cannot be performed. In other circumstances, an appropriately sized vein may not be present for an end-to-end anastomosis in which case an end-to-side anastomosis may be performed.

50.5 Preoperative Considerations

While most perform the LVA under general anesthesia, others have been successful in performing the operation using local anesthesia; however, given the majority of supermicrosurgeons use general anesthesia, all patients should have a complete workup anticipating surgery under general anesthesia. A thorough preoperative history is also critical to establish the underlying cause of the lymphedema, which is most commonly secondary to treatment for cancer in the Western world. The history should include details such as the etiology of the lymphedema, as some patients have a congenital form of primary lymphedema, onset and duration of symptoms, prior adjuvant therapies such as chemotherapy and radiation therapy, number and severity of prior infections, and hand dominance for upper extremity lymphedema. The physical examination should assess the degree of edema and quality of the skin, which allows for staging based on the **International Society of Lymphology** staging system. However, others have opted to use a different staging system using ICG lymphangiography imaging, which conveys an assessment of both the severity of the lymphedema and an algorithm for the treatment.[3]

The preoperative evaluation should also include imaging studies in cases where the diagnosis is unclear or if the history is inconsistent with the diagnosis of lymphedema. All patients should undergo a standard ultrasound duplex to confirm there is no evidence of a deep vein thrombosis as an alternative etiology for unilateral extremity swelling. **Lymphoscintigraphy** is also an important adjunct to evaluate the lymphatic drainage and lymphatic anatomy of the limbs. Others have also employed the use of **magnetic resonance lymphangiograms** in order to more clearly delineate the lymphatic channels that may serve as targets for an LVA.

All patients should also be seen and evaluated by certified lymphedema physiotherapists who are a critical component to the care, treatment, and management of all patients with lymphedema. Therapy including manual lymphatic drainage, compression garments, wrapping, and pneumatic pump devices are all integral to the treatment of lymphedema.[4] It is also important to have accurate objective measurements of patients preoperatively and during follow-up, the most common modalities are either circumferential measurements or perometer measurements.

50.6 Position and Skin Markings

The entire limb should be prepped and draped circumferentially to allow access to all potential targets for the LVA. The use of ICG has revolutionized the field and allows for visualization and marking of the potential lymphatic channels for the bypass procedure. Small aliquots (about 0.1–0.2 mL) of ICG are injected into the web spaces between the digits of the affected extremity subdermally (▶Fig. 50.1a). The room lights are turned off and the infrared imaging device is used to visualize the ICG being taken up by patent lymphatics. The current generation of imaging devices has allowed for penetration to nearly 1 cm; however, channels beyond that depth will not be visualized (▶Fig. 50.1b). It will usually take several minutes for ICG to travel through a lymphatic. The skin can be "milked" to help push the fluorescent dye through the lymphatic channels from distal to proximal. A skin marker is used to trace the fluorescent pattern of the lymphatic filled with ICG (▶Fig. 50.1c). Often, a vein can be visualized crossing over the lymph vessel, appearing as a linear dark shadow crossing over the fluorescent lymphatic. New technologies for identifying venous recipient vessels have also proven useful in marking the locations for the anastomosis.[5]

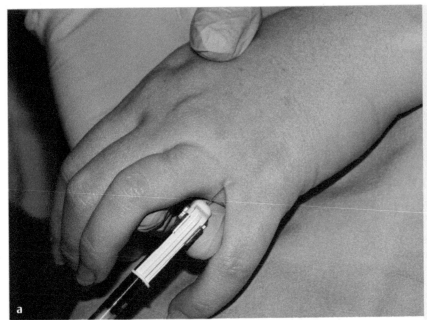

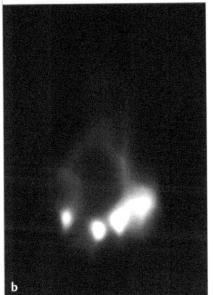

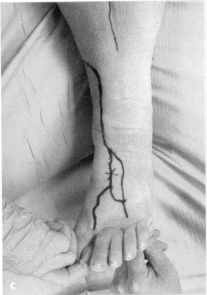

Fig. 50.1 (a) Subdermal injection of a small aliquot of indocyanine green (ICG) dye. (b) ICG lymphangiogram of an affected left foot. A linear pattern can be discerned representing uptake of ICG from the toe web space injection site into a patent lymphatic. (c) Skin markings on the left foot corresponding to linear ICG uptake patterns found during lymphangiography. (Part a image courtesy of Matthew M. Hanasono.)

50.7 Operative Technique

Following the ICG lymphangiography to identify the location of the lymphatic channels, it is also important to localize potential recipient veins. The location for the skin incision is determined over a point of intersection between the lymphatic vessel and the vein. Local anesthetic with epinephrine is injected along the length of the incision for hemostatic purposes. Approximately 2 cm distal to the anticipated incision, it is helpful to inject some lymphazurin dye in the dermis that will help to visualize the lymph channels. A skin incision is then made and should not cut full thickness through the dermis. The last layer of the deep dermis should be divided under high magnification using dissecting microscissors. At this time, a careful meticulous dissection is performed to identify the lymphatic channels (▶ **Fig. 50.2**). During this dissection, careful attention should be paid to preserve any veins that can serve as recipient vessels for the LVA.

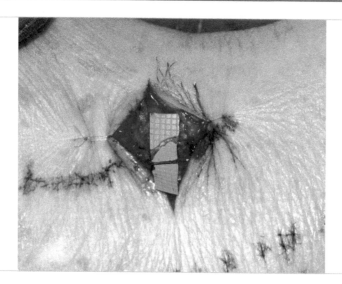

Fig. 50.2 An incision is made in the skin and a dissection is performed under high magnification to isolate a lymphatic vessel filled with lymphazurin blue dye and adjacent vein. (Image courtesy of Matthew M. Hanasono.)

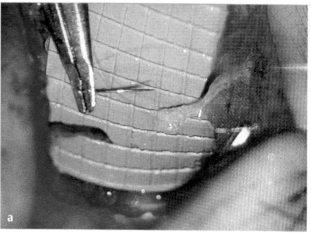

Fig. 50.3 (a) An 11–0 suture being used to perform a lymphovenous anastomosis (LVA), sewing in the direction from the vein to the lymphatic under high magnification. (b) Completed LVA in which lymphazurin blue dye can be seen filling the proximal vein, indicating a patent anastomosis. (Part b image courtesy of Matthew M. Hanasono.)

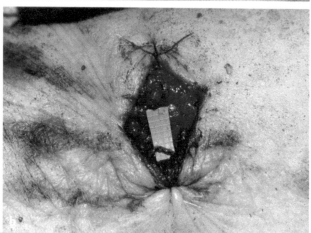

Once a suitable lymphatic and recipient vein has been identified, the anastomosis can be performed. Both vessels are divided and the anastomosis is completed using 11–0 nylon sutures connecting the distal end of the lymphatic to the proximal end of the recipient vein (▶ **Fig. 50.3a**). While some have performed the anastomosis of the proximal end of the lymphatic to the proximal recipient vein, most perform the anastomosis in the opposite orientation. The author uses microvascular hemoclips to ligate the proximal lymphatic and the distal vein. The number of sutures that are placed is dependent on the size of the vessels, but only the necessary number of sutures should be placed which may be as few as three in some anastomoses (▶ **Fig. 50.3b**).

Following completion of the anastomosis, it is critical to confirm the anastomosis is patent. This can be performed using a number of different modalities, either demonstrating drainage of lymphazurin dye into the vein or using fluorescent angiography to confirm passage of ICG into the vein. The incision is then closed as described in the following section.

50.8 Donor Site Closure

The incisions made to perform the LVA are typically about 1-2 cm in length and are closed primarily using any technique the surgeon prefers. The author prefers using an absorbable monofilament suture to close the deep dermal layer and a skin adhesive to close the superficial skin. Alternatively, simple interrupted permanent sutures can also be used to close the skin incision.

50.9 Pearls and Pitfalls

- For vessels that are too small to visualize the lumen without risking a back wall suture, the use of a cut piece of a 6–0 or 7–0 nylon or polypropylene suture as a stent will minimize the risk of this complication and ensures a patent anastomosis. Vessels that cannot be stented using a suture often are not amenable to an LVA.
- The use of lymphazurin dye is useful in visualizing the lymphatic vessels; however, there are some instances when the lymphatic channel does not have any dye in the lumen so the operating microsurgeon needs to be cautious and diligent in identifying lymphatic vessels, which are otherwise translucent.
- It is often easier to suture from the vein to the lymphatic, as it is easier to pass the needle tip into the lumen of the lymphatic, which is typically thin walled. Passing the needle into the lymphatic vessel first is challenging and can result in inadvertent back walling of the lymphatic.

References

[1] Paskett ED, Dean JA, Oliveri JM, Harrop JP. Cancer-related lymphedema risk factors, diagnosis, treatment, and impact: a review. J Clin Oncol 2012;30(30):3726–3733

[2] Suami H, Chang DW. Overview of surgical treatments for breast cancer-related lymphedema. Plast Reconstr Surg 2010;126(6):1853–1863

[3] Chang DW, Suami H, Skoracki R. A prospective analysis of 100 consecutive lymphovenous bypass cases for treatment of extremity lymphedema. Plast Reconstr Surg 2013;132(5):1305–1314

[4] Dayes IS, Whelan TJ, Julian JA, et al. Randomized trial of decongestive lymphatic therapy for the treatment of lymphedema in women with breast cancer. J Clin Oncol 2013;31(30):3758–3763

[5] Mihara M, Murai N, Hayashi Y, et al. Using indocyanine green fluorescent lymphography and lymphatic-venous anastomosis for cancer-related lymphedema. Ann Vasc Surg 2012;26(2):278.e1–278.e6

Index

Note: Page numbers set in **bold** or *italic* indicate headings or figures, respectively.